VIRAL FRICTIONS

MEDICAL ANTHROPOLOGY: HEALTH, INEQUALITY, AND SOCIAL JUSTICE

Series editor: Lenore Manderson

Books in the Medical Anthropology series are concerned with social patterns of and social responses to ill health, disease, and suffering, and how social exclusion and social justice shape health and healing outcomes. The series is designed to reflect the diversity of contemporary medical anthropological research and writing, and will offer scholars a forum to publish work that showcases the theoretical sophistication, methodological soundness, and ethnographic richness of the field.

Books in the series may include studies on the organization and movement of peoples, technologies, and treatments, how inequalities pattern access to these, and how individuals, communities, and states respond to various assaults on well-being, including from illness, disaster, and violence.

For a list of all the titles in the series, please see the last page of the book.

VIRAL FRICTIONS

Global Health and the Persistence of HIV Stigma in Kenya

ELIZABETH J. PFEIFFER

RUTGERS UNIVERSITY PRESS
New Brunswick, Camden, and Newark, New Jersey, and London

Library of Congress Cataloging-in-Publication Data
Names: Pfeiffer, Elizabeth J., author.
Title: Viral frictions : global health and the persistence of HIV stigma in Kenya /
    Elizabeth J. Pfeiffer.
Description: New Brunswick : Rutgers University Press, 2022. | Series: Medical
    anthropology | Includes bibliographical references and index.
Identifiers: LCCN 2021039375 | ISBN 9781978822320 (paperback) |
    ISBN 9781978822337 (hardback) | ISBN 9781978822344 (epub) | ISBN 9781978822351
    (mobi) | ISBN 9781978822368 (pdf)
Subjects: LCSH: HIV-positive persons—Kenya—Social conditions. | HIV-positive
    persons—Kenya—Public opinion. | AIDS (Disease)—Patients—Social aspects—
    Kenya. | HIV infections—Social aspects—Kenya.
Classification: LCC RA643.86.K4 P44 2022 | DDC 362.19697/9200096762—dc23
LC record available at https://lccn.loc.gov/2021039375

A British Cataloging-in-Publication record for this book is available from the British
Library.

In loving memory of Henry Kamau Muitiriri

CONTENTS

SERIES FOREWORD

LENORE MANDERSON

The Medical Anthropology: Health, Inequality, and Social Justice series is concerned with the diversity of contemporary medical anthropological research and writing. The beauty of ethnography is its capacity, through storytelling, to make sense of suffering as a social experience and to set it in context. Central to our focus in this series, therefore, is the way in which social structures, political and economic systems, and ideologies shape the likelihood and impact of infections, injuries, bodily ruptures and disease, chronic conditions and disability, treatment and care, and social repair and death.

Health and illness are social facts; the circumstances of the maintenance and loss of health are always and everywhere shaped by structural, local, and global relations. Social formations and relations, culture, economy, and political organizations as much as ecology shape variations in illness, disability, and disadvantage. The authors of the monographs in this series are concerned centrally with health and illness, healing practices, and access to care, but in these different volumes the authors highlight the importance of such differences in context as expressed and experienced at individual, household, and wider levels. Health risks and outcomes of social structure and household economy (for example, health systems factors), as well as national and global politics and economics, all shape people's lives. In their accounts of health, inequality, and social justice, the authors move across social circumstances, health conditions, geography, and their intersections and interactions to demonstrate how individuals, communities, and states manage assaults on people's health and well-being.

As medical anthropologists have long illustrated, the relationships between social context and health status are complex. In addressing these questions, the authors in this series showcase the theoretical sophistication, methodological rigor, and empirical richness of the field, while expanding a map of illness, social interaction, and institutional life to illustrate the effects of material conditions and social meanings in troubling and surprising ways. The books reflect medical anthropology as a constantly changing field of scholarship, drawing on research in such diverse contexts as residential and virtual communities, clinics, laboratories, and emergency care and public health settings; with service providers, individual healers, and households; and with social bodies, human bodies, biologies, and biographies. While medical anthropology once concentrated on systems of healing, particular diseases, and embodied experiences, today the field has expanded to include environmental disasters, war, science, technology, faith, gender-based violence, and forced migration. Curiosity about the body and its vicissitudes remains a pivot of our work, but our concerns are with the location of bodies in social life and with how social structures, temporal imperatives, and shifting exigencies shape life courses. This dynamic field reflects the ethics of the discipline to address these pressing issues of our time.

Globalization complicates influences on health outcomes: it (re)produces social and economic relations that institutionalize poverty, unequal conditions of everyday life and work, and environments in which disease prevalence grows or subsides. It shapes health experiences and outcomes across space, informing and amplifying inequalities at individual and country levels. In *Viral Frictions: Global Health and the Persistence of HIV Stigma in Kenya*, Elizabeth Pfeiffer expands on these complications, illustrating how local, regional, national, and global programs and actors rub up against local populations and services impacted by HIV (human immunodeficiency virus).

As the subtitle of this series indicates, we are concerned with questions of social exclusion and inclusion and of social justice and repair, again both globally and in local settings. The books challenge readers to reflect not only on sickness and suffering as well as deficit and despair, but also on resistance and restitution—on how people respond to injustices and evade the fault lines that might seem to predetermine life outcomes. The aim is to widen the frame within which we conceptualize embodiment and suffering.

Viral Frictions: Global Health and the Persistence of HIV Stigma in Kenya takes place in the Rift Valley region in the western part of the country, in a small town pseudonymously called Mahali that is near the regional capital, Eldoret. In this setting, HIV was always "general"—that is, it occurred among members across populations, including both sexes—but it affected more women than men. Nongovernmental organizations (NGOs) had introduced antiretroviral therapy (ART) starting in the late twentieth century, and public health centers began providing the same treatment a few years later. After a decade or so of denial, multilateral programs, donors, international and national organizations, and churches were immersed in the challenges of behavioral change, while concurrently identifying people at possible risk of infection, implementing comprehensive testing and counseling, and then starting people of all ages on ARTs to reduce the risk of transmission and prevent serious illness and death from acquired immune deficiency syndrome (AIDS), with the goal of ensuring that people would have lives of quality and duration. When Pfeiffer began the fieldwork on which this book is based, the town of Mahali and its region, like Kenya as a whole, had had over twenty-five years of experience with HIV. HIV/AIDS dominated donor activity, national discourse, and local economies.

Beginning in the mid-1980s, as HIV infection spread in eastern and southern Africa, towns like Mahali, scattered along major transport routes, gained reputations as hot spots of HIV infection associated with sex work. In Mahali, then and now, trucks pass from Mombasa, Kenya's largest port, through the far west of the country to Uganda and Sudan, and they return along the same routes. In Mahali, truck drivers take the opportunity to drop off trade goods such as coffee, tea, oil, and cement and to pick up other goods such as maize, wheat, dairy products, and vegetables. They refuel their trucks and check the tire pressure, oil, and water; they eat, drink in bars and nightclubs along the roadside, relax, and sleep. They are passersby. The residents of the town and its environs, as well as the members of the various NGOs and community groups based there, work to maintain these services, but at the same time their lives are troubled by sporadic intercommunal violence, forced migration and resettlement, political instability, drought, and competition for land. On an everyday basis, people struggle to maintain employment and to ensure that they have food and economic security. HIV is simply one factor in a mix of immediate and longer-term challenges.

Some two decades after ARTs were rolled out, Mahali and Kenya as a whole still deal with persistent new infections and deaths from AIDS. In attending to the competitive environment in which multiple agencies and actors seek to prevent HIV and deliver care, Pfeiffer seeks to explain why this is so and ties the incongruity of persistent HIV to stigma. In her compelling account of HIV and its entanglement with everyday local struggles in Mahali, she highlights how friction derails public health investment and programs at multiple scales. Global health initiatives and HIV-related stigma, she illustrates, interact with existing, entrenched inequalities in Mahali that reflect the intersections of race and ethnicity, gender and sexuality, and generation and class. Women's excess rates of infection are unsettled by these divisions: their care work and their limited options for generating income result in all women living with the potential stigma of putative sex work. Institutional instability, social change, and class status undermine social relations, reflected in the unwillingness of local residents to interact with state structures and services. Stigma and discrimination fan suspicion and erode trust. In this unhappy mix of tensions, Pfeiffer illustrates that people's mental health is also at risk. Meanwhile, HIV's social life fans out and splits into tributaries. The virus, its institutions and infrastructures, and its technicians and targeted populations are all marked by association and shame.

Stigma is often used to explain why people resist screening, diagnosis, treatment, disclosure, and continued care, even when there are obvious benefits in following this pathway. This book unravels what that means. As Pfeiffer shows, with compassion and care, frictions characterize HIV interventions and enflame the stigma of infection. She takes us to one town and opens up the social and economic complexities of people's lives. In doing so, *Viral Frictions: Global Health and the Persistence of HIV Stigma in Kenya* explains how social tensions fuel inequalities of risk, vulnerability, and life chances and thus continue to trouble the work of controlling HIV infection and AIDS.

PREFACE

SENSING MAHALI: A COMMUNITY IN MOTION

Mahali is a highway trading center, which means that it is a porous community: people, knowledge, and words are in motion, and frictions occur. It is located in the Rift Valley region of Kenya and would be considered a "town" in the United States, but it is referred to here as a "trading center" or a very small "urban center." Consisting of a short row of small businesses, shops, restaurants, hotels, and roadside kiosks and surrounded by lush, rolling hills and agricultural landscapes, Mahali has frequently been described simply as a truck stop, implying that it is also a place known to exist primarily to cater to the needs of the hundreds of truck drivers who passed through every evening. It also serves the needs of those living in several surrounding rural farming communities and is known to host a substantial number of sex workers. As one interlocutor told me rather bluntly, it was seen as "a place where men can eat sweet meat—both kinds—to satisfy the two stomachs: the *nyama choma* (roasted meat) for the eating stomach and the sexual one." Hardly a final destination for most Kenyans, Mahali is quite literally a place in the middle of things.

Located along a busy highway, Mahali is like one of many other centers similarly situated between the port of Mombasa to the southeast and the interior of Africa to the northwest. It is a convenient short stop on the way to many other places. It would be quite easy for a traveler to miss the community altogether, except for a series of extreme speed bumps placed on the road in front of the town's urban center, which force passersby to slow down and at least glance around. The community boasts ample parking for every size of vehicle, an ideal climate for sustaining a productive agricultural base, places to spend the night, churches of varying denominations, an entertaining nightlife, a gas station, a large market, and an HIV (human immunodeficiency virus) clinic (made possible by collaborations between various foreign entities and the Kenyan state) that provides free HIV testing, treatment, and care. With these attractions, the community beckons visitors passing through to stop in. Anna Tsing (2005, 10) writes of friction and roads: "Friction is not just about slowing things down. Friction is required to keep global power in motion. It shows us where the rubber meets the road. Roads are a good image for conceptualizing how friction works. Roads create pathways that make motion easier and more efficient, but in doing so, they limit where we go. The ease of travel they facilitate is also a structure of confinement. Friction inflects historical trajectories, enabling, excluding, and particularizing." In this book, I imagine that stories are like roads: produced by people to generate connectivity, exclusions, intersections, action, and impact, while also shaping and restricting what we know, see, and understand.

One does not have to be in Mahali very long before all one's senses become overwhelmed by the constant movement of people and products into and out of this center. People are busy. Bodies, knowledge, things, and stories are literally on the move. Sometimes this motion is strategic, as in the case of a job opportunity or a marriage. Some people come to or go away from the area in the hope of starting a new life or escaping a past, an experience, or a reputation. Others might flow through to be tested for HIV or for their monthly clinic appointments and to refill their prescriptions for antiretroviral therapy (ART). At other times, the movement is forced, as when a woman is chased away by her husband or in-laws. Historically, some people were thrust into motion when running away in terror from a burning home, business, or *shamba* (farm) whenever ethnic, economic, and/or political tensions erupted into violence and chaos. But even in moments of peace, there is a steady flow of bodies, technologies, and goods—and along with them (though less observable) a diversity of ideas, beliefs, knowledge, emotions, moralities, gossip, and HIV statuses. Many people living in or passing though Mahali are engaged in a variety of formal and informal (as well as legal and illegal) activities, with a wide range of agendas and purposes. By day and night, people from the urban center travel by foot, car, or motorbike to surrounding villages and neighboring towns and vice versa to sell or purchase a variety of goods including milk, agricultural produce, secondhand clothing, *chang'aa* (a strong, traditional, illegally home-brewed spirit), companionship, and sex. Other people—including global health experts, NGO workers, entrepreneurs, and development specialists from the United States, European countries, India, and China—travel by car, truck, or *matatu* (a fourteen-seat public transportation minibus) from other parts of Kenya, Uganda, the Democratic Republic of the Congo, Burundi, and beyond. Sometimes it is not a person but rather a new policy, program, research project, or evidence-based approach for HIV prevention and treatment that comes into Mahali from the Kenyan state, working in partnerships with international agencies, the private sector, and local governments.

All of this attracted me to Mahali as the place for my research. Throughout my years of fieldwork, I not only saw but also heard, felt, smelled, and even tasted the motion. I was regularly overwhelmed by it and found it difficult to keep pace with the trajectories of people's lives that sent them moving around the country and across the continent (and beyond), as people used excerpts from their lives to explain who they imagined themselves to be. When I conducted open-ended interviews in buildings or houses close to the road, I could feel a rumble deep inside my chest that matched the sound and speed of passing vehicles as they raced, slowed, and then bumped and rattled across the speed bumps. This motion was even captured on my audio recordings. As I transcribed interviews at home,

I relived my experiences in Kenya as the steady flow of trucks and cattle or the flapping wings of chickens sometimes temporarily engulfed the voices of the people talking in the recordings. At the peak of the annual drought in February, the air was hot, dry, and windy, a combination that caused dust to burn my eyes. These conditions also changed the lush green landscape to a bland brown and made the cows unable to produce milk, leaving locals to serve tea made from water instead of the preferred local chai made from milk. I could feel and taste the motion of passing seasons.

The area hosted a broad mix of people from Kenya's forty-six diverse ethnic groups, including individuals identifying themselves as Kisii, Luo, Kamba, Embu, Meru, and Luyha. However, it was predominantly home to people who described themselves as either Kikuyu or Kalenjin, political and sometimes linguistic categories that incorporated and referred to members of several ethnically distinct cultural groups (see Lynch 2011). Most people first learned to speak their ethnic language, or mother tongue, but the two official languages of Kenya are English and Kiswahili, the latter serving as the lingua franca in Mahali and across the country. Both languages are taught as formal subjects in primary schools that are free and compulsory up through standard 8 (the equivalent of eighth grade)—the level at which, in late October, students take the Kenya Certificate of Primary Education exam that helps determine their placements and options for secondary education.

In 2019, an estimated 52.6 million people were living in Kenya (World Bank 2021), and the local, freestanding HIV clinic put the number of people in Mahali and the surrounding rural areas at approximately 11,000. The clinic needed to determine the population size to carry out an intensive HIV home counseling and testing (HCT) program that was implemented on several occasions across communities in the Rift Valley in 2011, 2012, and 2014 while I was doing fieldwork. HCT was intended to help people, but it also created frictions. The porous boundaries of Mahali also contributed to many frictions. This was an important aspect for understanding and making sense of the complexities of HIV stigma, as well as the widely diverse stories that I heard while I conducted research.

Despite the hustle and bustle of life in the day and night, if one knew where to go or what to look for, things slowed down in Mahali in some spaces and at some moments. The speed bumps were the most obvious places, but others were out of sight of the main road. I came to experience and sense these other places personally. For example, when I was riding on the back of a *boda boda* (motorbike taxi) but did not beat the afternoon rain, I got stuck in the deep mud that had only moments earlier been a dirt road and I had to walk, my own movements sluggish from the heavy accumulation of mud on my shoes.

Things slowed down in other places, too. During church services and various ethnic rituals—engagement parties and circumcision celebrations, for instance—people joined together, sometimes sitting in large circles. They danced, celebrated life, sang (sometimes in a multitude of languages), performed, and gave speeches that almost always included educational information about HIV. People also slowed down in houses, compounds, slums, illegal brew houses or "dens," clinics, and open fields outside the urban center, as they ate, drank, smoked cigarettes or *bhangi* (marijuana), and socialized with one another, sitting and waiting to see what might happen next. Some people were waiting in the hope of something, anything. Others were waiting in the long queues in the (sometimes chilly) cement hallways at the HIV clinic in anticipation that a health professional might ease their suffering or solve the health problem of a child or other loved one. On rare occasions, things almost came to a halt. For example, when a person (frequently a man) had delayed getting medical care and treatment for an HIV infection, his body, emaciated by this virus, was still and awaiting the so-called Lazarus effect of ART. With very few available jobs and a weak economy, some people sat around idle, drunk, and often demoralized. But in all these places and the activities that occurred in them—formal or mundane—I encountered and witnessed profound warmth, kindness, comfort, and patience demonstrated through very fine acts of generosity and hospitality.

Mahali has been a site of considerable historical and continuing tensions over land, epitomized by the fact that ethnic and political violence has erupted with nearly every democratic presidential election since 1992. However, the worst destruction in Mahali occurred following the perceived rigging of the 2007 presidential election. During my research, scars of the violence—physical across the landscape and emotional in conversations—remained with local residents as constant reminders of the interethnic, intercommunity violence that had once taken place and might recur, and anxieties and tensions were high whenever the country approached elections.

I was told a few times that the abandoned ruins of buildings were strategically kept "to remind us that we used to be modern—and that we didn't all used to be the same." Other artifacts, such as the newly erected houses provided by humanitarian agencies, evoked the idea among locals that the people of Mahali had experienced a reversal of time, and that development had moved backward. After the 2007–2008 postelection violence, locals could not rebuild the community by themselves: they had to rely on outside entities, aid organizations, and the good intentions of "well-wishers," as they sometimes referred to individual foreign donors. While local people were grateful for the assistance, they also sometimes interpreted this dependence as shameful and as evidence that they had been cast into the "margins of the state" (V. Das and Poole 2004). Some key interlocuters shared a nostalgic sense of longing for a return to an imagined ideal past when people had been self-sufficient and did not have to depend on outside assistance.

Given all the motion, stillness, and frictions that people in Mahali had experienced and endured, I found that it was simultaneously a place of celebration, hope, frustration, destruction, disparities, insecurities, and contradictions. And it was never lacking in possibilities. While I witnessed moments of great despair within and between people, as well as violent outbursts of anger and aggression, I was always struck by the contagious sense of hope. Sometimes I would cry with people as they talked to me, unsure how I might best comfort them (and myself) in their sufferings and/or their desperate requests for help with problems so complex and troubling that I (or anyone else) was completely powerless to solve. At other times, tears would fall from an otherwise emotionless and numbed face, hardened by the painful passage and trajectories of time. But at the same time, Mahali was filled with tremendously warm smiles, laughter, and joy. I shared countless hours of laughter with people, occasionally erupting from unantici-pated incidents of happiness, silliness, and amusing moments. At other times, the laughter emerged from the most ironic circumstances or awkward engage-ments. This kind of laughter was often at my expense and erupted alongside the many cultural and linguistic blunders I made along the way. At still other moments, the laughter came "from the bottom of the chest" (Mbembe 2001, 167), the place of sufferings from the horrors, insecurities, and terrors of life (Janz 2002). In these instances, our laughter was really "out of place": it indexed the absurdities, contradictions, injustices, and ironies of living in our shared world with its chronic violence and gross inequities (Donna Goldstein 2003).

I used all of my senses as an ethnographer to collect the stories I tell about stigma in the pages that follow, including those I participated in and thus helped construct. The stories evoked all of these emotions and responses and offer a snapshot of the complexities of our globalized world. I examine the social con-tradictions and ongoing relational tensions produced by HIV—the infection and intertwining local, national, and global responses to it—that fuel and sustain processes of stigma, as well as the simultaneous possibilities for some people and potential perils for others. For a select minority of researchers, scientists, and practitioners, HIV brings huge rewards, prestige, and attention as they study, learn, and apply the most rigorous and up-to-date scientific knowledge and bio-medical technologies to treat people with the virus and prevent it from spread-ing. Yet knowledge is always partial, and thus policies, programs, and funding priorities frequently shift. As we shall see, this aggravates processes of stigma because those changes are felt, experienced, and interpreted and therefore must be negotiated by those living in regions (like eastern Africa) where the disease burden is high and everyday living conditions are marked by uncertainty and insecurity. Consequently, for many people, knowledge about someone's HIV seropositive status can at times become political, and an HIV diagnosis has to be managed and handled with skillful precision. Throughout my research, however, this latter form of expert knowledge was rarely acknowledged or taken into seri-ous account by global health workers. Yet when the social and political realities facing people are not acknowledged or addressed, the lifelong management of

ART becomes challenging, at best. In this book, I suggest that this sort of so-called local knowledge must be considered if AIDS and stigma are to be eliminated.

VIRAL FRICTIONS: AN ETHNOGRAPHY OF THE PERSISTENCE OF HIV STIGMA

The ethnography of stigma is both a process and a product. As Catherine Riessman (1993, 1) puts it, "story telling is what we do with our research materials and what informants do with us." Sociocultural anthropologists spend much of their time listening to the stories, talk, and gossip of other people. I became intimately engaged in the social and narrative processes in Mahali by using the classic anthropological technique of participant observation. I lived, worked, and hung out with, as well as observed, the people I wanted to learn more about for extended periods of time from 2010 to 2019. I further gleaned insights into the social and structural processes of HIV-related stigma and discrimination by collecting and triangulating data derived over the years from more than 150 semistructured interviews with individuals and small groups and a series of life-history interviews. At my request, ten local residents compiled conversational journals for a period of six months in 2012. This latter methodology was developed by sociologists to study local gossip and as a method of collecting data on responses to new biomedical interventions in sub-Saharan Africa (see Watkins, Swidler, and Biruk 2011). I also engaged in ongoing informal conversations with key interlocutors, people I got to know well over the years. I was trained and inspired by a mentor who works collaboratively with the people being studied across the entire research process—from determining the research questions and developing the research design to analyzing, interpreting, and disseminating the data (Lassiter 2005).

Each day in the field, and through several different projects related to the social aspects of HIV, I rotated working independently or alongside Irene, Emmah, Beatrice, and Henry, my four well-connected and trained research assistants. They had been selected to collectively reflect some of the social, linguistic, and ethnic variability found in Mahali. Employing and collaborating with local residents from various backgrounds helps ensure that the entire research process is rooted in local concerns and perspectives. This method also helped me reduce the biases that are inherent in ethnographic data collection processes, especially when it comes to documenting and studying sensitive topics such as HIV, AIDS, and stigma in postcolonial contexts. As a group, we worked together to conceptualize the projects and socially and linguistically revise interview protocols and study instruments. Local expertise was crucial for developing the rapport necessary to carry out community-based, HIV-related research and for identifying and recruiting interlocutors across the social spectrum, as well as for interpreting and translating during and after interviews and participant observation sessions.

When I was in Kenya, my research assistants and I met regularly as a group to discuss and analyze data using an iterative thematic coding approach commonly used in ethnographic analysis (Ryan and Bernard 2003) and to guide subsequent areas of investigation. Throughout our years of research, we also developed routines that carved out extra, more relaxed time together following formal group meetings. For example, about an hour or two before we anticipated finishing our work, Henry would call his favorite restaurant butcher and order one or two kilograms of either potatoes and boiled meat or *nyama choma*—usually mutton, sometimes goat, and only rarely beef. Once we completed the activities on our research agenda, we would slowly make our way through the congested trading center, dodging motorbikes and plumes of diesel smoke and stopping to greet people we knew along the way, until we reached the *hoteli* (restaurant) where our meal was waiting. After shaking hands with several men who were inevitably standing out front, we would pass through the cold cement brick building (containing large cuts of meat hanging on one side and a huge poster advertising Tusker, a popular East African Breweries beer brand, on the other side) and into the small, open-air, dirt courtyard behind it. There, we would find an eclectic group of individuals, people I came to recognize and know over time—(wealthier) sex workers, local politicians, health workers, business owners, and civil servants (e.g., police officers, postal workers, and public school teachers). The courtyard was scattered with light-blue picnic tables with chipped and peeling paint, under which the occasional cat begged for scraps. Lining each side of the courtyard was a long and slender room with an open front made of loosely constructed boards and a corrugated tin roof. Inside the room on one side were additional tables encircled by plastic chairs or lined with wooden benches, sheltered to provide relief from the rain or sun. The room on the other side was divided into several stalls, each with a grill and wood stove that constantly billowed smoke as food was cooked to order over open flames and coals. At the back of the courtyard was a fence that butted up to several *chang'aa* dens, where people who could not afford expensive, officially bottled forms of alcohol sold in bars drank strong local brews, socialized, and sometimes (if they were visiting a place with electricity) watched television, including sporting events and the latest popular telenovelas.

After finding a place to sit, we would take turns visiting a metal tank of steam-heated water, turning the wobbly knob of a spigot until it began to drip, lathering our hands with a small chip of bar soap, and rinsing them using a trickle of nearly boiling water. Even at the finer establishments in Mahali, electricity was intermittent, and there were limited places with running water. Wealthier homeowners had pit toilets at the backs of their homes; working flush toilets were rare. Servers at the restaurant we frequented were young men who wore white coats that resembled those worn by physicians, and one of them always delivered us the same order: two bowls of *ugali* (a thick, white dough-like starch made from maize flour that is a staple food and eaten with one's hands), a plate of *kachumbari* (a salsa-like salad made of uncooked fresh tomatoes and onions), and our meat on a cutting board with a small pile of salt in the corner (for dipping). The server cut the meat in front of us so we knew it was fresh, and just as he turned to leave, Emmah and Henry would always request *pili pili*, a hot red pepper, and we would laugh when they referred to a fondness for "tear gas." We spent hours talking and laughing over the food we shared in this courtyard, and the time always ended with each of us drinking a glass bottle of soda—Fanta, Coke, Sprite, or Krest.

I spent a significant amount of time with my research assistants, and as a result they regularly offered supplemental insights into the meanings or larger stories behind what was stated during interviews and supplied me with seemingly endless interpretations (sometimes a running commentary) of the various happenings at the *hoteli* we frequented, as well as community-wide events, celebrations, and incidents. Irene, Emmah, Beatrice, and Henry helped keep me up-to-date on the latest local gossip and were always willing to offer me between-the-lines readings of what otherwise required a tacit social knowledge that only a person entrenched in the local politics and history might have. They also became my close and trusted companions, and for their ongoing friendship and family-like support, I remain exceedingly grateful. While I am the lone author of this book, the stories presented and ideas that shaped the basic premise of the arguments in it might be described as taking form through a process of "polygraphy" (Whyte 2014). The stories told throughout this book are from multiple collaborative voices, and thus the work might be considered multisited: over the years, five people situated in a wide variety of positions, places, sets of concerns, and experiences worked together to tell about viral frictions.

Like all anthropologists, I have ethical concerns and worry about protecting the confidentiality of all participants. Therefore, while I illuminate the lives of and words spoken by real people who were navigating and negotiating real circumstances that occurred in real places, I describe them as composites of the many interactions and conversations—formal and informal—that I had with a wide range of people, as well as of the observations I made working in the Rift Valley over the past decade. In other words, I have restructured some of the events, as well as blended and blurred some of the descriptive characteristics, as a way of protecting the identities of people. Like Jason De León's (2015, 43–44) description of undocumented migrants attempting to cross the U.S.-Mexico border through the Sonoran Desert—drawing on the work of Michael Humphreys and Tony Watson (2009)—the viral frictions presented throughout this book might be considered an account of "semifictionalized ethnography, or a 'restructuring of events occurring within one or more ethnographic investigations into a single narrative.'"

Ethnographers ultimately retell the stories they have heard, and the "listener becomes the speaker" (Bakhtin 1986, 68) in the production of the ethnographic account, which is what you will read in this book. Anthropologists are no longer shy about admitting that they do not tell *the* story about a person or group of people at one particular place and time but rather tell *a* story, as they came to understand things from their own limited and biased position as a researcher (Marcus and Fischer 1999). This book tells an ethnographic story about the stigma associated with chronic HIV infection and AIDS using the stories that my Kenyan research assistants and I—a white, middle-class, American mother with a PhD in sociocultural anthropology—collected through rigorous and intensive field research. Another set of researchers might experience and tell this story differently.

In *Stigma: Notes on the Management of Spoiled Identity*, the first book written on the topic of stigma, Erving Goffman (1963, 138) imagined that every person had occupied the stigmatized role, and he conceptualized stigma as "a two-role social process in which every individual participates in both roles." These roles were enacting processes of stigmatization and feeling social stigma in some aspect of life. I draw on these ideas, and while the contexts and settings described in this book might be new and unfamiliar to some readers, I hope that the stories presented about stigma—feelings of shame, not being "normal," or being left out or excluded—may not be totally foreign. I therefore join Annemarie Mol's (2008, 11) practice of taking seriously the charge to "no longer marginalize" those living with disease since "none of us [is] immune" and "normality is not presupposed," and I hope that readers are able to imagine themselves as "involved in the situations described."

ACRONYMS AND ABBREVIATIONS

ACP	AIDS Control Programme (WHO)
AIDS	acquired immune deficiency syndrome
ART	antiretroviral therapy
CDC	Centers for Disease Control and Prevention (United States)
CSW	commercial sex worker
Global Fund	Global Fund to Fight AIDS, Tuberculosis and Malaria
GNP+	Global Network of People Living with HIV
GPA	Global Programme on AIDS (WHO)
HCT	home counseling and testing
HIV	human immunodeficiency virus
HIV−	HIV negative
HIV+	HIV positive
IDP	internally displaced person
KANU	Kenya African National Union
MAP	Multi-Country HIV/AIDS Programme for Africa
MSM	a man who has sex with a man
NACC	National AIDS Control Council (Kenya)
NGO	nongovernmental organization
PEP	postexposure prophylaxis
PEPFAR	U.S. President's Emergency Plan for AIDS Relief
PEV	postelection violence
PIT	provider-initiated HIV testing and counseling
PLWHIV	people living with HIV
PrEP	pre-exposure prophylaxis
PWID	a person who injects drugs
SDG	Sustainable Development Goals (United Nations)
SPA	Special Programme on AIDS (WHO)
TAC	Treatment Action Campaign (South Africa)
TasP	treatment as prevention
U=U	undetectable and untransmittable
UKIMWI	*upungufu wa kinga mwilini* [immune deficiency]
UNAIDS	Joint United Nations Programme on HIV/AIDS
UNICEF	United Nations Children's Fund
USAID	United States Agency for International Development
VCT	volunteer counseling and testing
WHO	World Health Organization

VIRAL FRICTIONS

INTRODUCTION

"She died of shame—that stigma! The family members, especially the husband, could not be associated with her after the doctors revealed her [HIV+ (human immunodeficiency virus positive)] status, so she refused to eat, pretending a toothache." This was the brief aside I was quietly offered after the mood of the conversation suddenly shifted from lighthearted to somber among the other guests in the house I was visiting. A woman had been buried the previous day, leaving locals to decipher the meanings of the various elements of her biography that had been exposed during her funeral. It was at the beginning of one of my fieldwork trips to a Kenyan community located along a busy highway, a very small town or urban trading center that I refer to as Mahali,[1] meaning "place" in Kiswahili. I had arranged to undertake ethnographic research there to explore the social and structural roots of stigma and discrimination related to HIV and acquired immune deficiency syndrome (AIDS).

A standard practice at funerals in sub-Saharan Africa is for groups of friends, church members, relatives, and colleagues to come together to share different aspects of their relations with and circulate stories about the deceased, both formally through eulogies, mourning rituals, and photographs, and informally through gossip. Through these processes, listeners gain a fuller portrait of the person and his or her relationships, and "a life took shape from its shards" (John Comaroff and Comaroff 2001, 276). I did not attend the funeral of this woman, nor had I ever met her, but through the collaborative narratives of people I encountered during my time in Mahali, various details about her life were revealed to me.

Struggling to put together the tiny pieces of the stories I was hearing, I was struck by the messiness of both social life and fieldwork in the modern interconnected world. I had immediately become entangled within the complex webs (Geertz 1973) of unfamiliar cultural, political, economic, and historical contexts, and I felt very much "in the middle of things" (Tsing 2005, 2). The gossip and rumors that had circulated among attendees at the burial of the woman were being used by people across the community to derive meaning, using distinct and tacit cultural logics (Bahktin 1986). As an outsider, I did not yet have the perspective to fully contextualize or understand the history and complexity of the stories, but I began to listen. I became privy to a local circuit of talk that I later realized served to link HIV infection and AIDS disease to broader forces that continued to (re)shape the community; people's lives, deaths, and identities; and the interpersonal and intrapersonal relationships being negotiated and experienced between people living in and passing through Mahali.

Later that night, and in the privacy of my room, I jotted down some of the "utterances" and "discourses" (Bakhtin 1986) of the accounts I had heard, as well as some of my initial impressions. The woman was characterized as an older, respected, wealthier community member who had been married for years to an elder of a local church congregation. It seemed to me that people thought one of the most impressive aspects of her biography was that she was suspected of having kept her HIV+ status and use of antiretroviral therapy (ART) secret. Anxieties about this kind of secrecy were made possible in Mahali in part through complex partnerships among national and international government agencies and public and private donors—the United Nations (UN); nongovernmental organizations (NGOs); development organizations; domestic and foreign global health institutes; medical researchers and practitioners, students, and volunteers—and the World Health Organization's (WHO) recommendations and guidelines, which had been created to achieve and were united around the common goal of ending the AIDS epidemic in Kenya. These partnerships constituted what some scholars have referred to as the global "AIDS industry" (Patton 2002; Nguyen 2010).

People were ambivalent about the woman's allegedly secret use of ART. On the one hand, they appeared impressed that she had kept such information private, a goal not only idealized, valued, and considered respectable but also recommended as a general practice for preserving one's moral reputation and social networks. On the other hand, some of the residents of Mahali with whom I spoke were astounded that the woman had duped so many people who had imagined her to be a person of high moral integrity and for whom HIV infection was unthinkable. This tension seemed to be accompanied by resentment, as well as unspoken anxiety, tension, and insecurity, for reasons that I did not yet understand. Still, many community members took "gossipy note" (Goffman 1963, 27) of their observations made during the funeral, an event that church leaders did not perform or attend. This central, but missing, component of her burial ceremony cemented the local story that she had been secretly living with HIV. Still trying to make sense of this story several months later, I asked Ruth—a church friend of the woman and one of my key interlocutors—for an explanation of how the church's clergy could possibly have known she was infected, if she had indeed successfully kept her seropositive status private. Sitting outside on tiny wooden stools in the plot of land Ruth owned a few miles from Mahali's urban center, we were sorting recently harvested potatoes, putting the best-looking ones in a burlap sack to be sold at the market and the remainders in a bag to take home to feed her husband, three children, and neighboring households. Ruth explained matter-of-factly how the woman had suddenly come to be a "discredited person" (Goffman 1963, 41) and thus treated as such in death: "She became very ill and weak and was admitted to [a national referral hospital] where [provider-initiated HIV] tests are done automatically. She was found [to be] HIV+, so her marital partner had to be contacted and tested. When the husband learned that he was negative, he went to the church and told the pastor and church elders. When she died, they treated her as a prostitute and refused to perform the ceremony."[2] HIV infections were predominantly acquired through heterosexual sex in Kenya, and 44 percent of HIV cases occurred among discordant marital or primary partners—that is, the HIV+ person's partner was HIV negative (HIV−) (NACC 2005, 2009; WHO/UNAIDS/UNICEF 2011; NASCOP 2012; Avert 2020). In response, and throughout my research trips, the AIDS industry heavily pushed HIV testing, counseling, and partner disclosure among couples as part of a national strategy to reduce HIV infections ("Putting HIV-Positive People at the Centre of Prevention" 2010; NASCOP 2013; Avert 2020) that prioritized the rights of people to know if their sex partners were infected with HIV over patients' right of privacy (Hardon et al. 2012). These globally and nationally funded strategies collided with already existing gender inequalities and politics in Mahali to produce unanticipated outcomes. Circulating global, national, and local stories and practices associated with HIV intertwined to give shape to the explanations of the tragic, untimely death of one community member and reinforced already familiar and moralizing messages about HIV—the infection, responses to it, and those living or associated with it during a period of uncertainty and social change.

Fragments of the (re)telling of versions of this story about the burial of the woman (and others who were later linked with it; see chapter 2 for details about "the List") continued to percolate and surface throughout this year-long research trip—including weeks after the funeral, when my research assistants and I began to pilot a series of open-ended interview questions in the home of one of the assistants. James, the bookkeeping clerk at a Catholic school, and I were seated at opposite ends of a couch, our bodies wrinkling the light-blue embroidered cloths (which could be easily removed and washed) that covered the seats so they would not get dirty. In response to a question about the last time he had heard someone talking about HIV or AIDS, James remarked that community members continued to be "shocked" by this still circulating news:

> The last time I heard about HIV was just yesterday. You see, in this community we all recently attended a burial—a wife had passed on. People are still very much talking about [her]. I heard that she became sick and was taken to [a nearby public] hospital, but almost instantly, she came back home. The following day, she fell

down and died. Just suddenly. When the husband came home, he found his wife dead. The wife was taken to the mortuary so that a postmortem could be done. But I heard that they never did [the postmortem], and when I asked why, I was told that it was because the woman was HIV+ and was hiding [her HIV status from everyone]. It was only the sister who [had known her status]; even the husband had not known the wife was HIV+! So, you see, everyone in the community is very shocked by this news, so every person is talking about it. It is very shocking to us.

Fieldwork experiences like this one demonstrated the kinds of things people were telling each other about the HIV epidemic and underscored the social tensions and moral ambiguities produced by the virus during a period of increased access to global health technologies, including HIV tests and ART. This story of "partial secrets" (Squire 2015), nondisclosure, ART, shame, and ambivalence was generated by community members who were trying to make sense of HIV and resolve the dissonances produced by it in ways that overshadowed the life and death of a person. Furthermore, the story pointed to the persistence of HIV-related stigma in eastern Africa, the power of words to enforce that stigma, and the way this virus was still perceived and experienced as exceptional during the age of treatment (Moyer and Hardon 2014; Benton 2015; Reed 2018). The circulation of such a story raised a series of questions with which I grapple in this book: Why were stories of HIV stigma, discrimination, and prejudice traveling around the community during an age of unprecedented ease of HIV prevention and treatment? What might listening critically to stories of HIV discrimination—told by those who have experienced it and those who intentionally or unintentionally reproduce it—reveal about what global health initiatives feel like to people living in the communities where they are inserted? What do stories like this one teach us about the perceived and experienced effects and limitations of global health programs, policies, and protocols aligned with national governments' efforts to address health problems around the world? What do stories about HIV stigma expose about globalization, including the inequalities it (re)produces and its role as a force that shapes everyday experiences, life and death, relationships, power arrangements, culture, and social worlds? With this book, based on a decade of research in Kenya conducted from 2010 to 2019, I offer a critical ethnographic case study of stigma, using it as a microcosm to understand broader social processes, the complexities of globalization and health, and their profound impact on the persistence of HIV stigma.

Processes of globalization—the intense integration and global flows of economic capital, ideas, images, products, technologies, knowledge, bodies, and viruses—fueled the AIDS pandemic and other diseases and, by the late 1990s, had "invented" (Brandt 2013) a new response: global health care, which transcended national borders. Globalization, as presented here, included the rapid spread of global health stories, science and scientists, research and its technologies and training, funding, knowledge, advocacy, activism, and practice. AIDS and globalization changed the way governments and NGOs tackled the prevention and treatment of diseases. That combination also changed the lives of people in communities that hosted global health initiatives. There was an extraordinary increase in the number of public and private funding sources to tackle a wide range of high-profile vertical (disease-specific) programs, especially those related to HIV (Garrett 2007; Benton 2015). Many of these programs were composed of collaborations between elite North American or European research institutions and their resource-poor country partners. Their stated goals were often the same: to reduce health disparities within and between countries. Yet in practice, the programs were not equal partnerships or collaborations (Brada 2011; Crane 2013; McKay 2018), nor did the outcomes reflect a full investment in reducing the structural, political, and social determinants of health and inequalities: for example, discrimination, racism, and uneven access to education, housing, transportation, food and material security, physical and emotional safety, and the like (Wilkinson and Marmot 2003; Kalofonos 2010; Mendenhall et al. 2015; Goodman 2016; Moyer and Igonya 2018). Such factors are at the core of health disparities (Biehl and Petryna 2013) and spur efforts to improve global health (Geissler 2013).

After several decades of fierce debates about whether AIDS should be handled as an exceptional disease that required special attention and financial support above and beyond normal health interventions (Epstein 2007; Julia Smith and Whiteside 2010), there was a shift toward the normalization of HIV when highly effective treatments became more equitable and affordable in the Global South (McGrath et al. 2014; Moyer and Hardon 2014). This normalization first emerged as a possibility during the 1996 International AIDS Conference in Vancouver, British Columbia, where the discovery of ART was unveiled and set new treatment standards that effectively transformed the disease into a treatable condition in the Global North (Julia Smith and Whiteside 2010). With a sense of optimism, the Joint United Nations Programme on HIV/AIDS (UNAIDS) was established in the same year. UNAIDS' goals were to provide global leadership in response to the epidemic, promote global consensus on the best policies and programs, monitor the implementation of recommended strategies at country levels, and strengthen the capacity and political commitment of leaders of national governments to develop effective and comprehensive strategies (Bor 2007; Knight 2008). Under the leadership of Peter Piot, UNAIDS endeavored to improve and expand the intensive international efforts of those working for its predecessor, the WHO Global Programme on AIDS (GPA), which had operated as the Special Programme on AIDS (SPA) in 1987 and the AIDS Control Programme (ACP) in 1986. As early as 1986, experts from WHO had already established a Global Strategy for the Prevention and Control of

AIDS, a one-size-fits-all approach that outlined the official prevention and surveillance guidelines and strategies to be used across nations—and had deployed researchers to collect data and start creating a realistic portrait of the international scope of the pandemic. By 1988, WHO was providing international expertise, incentives, technical assistance, and resources to any country that requested collaboration (Mann 1987; WHO 1988). The WHO GPA was eventually criticized, and ultimately replaced by UNAIDS, for failing in its leadership role and lacking the ability to coordinate across partner organizations (e.g., the United Nations Children's Fund [UNICEF], the United States Agency for International Development [USAID], and the World Bank), which contributed to the loss of direction in national programs. The conclusion was that the GPA had focused too narrowly on medical perspectives, at-risk groups, and scientific education that did not adequately translate into the desired behavior changes. This focus neglected the acknowledgment and consideration of changes that needed to be made at social and global levels (Iliffe 2006). A unique approach of UNAIDS, when compared to the WHO GPA, was its vision of working across different sectors in ways that involved collaborating with people living with the disease, community-based organizations, and major NGOs working in the AIDS field, including the Global Network of People Living with HIV (GNP+), in efforts to bolster the creation of socially supportive and safe living environments (Knight 2008).

By 1998, UNAIDS had established an updated repository for global AIDS data that captured not only the global magnitude of the pandemic but also showed that the disease was already generalized and a leading killer across the eastern, southern, and central regions of sub-Saharan Africa (WHO 1999). This repository was the first officially acknowledged single source of reference for AIDS data (Knight 2008). At this point in Kenya, for example, although the first case of HIV had been officially diagnosed in 1984, little was being done outside the health sector, and the government remained steadfast in its silence, denial, and inaction while the epidemic grew for fifteen years (Boone and Batsell 2001). The early but limited work being done by international groups during the first two decades borrowed from and mirrored the work being done at the time in the Global North, where efforts were tightly focused on controlling the spread of the disease by targeting and encouraging behavior change among members of at-risk groups. In Kenya, this translated into an emphasis on female sex workers (see chapter 1), especially in major cities like Nairobi and Mombasa. The impact of these efforts was minimal, as evidenced by the fact that by the time the Kenyan government finally took concrete actions in the late 1990s, the disease was already a leading cause of illness in the country: 13.95 percent of the adult population was living with HIV (NASCOP 1999; UNAIDS 2000), and an estimated 700 people were dying every day from AIDS-related illnesses (HRW 2001). These deaths resulted in an estimated 730,000 orphans, because 75 percent of all

AIDS-related deaths occurred among adults during their reproductive years (between the ages of eighteen and forty-five) (UNAIDS 2000). The initial responses and outcomes in Kenya stood in stark contrast to those in neighboring Uganda where, by 1986, government leaders had already acknowledged the scope of the problem, asked WHO for help, and joined forces with entities like the GPA and UNICEF to roll out more comprehensive strategies for prevention (UNICEF-WHO 1989; Knight 2008). Likewise, by 1987, Ugandan activists such as Noerine Kaleeba had established the AIDS Support Organization to support families caring for people with HIV, educate the community and health care workers, and eliminate stigma and discrimination. Activists coined the phrase "living positively with AIDS" to confront and challenge global public health messages like "AIDS kills" that framed the disease almost exclusively as a death sentence (Knight 2008). Many people, including Kaleeba, have credited the early reduction of HIV prevalence rates in Uganda to the unique approach used by President Yoweri Museveni, who made it politically correct for all people to talk about AIDS.

Citing new data, other evidence, and knowledge, the leaders of UNAIDS and other activists advocated for increased funding for the rollout of ART and AIDS-specific programming in parts of the world most impacted by the epidemic in the Global South (Knight 2008; Levine et al. 2009). These ideas and efforts were amplified during and following the 2000 International AIDS Conference, held in Durban, South Africa. It was there that AIDS was framed not only as a medical condition but as an international human rights issue. This was a novel public health prevention tactic adopted from the one used in the Global North by AIDS activists, including those involved in the gay rights movement during the 1980s and 1990s. This new public health approach for tackling and containing HIV, a communicable disease, involved activists who were living with and speaking out about HIV. It prioritized individuals and their right to be free of stigma and discrimination over the broad public health protections that had historically centered on quarantining infected individuals (Bayer and Fairchild 2006; Knight 2008; Fisher, Kohut, and Fisher 2009). These ideas were adopted by health officials across North America and Western Europe, where there was concern that stigma would cause members of certain at-risk groups to resist HIV testing and avoid health care services if they were infected, which could spread the disease into the general population (Rosenbrock et al. 2000). This latter fear never materialized to the degree that it was anticipated in the Global North. Yet these strategies were still picked up and internationally amplified first by Jonathan Mann and later, more intensely, by Piot, who promoted health as a human right; played early, active, and influential roles in mobilizing international cooperation and donor support; and spearheaded the global strategies outlined by the GPA (Kim 2015). At the beginning of the twenty-first century, AIDS conference attendees in South Africa used a human rights framework to confront deeply rooted racist discourses about the lives of poor and uneducated Africans who could not tell time or adhere to biomedical regimens (Crane 2013). Humanitarian organizations, such as Médecins sans Frontières, successfully challenged such racist claims by demonstrating that people in the Global South could adhere to ART treatment just as well as, if not better than, those in the Global North (MSF 2009). Still, the cost of ART remained prohibitively high and was out of reach for people living in countries that had both a high burden of disease and a lack of health resources (Julia Smith and Whiteside 2010). Activists called for the prices of ART to be reduced so government-provided treatment programs could be rolled out across the Global South in the name of human rights (Julia Smith and Whiteside 2010). Government leaders in India and Brazil took on powerful institutions such as the World Trade Organization, demanding compulsory licensing that would allow them to manufacture affordable, generic medications (Biehl 2007, 2008). And in the United States, activists applied pressure on the U.S. government in its support of patent legislation among pharmaceutical companies (Julia Smith and Whiteside 2010, 4; see also Engel 2006).

AIDS activists, scholars, and professionals from South Africa, India, Brazil, the United States, European countries, and beyond thus launched aggressive campaigns that mobilized substantial resources, which in 2002 resulted in Botswana's implementing the first universal-access treatment program in sub-Saharan Africa. An especially influential voice was the Treatment Action Campaign (TAC), established by the South African activist Zackie Achmat. TAC took the South African government to court for refusing to provide the drug nevirapine, which prevents mother-to-child transmission of HIV. In a landmark ruling in 2002, the Constitutional Court ordered the government to provide nevirapine and expand HIV testing and counseling services (Knight 2008). The following year, facing pressure from TAC and the international community, the government followed Botswana's example and announced that it would offer public treatment programs for HIV in 2003 (WHO/UNAIDS/UNICEF 2009). It continues to do so.

At the same time, world leaders framed AIDS as a "global emergency," using the rhetoric of globalization to underscore the potential threats to processes of securitization, democratization, and peacemaking imposed by this disease (Julia Smith and Whiteside 2010, 3). For example, UN secretary general Kofi Annan called for a "war chest" of $7–$10 billion per year from donors to help in the global "battle" against AIDS (Knight 2008, 128–129). Likewise, the high volume of AIDS orphans roused international concerns about potential social unrest as people imagined vulnerable children to be ideal recruits for militant rebel and terrorist groups (Barnett and Whiteside 2006). To tackle issues of global concern, such as those related to communicable diseases, poverty, and debt relief, donor countries scaled up international aid contributions (see chapter 1). International leaders and funders pushed the use of HIV testing and emphasized a behavioralist approach—the ABC model, to practice Abstinence, Be faithful, or use Condoms—of HIV prevention in sub-Saharan Africa (see chapter 1). The adoption of this controversial approach was based on an early, successful model from Uganda, where early government-driven efforts, with the support of WHO, had stressed the reduction of the number of sex partners (especially among men) through a campaign called Zero Grazing (Green 2003; Shelton et al. 2004; Green et al. 2006), which has been credited for the country's reduction of HIV infection rates by two-thirds from 1990 to 2001 (Epstein 2009). While donor countries promoted the ABC model for AIDS prevention in sub-Saharan Africa, WHO launched a massive global treatment campaign, and by 2006, the governments of 111 countries had committed to achieving universal access to HIV prevention, treatment, and care by 2010 (WHO/UNAIDS/UNICEF 2009). At that time, I began conducting the HIV-related research in Mahali on which this book is based.

Global health efforts targeting HIV have since turned to an approach that relies heavily on using routinized, biomedical models, surveillance, and technologies such as HIV testing, ART, and, more recently, pre-exposure prophylaxis (PrEP) to treat and prevent HIV. Accordingly, the framing of global health narratives switched from one presenting AIDS as a deadly global health crisis in the 1980s, 1990s, and early 2000s to one claiming that HIV was a chronic condition, manageable through promising technological solutions and biological knowledge about healthy, responsible living across the Global North and South (Hardon and Moyer 2014; McGrath et al. 2014; Prince 2014). Specifically, while there is still no vaccine or cure for HIV, treatment as prevention (TasP)—prevention through increased access to medical testing and medication—made it possible to imagine the idea of eradicating this disease from the globe. TasP fueled new discourses about the possibility of using medications to bring about the end of AIDS and an AIDS-free generation, and spurred UNAIDS to set ambitious, fast-track goals. In 2014, UNAIDS established the two-stage program of 90-90-90 by 2020 (referring to 90 percent of people infected knowing that they are seropositive, 90 percent of those people taking ART, and 90 percent of that group achieving viral suppression and thus being unable to transmit the virus to anyone else), followed by 95-95-95 by 2030 to end AIDS by 2030 (UNAIDS 2017; Kenworthy, Thomann, and Parker 2018). With the goal of eradication in mind, the concept of the HIV cascade of care (or the HIV cascade, the standard model for quantifying, describing, and analyzing patient behavior in terms of the management of lifelong HIV care) has emerged and shaped the research and treatment agendas of global and public health scholars and professionals. New forms of statistical calculations and evidence, as well as constantly shifting funding priorities, regularly unveiled the latest hard-to-reach or key populations that were imagined by global health experts (Moyer and Igonya 2018) and subsequently were transformed into novel, often fleeting, targets of HIV interventions, projects, and programs (Adams 2016; Biruk 2018). The successes of these kinds of interventions were measured by the number of "services provided" and "lives saved" (PEPFAR 2008, 8).

Little scholarship has been devoted to a global update on the successes and failures of UNAIDS to reach its 90-90-90 targets by 2020. In July 2020, UNAIDS (2020b) reported that only fourteen countries were on track to meet the targets by the end of the year, and evidence from one systematic review suggested that while high-income countries had generally met their UNAIDS targets, low- and middle-income countries had failed to do so (Karatzas et al. 2019). For example, reports from Kenya revealed that while the country was headed in the right direction, it had not yet reached the 90-90-90 targets (UNAIDS 2019, 2020b). The inability of resource-limited countries to reach the UNAIDS targets was attributed to a lack of adherence to global health HIV policies and guidelines and the lack of both supportive infrastructure and the active engagement of all stakeholders (Karatzas et al. 2019). These conclusions are based on the assumption that global health efforts are neutral and inserted into places with social, cultural, moral, and structural conditions that are similar to those where the guidelines and policies were created. Failures were thus construed as compliance problems rather than problems with undemocratic and panacean guidelines, protocols, policies, and interventions for treatment—all of which introduce baggage that, when inserted into new places with distinct historical, cultural, and political realities, inflict social and institutional changes (Hardon and Dilger 2011; Hardon and Moyer 2014; Kenworthy 2017; Winchester et al. 2017). Furthermore, globally circulating interventions, policies, and guidelines (firmly anchored in individualistic human- and sexual-rights frameworks and norms) are not identically interpreted across cultures or evenly embraced by all stakeholders, which sometimes results in national and local adaptations (Angotti 2012), unintended consequences (Patterson 2018; Hershey 2019), and "misaligned priorities" among the many actors involved in the responses to AIDS (Dionne 2017).

Other studies of the barriers for people as they are exposed to HIV cascade programs reveal that people still continue to refuse testing, resist treatment, and do not stay in care (see, e.g., Manderson, Cartwright, and Hardon 2016)—even in places like Mahali, where free and comprehensive biomedical treatment and care have been available since 2004. Especially confounding to global health experts are data pointing to the persistent role that stigma plays in population resistance (UNAIDS 2003, 2017, 2019, 2020b; WHO 2021c). Such findings challenge assumptions made by medical professionals, public health planners, and AIDS activists that more equal access to HIV treatment, care, and knowledge would normalize, depoliticize, and destigmatize the disease (Castro and Farmer 2005). In this book, based on fieldwork carried out since 2010, I critically trace the HIV discourses that circulated among the subaltern, or those with little power to influence global health initiatives and efforts (Hardon and Moyer 2014) to explain how and why the stigma associated with HIV persists in the age of treatment. At the center of my analysis are the stories people tell, stories that allow me to foreground the everyday lives, concerns, cultural logics, perspectives, and health-seeking behaviors of people experiencing, interpreting, resisting, enacting, and/or negotiating processes of stigma and discrimination. While doing this, I have been mindful of the broader contexts shaping those processes, and I draw on this in my analysis of how people made sense of HIV and the stigma attached to the infection (as well as of the global health responses to AIDS and the stigma) in their lived realities and conditions.

MAKING SENSE OF HIV AND STIGMA NARRATIVES IN KENYA

During a six-week trip to western Kenya in 2019, I was struck by the many impressive and observable changes that had taken place since my last visit, in 2014. Roads had been expanded and freshly paved, making driving considerably less dangerous than in 2010, when I first began visiting the country and when it was common to see cars and trucks flipped over on the side of the road following often fatal accidents. This work included major improvements to the main highway that began in the low-lying coastal town of Mombasa, passed through the capital of Nairobi, and climbed gradually upward across the equator, going through ear-popping elevation changes and forests, as well as larger towns and numerous trading centers and truck stops across the Rift Valley. On any given day in 2019, elite Kalenjin runners—as well as other Kenyan and international world-class athletes—could be seen training alongside the road. Athletes travel to the region from all over the world to take advantage of the year-round temperate climate, the high altitude, and especially the running camps offered in places like Iten, a city 7,000 feet above sea level that is known as the City of Champions.

By 2019 in Mahali, schools had been provided with intermittent access to electricity, the internet, and mobile computer labs. The HIV clinic had received an impressive face-lift, and there was even a working ambulance for emergencies in the region. While I had been away from Kenya, I had received disconcerting text messages about accidents that had happened to friends, as well as relieving news that their lives had been spared because of the introduction of ambulatory services. In Eldoret, pedestrians filled an extensive network of newly paved sidewalks, where I was occasionally stopped and asked by strangers if I would pose for selfies with them on their smartphones. I could shop in expensive grocery stores and high-end shopping malls, eat at Kentucky Fried Chicken franchises, go to nightclubs where participants in a vibrant youth culture engaged in mobile journalism and performed in *kitenge*[3] fashion shows to tackle global causes such as ending rape culture. I could meet with friends and colleagues over cappuccinos at coffee shops offering free Wi-Fi. New hospital building renovations and fresh coats of paint complemented the expanded and improved services, technologies, laboratories, and consultation rooms that were filled with well-qualified staff members who had been trained in diverse national and international settings. There were new maternity wards; cancer, cardiovascular, and diabetes centers; and pediatric facilities.

Global health efforts had contributed substantially to development in the Rift Valley, which became possible in part because the HIV epidemic had had such a damaging impact on economic development and growth in Kenya, as in other countries in sub-Saharan Africa (Hecht et al. 2006). Global health interventions—considered as a set of tools to address the universal, if uneven, human problem of diseases—became linked to the promotion of economic development in low- and middle-income countries like Kenya. This was evident in the creation of and priorities outlined in the UN Millennium Development Goals (which expired in 2015) and subsequently through the adoption of the Sustainable Development Goals (SDGs) (Hammonds et al. 2019). In these goals, the health and well-being of populations were designated as a crucial area of intervention for economic growth.

Despite visible social and infrastructural improvements, the stories I heard by 2019 about HIV and stigma were surprisingly consistent with those I had collected during previous research trips and across a variety of projects with which I had been associated in various capacities. HIV and stigma narratives were not only persistent, they also seemed to be hegemonic. This was striking because global health efforts had done so much to address the disease through HIV cascade programming. While there were subtle mutations over the years, the 2019 version of the familiar story can be summed up in the following way: HIV was a disease of poverty, and HIV testing, treatment, retention in care, and rates of viral suppression were negatively impacted by stigma in Kenya, a country described as a hostile environment for people living or associated with HIV. The story continued: People living with HIV (PLWHIV) were rejected and experienced myriad forms of stigmatization at various (overlapping) levels—both intrapersonal (or within one's self or mind, referred to as perceived stigma and internal or self-stigma) and interpersonal (or at the hands of others, through felt, enacted, and courtesy stigma [Goffman 1963]), including at the community level (public stigma) and the institutional level (structural stigma)—all of which I describe in the following chapters (for a concise overview of the various forms of stigma, see Brewis and Wutich 2019, 207–208).

The suggested source of stigma was equally persistent across the everyday discourses of people with whom I spoke (see chapter 5), and it has continually been documented in media stories and peer-reviewed journal articles: Kenyans, especially poorer ones, lacked knowledge and had cultural belief "problems," harboring "persistent negative and inaccurate community beliefs about HIV"

(McHenry et al. 2017, 225). This understanding of stigma and the ways to address it had roots in early social psychological theories developed in the Global North, which interpreted stigma as a static, fixed characteristic of a person located within the minds of individuals (Parker and Aggleton 2003). According to this view, stigma persisted due to a lack of scientific knowledge, and it thus caused people to make poor choices and harbor unwarranted fears about HIV. The solution was simple: increasing the focus on HIV awareness and education based on individualistic notions of risk, prevention, testing, and treatment. Yet this approach has long ignored any consideration of the larger structural inequalities that contextualized the "choices" made by people (Castro and Farmer 2005, 54; see also Booth 2004; Fassin 2007; Marsland and Prince 2012) and the reality that all humans construct their identities, lives, desires, and goals in concert with other valuable, life-sustaining social relationships and according to a socially constructed, yet still very real, set of norms, roles, values, morals, expectations, obligations, and hierarchies that extend well beyond a biomedicalized view of life. Therefore, knowing that there is "danger" in telling a "single story"—not because it is wrong, but because it is incomplete (Adichie 2009; see also Mkhwa-nazi 2016)—the impetus for writing this book was my desire to offer a thicker (see Geertz 1973), more nuanced explanation for the persistence of HIV stigma.

During the past decade, I documented variations of these HIV and stigma narratives everywhere I looked and listened. Yet the continual conclusion that the root of the problem of stigma was faulty beliefs and a lack of scientific knowledge, especially among poor people, is one-sided and a simplistically thin description that obscures as much as it informs. The persistent story emerged under colonialism, when racist discourses and practices routinely centered on the idea of so-called diseased Africans with backward beliefs and cultures who needed to be saved by people who were more mature, educated, and cultured (Vaughan 1991; Karp 2002). Education is an essential cornerstone of global public health. However, the ways that messages and programming are imagined and framed make a difference. Thus, interventions need to be both recognized as potentially political actions and constructed carefully, using input from the people targeted by the interventions (Dionne 2017) and keeping the population's social, cultural, and political realities in mind. Programs such as those for sex workers, people who inject drugs (PWIDs), and men who have sex with men (MSMs) have been designed to target the most economically marginalized individuals within hard-to-reach or key populations as they are imagined by donors and international researchers (Moyer and Igonya 2018).

The enduring focus on the poorest members of at-risk populations in Kenya is tied to HIV scholarship and academic interest in risk-related behaviors and environments. An early, yet dominant theory from public health in the Global North was the notion that the spread of HIV was the result of bad and unhealthy choices made by people who were misinformed, which caused them to engage in risky behaviors and have irrational fears about HIV and those living or associated with it. Anthropologists offered a compelling political critique to this framing of HIV, arguing that broader forces, such as structural inequalities, were involved and created risk environments for particular populations (Parker 2001; Farmer 2004; Rhodes et al. 2005). Anthropologists thereby synthesized key public health ideas about education and risk through the explanatory mechanism of structural, especially socioeconomic, inequalities (Gilley and Pfeiffer 2017). This gave rise to the need to address not only the behaviors of people, but their vulnerability to HIV infections according to their socioeconomic position. A major factor identified was known as the "'poverty spiral': the impact of the epidemic on national development and of development on the epidemic" (Knight 2008, 63). This (re)imagining has had an important and significant influence on the way HIV and stigma are conceptualized and addressed in Kenya. Yet, as we shall see, these approaches inadvertently reinforce stigma and negative associations with the disease and limit the effectiveness of global health efforts (see chapter 5). This suggests that it is time to revise the way we think and talk about HIV and address stigma.

The constant claim that economically marginalized people lack proper knowledge about HIV ignores the fact that economic realities and global health programming, policies, and guidelines surrounding HIV—as a form of international development work that primarily targets sexuality and reproductive health—are fundamentally viewed in political and moral terms (Adams and Pigg 2005; Ferguson 2006; McCoy and Singh 2014). As global health efforts simultaneously promoted the normalization of the disease and pushed programs that heavily targeted the poorest members of still criminalized key populations for intervention, the subtle information sent to Kenyan citizens aggravated already existing social tensions and created new ones in the contexts of a generalized epidemic and extreme inequalities. Since HIV and its associated stigma remained linked to enduring socioeconomic inequalities, discourses about HIV infections evoked a strong sense of morality versus immorality and chaos (Dilger 2008). Moralizing discourses about HIV and AIDS are therefore as much about the broader contexts of globalization that (re)produce the social, structural, and systemic inequities fueling their spread as they are about an infection and a disease (Yang et al. 2007; D. Smith 2014). Global health information and programs thus inadvertently helped maintain the link between HIV and immorality in addition to aggravating stigma, fear, and shame among members of the middle class and others who became infected but, understandably, did not want their social statuses or reputations tainted or damaged (Moyer and Igonya 2018). Likewise, a singular focus on HIV awareness and education disregarded the broader relationships and factors that fuel and sustain the processes of stigma but were set aside in favor of using a rigid biomedical treatment regime and the chronic disease paradigm (Mattes 2011; McGrath et al. 2014). Using Michael Taussig's ideas of "public secrets," Paul Geissler illustrates how global health research in East Africa frequently demands "unknowing" the very inequalities that facilitate it: "Unknown knowns—or 'public secrets'—may play an integral part in publicly funded medical science. . . . [S]uch unknowing pertains to vital material inequalities across the relations of scientific production. These inequalities are open to experience but often remain unacknowledged in public speech and scientific texts. . . . Unknowing [inequalities], then, facilitates research; and it shapes the resulting work and perpetuates the political and economic contradictions that pervade the context and the research endeavor itself" (2013, 13).

Global health, viewed as an "imaginative project" (Tsing 2005, 32), frequently screened out conflicts, contexts, and inequalities, including those necessary to explain and address the persistence of HIV stigma. Efforts to address stigma have thus centered on the problem of beliefs and a lack of proper knowledge since at least 2010, when I began formally studying the topic and observed anti-stigma campaigns at work across Mahali. But HIV stigma persisted in spite of education and awareness programs (Mattes 2014; Niehaus 2014), and instead, the logics that fostered stigma were altered through these campaigns (see chapter 5). While programs created using this premise may legitimate "a potentially endless horizon of intervention" (Brada 2011, 290), they fail to achieve the intended outcome of eradicating stigma and, ultimately, AIDS. At worst, they inadvertently perpetuate the social tensions and inequalities that support and increase such processes.

Stigma, classically conceptualized by Erving Goffman (1963, 3) as an "attribute that is deeply discrediting," is central to the social construction of the identity of a person. For Goffman, discrediting attributes were wide-ranging, context specific, and sometimes detectable, such as skin color, language or accent, or physical deformity or difference. They could also be hidden but damaging if exposed in the wrong place or time, such as through the disclosure of an HIV status—as exemplified through the story at the beginning of this introduction about the damaged reputation of the woman who was buried. Goffman emphasized stigma as an unavoidable part of social life that shaped and complicated human interactions and yielded exceptional, health-demoting consequences for some people. To recognize and understand the processes through which certain attributes become discredited, Goffman (1963, 3) stressed a contextual focus on "a language of relationships" that set up the boundaries around and through which members living in any given society learned to assess whether people (themselves and others) were normal or not. It is only in relation to a socially constructed concept of normal that those who cannot conform are stigmatized, denied full social acceptance, and deemed "not quite human" (Goffman 1963, 5). According to Goffman, both the normal people and the stigmatized learn through messages—communicated, often subtly, through their daily living— and become aware of their own statuses in relation to one another, especially during mixed contexts or moments when multiple people are in the same social situation, where they (inter)act accordingly. Building on this seminal work, a significant body of literature emerged, and stigma is now acknowledged as a fundamental driver of global health disparities (Hatzenbuehler, Phelan, and Link 2013). It has been theorized by social scientists in various, discipline-specific ways, including as a moral issue in which a stigmatizing condition reveals what is most at stake and threatened among both those who are stigmatized and those who do the stigmatizing and share a local social world (Yang et al. 2007).

VIRAL FRICTIONS: UNDERSTANDING THE PERSISTENCE OF STIGMA THROUGH STORIES

Social scientists posit that while processes of stigma are universal human experiences, they are always locally distinctive and contingent because they are situated in already existing and shared moral logics and social rules (Yang et al. 2007), specific forms and histories of violence (Castro and Farmer 2005), and other social and structural inequalities around which lines of differences are drawn in particular places (Parker and Aggleton 2003). Therefore, scholars argue that to address stigma, it is essential to understand the underlying roots of it in a particular place (Pescosolido et al. 2008). Yet the central component of Goffman's original theory that specified the importance of centering "a language of relationships" to understand such processes remains narrowly conceptualized both by global health experts and anthropologists. Global health policies and programs committed to eradicating AIDS are often premised on the notion of a universality of experiences with HIV and stigma and thus the idea that universal scientific knowledge, education, and health practices and policies can adequately address these problems across the world's wide range of social experiences and identities (Booth 2004, 8–11). But this approach neglects any serious consideration of how a normal person is constituted in a given setting and dismisses the possibility that the biomedical requirements of ART and other aspects of living with HIV may actually place a person outside the bounds of what is considered normal in some places, especially among populations living in conditions of uncertainty, violence, and limited resources (see chapters 5 and 6). At the same time, ethnographies, like contemporary social-scientific theories about stigma, often depend on the idea that clear borders can be neatly drawn around a locality. However, the notions of *universal*, *global*, and *local* contain many assumptions, and little scholarship has paid serious, critical attention to the relationships among them to consider how they might be working together to build and maintain the social tensions at the heart of persisting processes of stigma. In fact, anthropologists have recently engaged surprisingly little in generating theory about the relationships among stigma, globalization, and health during the age of treatment in the Global South. This neglect is striking because anthropologists have long understood globalization as a complex set of relationships (Massey 1994; Gupta 1998), and anthropology has had much to say about globalization and HIV in Africa (Booth 2004; Farmer et al. 2006; Nguyen 2010; Crane 2013; D. Smith 2014; Benton 2015).

The metaphor of friction, used by the anthropologist Anna Tsing to conceptualize globalization, aptly characterizes a language of relationships and the unanticipated tensions produced between the local and the global. For Tsing (2005, 5), universal sets of knowledge are tools—such as those associated with vertical global health HIV programs—that link geographically scattered communities and collide with other systems of knowledge to produce friction, or unexpected outcomes that help keep "global power in motion." While Tsing emphasizes friction as a product of collisions between global and local knowledge, in this book, I focus on the frictions produced within and between local, regional, national, and global scales that intersect to form the roots of HIV-related stigma in Kenya. As Kim Dionne (2017, 8), who has previously explained why AIDS interventions frequently fail in sub-Saharan Africa, rightly notes, "success depends on each link in a global hierarchy." Without careful, critical examination and analysis of the frictions produced within and between these scales, we risk contributing to the (re)production of the social and structural processes that help maintain persisting forms of intersecting stigmas.

Understanding the positioning of a local community in relation to the larger region and nation-state, as well as the relationships between Kenya and other countries, is critical for understanding persisting processes of stigma. While so-called local beliefs, perspectives, experiences, and frictions are certainly (re)shaped by relatives, friends, employers, neighbors, rivals, and others living in close proximity to each other, they are also influenced by doctors, international workers, students, volunteers, NGO workers, pastors, social workers, and other people who are responsible for promoting and implementing (or neglecting to promote and implement) programs at the community level. Local ideas about who is normal (or not) are further molded by the larger nation-state within which a community is embedded. This is because, for example, African NGOs, politicians, government officials, and other leaders are active agents in global health governance and often help determine where, what, when, and how development initiatives, messages, programs, and policies are implemented, or even if they are put into action at all (Patterson 2018; Hershey 2019).

Yet political leadership never happens in a vacuum, and a country's place in the global economy shapes the nature of state governance (Bor 2007). Specifically, delicate relationships and collaborations were produced between NGOs and governments of countries in sub-Saharan Africa after foreign development donors and funding agencies shifted to channeling money into NGOs—claiming that governments were corrupt—throughout the 1990s (Bratton 1989; Chege 1999). These historical actions gave rise to the governance of HIV-related service delivery systems and programming in Kenya, where it was "difficult to tell where the government [ended] and the NGO [began]" (Brass 2016, 12). Local subjectivities and frictions are thus further (re)constructed by international governments, corporations, donor funding contingencies, and policies that are designed and determined in collaborations between national and foreign medical researchers and practitioners, development experts, politicians, and leaders from around the world. As funding for HIV-related programs became available and as world health guidelines and evidence-based approaches shifted, they had very real impacts (both positive and negative) on people's lives, relationships, bodies, and psyches. This was true even though the people designing the recommendations, policies, and interventions never actually met or directly consulted with the people they intended to benefit (Booth 2004, 11; Dionne 2017).

While Goffman did not conceptualize stigma with the HIV epidemic in mind, anthropologists and sociologists have done so to advance understandings of stigma as a complex social process dependent upon social, economic, and political powers (Link and Phelan 2017) and as part of an ongoing struggle over the maintenance and legitimization of myriad forms of inequalities, including those associated with class, race, ethnicity, gender, and sexuality (Parker and Aggleton 2003). "Stigma power" is used by those who stigmatize others at all levels as a way not only to keep people in line, but also sometimes to keep individuals and populations "down, in or away" (Link and Phelan 2014, 24). Disease stigma is often just the tip of much deeper and enduring social, political, structural, systemic, and global inequalities (Yang et al. 2007). As we shall see, in Kenya, moralizing discourses about HIV and processes of stigma springboarded both into and out of deeply rooted national politics, conflicts, and inequalities (across lines of ethnicity, gender, sexuality, and class) that were fiercely debated, thereby keeping them all in motion during a period of rapid social change.

Global health experts contend that one of the most significant barriers to ending AIDS is stigma (UNAIDS 2016, 2020b). Likewise, medical anthropologists claim that HIV-related stigma contributes, in part, to the continuation of HIV exceptionalism (Moyer and Hardon 2014; Mattes 2019). In this book, I want to flip these arguments to suggest that both AIDS eradication efforts and HIV exceptionalism aggravate processes of stigma and intertwine to fuel and sustain its persistence. My primary argument is intentionally straightforward in discussion but complex in application: HIV-related stigma persists through complex processes of globalization, or what I call viral frictions. In the pages that follow, I demonstrate what stigma is and does. I emphasize the global processes through which the rationale behind the "deeply discredited attribute" (Goffman 1963) of HIV is morphed but maintained like a virus, rather than eliminated, through frictions produced by virally circulating and colliding global, national, and local health-related knowledge, discourses, and practices. Globalized efforts, associated with normalizing HIV and ending AIDS, will not work effectively in a community characterized by extreme social, economic, and political tensions and uncertainties (see chapter 2), where the virus is still perceived and experienced as exceptional (McGrath et al. 2014; Moyer and Hardon 2014; Benton 2015). I therefore imagine HIV stigma as a linguistically and socially constructed cultural process produced at the nexus of local, national, and global relationships and storytelling about and practices associated with HIV, which is where this book locates the root of its persistence in the age of treatment. I discuss moments when stigma erupted at the intersecting pushes and pulls of HIV exceptionalism and normalization and was used as a human device for a variety of purposes, logics, power struggles, and agendas. A central message in this book is that colliding stories, as they play out in particular contexts, can help create, transform, and perpetuate processes of stigma. Words, metaphors, images, statistics, and silences used to speak of, explain, temper, or ignore viruses shape the ways in which people understand, respond to, and experience diseases (Sontag 1989; Treichler 1999; CDC 2021) and, consequently, inform processes of stigma. Put another way, narratives that are told, (re)told, or silenced about HIV are powerful and "just as real as germs" (Briggs and Mantini-Briggs 2003, 7) and medications (Diane Goldstein 2004).

To theorize and help explain the persistence of HIV-related stigma, I develop the concept of viral frictions by engaging with and contributing to anthropological theories and debates on narrative, globalization, critical development studies, and HIV in eastern and southern Africa. I use *viral* to evoke several ideas. The first and most obvious reason is because the stories with which I critically engage are, in part, about a disease that is spread by a virus. But the term primarily refers to the sudden and rapid movement of a story—as a universal—around the globe. People with the power to make stories "go viral" are envied, praised, rewarded, and imitated (Elie 2020). By using the term *viral*, I illuminate the centrality of narratives as a force that shapes the human experience. I also show the enormous successes that global health storytelling—about the science, knowledge, and technologies (e.g., rapid tests and ARTs) of HIV and stigma—has had in spreading rapidly, or virally, around the globe to become received as wisdom and truth.

The viral storytelling and practices of global health experts that are described in these pages are related to those that normalize and promote HIV as a primarily biological, chronic condition to be remedied through biomedical interventions, technologies, and scientific knowledge. This tactic gives no serious consideration to the deeply social nature of maintaining lifelong ART adherence, especially in contexts where food scarcity, insecurity, poverty, and politically violent conditions are a constant part of normal daily living for everyone (Kalofonos 2010; Prince 2012; Mattes 2019). Normalization efforts through TasP are thus at odds with what PLWHIV require to live a normal life on ART

(McGrath et al. 2014), and unanticipated consequences, differences, disjunctures, and frictions are produced when global health efforts mute and ignore the structural conditions that embed and give shape to the social and personal care needs of the people they intend to benefit. This neglect helps preserve HIV exceptionalism (Moyer and Hardon 2014; Benton 2015) and the enduring mark (Goffman 1963) attached to a person living with or associated with HIV, thus keeping stigma firmly in place despite the uneven availability of treatment.

With the biomedical turn in HIV treatment and care in mind, I frame global health as an "anti-politics machine." This concept was developed by James Ferguson to explain the language and practices used by development experts in Lesotho that disregard the political, social, and historical factors that actually explain how and why poverty exists and persists in the Global South. Ferguson (1994, 256) argues that while development initiatives routinely fail to achieve their planned goals and are not "a machine for eliminating poverty," they produce unanticipated "instrument-effects" that inadvertently become a "machine" for strengthening and expanding the power of politically self-serving state bureaucracies:

> By uncompromisingly reducing poverty to a technical problem, and by promising technical solutions to the sufferings of powerless and oppressed people, the hegemonic problematic of "development" is the principal means through which the question of poverty is depoliticized in the world today. At the same time, by making the intentional blueprints for "development" so highly visible, a "development" project can end up performing extremely sensitive political operations involving the entrenchment and expansion of institutional state power almost invisibly, under cover of a neutral, technical mission to which no one can object. The "instrument-effect," then, is two-fold: alongside the institutional effect of expanding bureaucratic state power is the conceptual or ideological effect of depoliticizing both poverty and the state. (Ferguson 1994, 256)

Global health efforts in Kenya have failed to reach UNAIDS targets set to end AIDS. However, the Kenyan government, which initially delayed addressing the epidemic, has implemented one of the most impressive responses to HIV over the past decade, as I describe in greater depth in chapter 1. The state gained "instrument-effects" (Ferguson 1994, 256) when it became attached to global health entities and funds and by making public claims and mobilizing intensive efforts to normalize and tackle HIV to end AIDS. These actions served as a marker—to citizens and the international community—of morally good and responsible governance (Benton 2015), produced more accountable public services that boosted the legitimacy of the state (Brass 2016), and enhanced processes of democratic consolidation (Wambuii 2006). HIV and the global response to it thus unwittingly increased the power and influence of the state and the agency of African leaders (Patterson 2018) in Kenya, as well as their ability to exploit, manage, control, and reinforce old hierarchies of people and communities and create new ones through the implementation of allegedly depoliticized actions. For example, a select group of elite Kenyan nationals held and still hold high-ranking positions in HIV-related NGO and government global health initiatives and academic research partnerships across the country and beyond. Mirroring that fact, ironically while HIV continued to be perceived and experienced as a stigmatizing condition, knowing about HIV brought value to people across the socioeconomic spectrum. This happened as they struggled to gain access to resources, prestige, social networks, and capital (financial, social, and cultural) and competed for meagerly paid employment and unpaid volunteer positions as a strategy to gain attachment to the AIDS industry (Prince 2014, 73). Over the years, possessing officially sanctioned global health knowledge about HIV—as mediated by the state and constantly changing funding demands and policies—came to evoke the sense of a person with a modern identity who was an enlightened, empowered, and morally good citizen with the potential for upward mobility (Prince 2014). As global health efforts boosted the chronic illness paradigm and pushed biomedicine as the solution, they advantaged elite Kenyans working in high-ranking jobs but marginalized those with less formal education, because lower-skilled, community-based positions, which were focused on the social needs and support of PLWHIV, came and went as funds dried up and priorities shifted (Prince 2014; Reed 2018).

The significance of global health's success in drastically reducing HIV infection rates and bringing relief to people from the burdens of and suffering from AIDS-related deaths in Kenya cannot be overstated: the lives of many people have been spared and improved because of global health knowledge, technologies, and resources. At the same time, it is difficult to exaggerate the intensity through which global and national public health efforts endeavor not only to normalize and biomedicalize HIV but also to exert power and surveillance over people—especially those living with HIV and those living in poverty. The intent is to (re)fashion their thinking, behaviors, and lives around new forms of individual self-care (de Klerk and Moyer 2017), the rules of positive living (Rasmussen 2013), and other rigid (and often forceful) regimes of biomedical knowledge and treatment (Mattes 2011) with the goal of persuading people to be responsible, well-informed, empowered, and healthy Kenyans (Prince 2014, 79). As Adia Benton (2015, 7) notes of "ideologically vertical" global health programs in Sierra Leone, they are also "methodologically horizontal" in that their discourses, practices, and logics have a "tendency to creep and seep" into development programming, politics, the media, subjectivities, concerns, moralities, and the like to produce particular kinds of citizens. The "creep and seep" of the biomedicalization of HIV and life in the context of an epidemic that is still experienced and perceived as exceptional open up new spaces in which tensions, contradictions, inequalities, power, and justice are fiercely negotiated (Benton 2015). Although this "epidemic of knowledge" (Boellstorff 2009, 356) was not intended by global health policies, researchers, or programs to produce palpable transformations in the ways people construct their lives, identities, hopes, desires, sense of belonging (or lack of belonging), local social worlds, and who is considered normal and who is not, it has transformed them. Furthermore, the transformations have mutated rather than ameliorated processes of HIV stigma in communities where eradication efforts are underway. It is in these ways that I imagine global health stories work virally and produce unanticipated frictions in Mahali.

To demonstrate how viral frictions contributed to the persistence of HIV stigma, I pay critical attention to the circulation of voluminous information about HIV and AIDS—from statistics, biomedical knowledge and technologies, media reports, illness narratives, eulogies, memories, local gossip and rumors, and so on—that worked their way into the local narratives I collected through a wide range of qualitative research methodologies, techniques, and projects over the years (see the preface). Mikhail Bakhtin draws attention to the ways in which statements are never independent because people are always speaking the words of others. As he writes, "Any utterance is a link in the chain of speech communication" (1982, 91). Words about HIV stigma, science, technologies, and knowledge came into Mahali through national campaigns aired on radio and television, printed in newspapers and on posters, billboards, and vehicles, and displayed on individuals wearing T-shirts advertising the latest HIV campaigns and slogans. Global health testing and counseling efforts to normalize HIV and promote living positively, as well as NGO programming centered on those most at risk, also spread the information. As people learned more, they began to circulate, repeat, and/or resist this overload of knowledge in distinct yet coherent patterns rooted in their own memories, knowledge, experience, and moral, cultural, and political logics (Pigg 1992; Stoeltje 2009). These stories help reveal the collisions of, as well as the frictions produced at the intersections of, multilevel knowledge, practices, and agendas. At the same time, words and narratives—broadly defined as a form of metaculture (Ochs and Capps 1996)—help (re)shape social and structural forces that move culture along (Urban 2001). The virality of global health storytelling illuminates the social and structural changes (re)produced by and through them.

I explore the effects of globalization and development, including through global health initiatives, on those living in a community plagued by chronic uncertainty, corruption, major social change, and other cascading inequities. In the pages that follow, I also demonstrate how violent structural and political conditions engulf the lives of people, deny many people social justice, and continue to intersect with and fuel processes of HIV-related stigma. Furthermore, I highlight the limitations and unintended consequences of the most recent global biomedical and technical turns in HIV initiatives and their accompanying discourses and practices around the normalization of HIV. Eradicating AIDS and the stigmas associated with it by using medications and proper knowledge is very challenging if little attention is paid to the underlying economic, moral, political, and social relationships, concerns, anxieties, and chronic inequalities that cannot be fixed with biomedical technologies. Understanding how social actors describe themselves and their lives, experiences, and desires—as framed through global, national, and local health discourses about HIV and AIDS—is required if HIV and stigma are to be understood and eliminated worldwide.

PLAN OF THE BOOK

In the chapters of this book, I emphasize different forms of stigma (e.g., structural, public, intrapersonal, and interpersonal) to reveal how such processes reinforced each other through the frictions produced between local, regional, national, and global levels. I especially focus on intersectional stigma, or how global health initiatives and HIV-related stigma interacted with the already existing inequalities being fiercely negotiated in Mahali and nationally in Kenya across lines of race and ethnicity (chapter 2), uncertainty and social change (chapter 3), gender and sexuality (chapter 4), mental health and class status (chapter 5), and generation and moral personhood (chapter 6). In sections of the chapters, I reflect on exceptional moments of fieldwork as well as my own positionality, drawing on a combination of field notes, casual conversations, and interactions with other people (including my research assistants). These moments reveal the complexities of social life, fieldwork, and global health efforts in the modern interconnected world, and they point to important insights about the persistence of stigma that can be gleaned only by "being there" as an ethnographer (Borneman and Hammoudi 2009). These kinds of insights are often missed by the larger epidemiological studies that dominate contemporary global health research and practice, and thus they add value to those studies.

Chapter 1 contains an anthropological history of HIV, as well as a broad overview of international funding, programs, policies, and guidelines that have flowed through Kenya. Chapter 2 opens with locally circulating stories about a rumored list of the names of women who were allegedly living with HIV. To provide context for readers to further understand stories about the List, I offer an abbreviated social and political history of Kenya. Then I examine the ways in which national narratives about political violence, ethnic conflict, and HIV—perceived and experienced as catastrophes fueling local discontents—have blended to create and sustain (de)moralizing discourses about place, ethnic animosities, and stigma. In this chapter, the perpetuation of stigma is portrayed as intimately linked to and springing into and out of the legacies of racism and existing national and political ethnic inequalities and regional hostilities. In chapter 3, I continue to focus on Kenya in relation to the global community by highlighting the content of a range of media articles that people discussed with me over the past decade, which helps situate my more contemporary study of stigma in the contexts of extreme uncertainty that, I argue, color the ways in which people living in Mahali make sense of and experience HIV, AIDS, and global health initiatives. In this chapter, I demonstrate how stories about HIV and AIDS knitted global health knowledge together with local knowledge about how to manage HIV to produce what I call the politics of uncertainty and to (re)shape manifestations of HIV-related public, institutional, and interpersonal forms of stigma and local socialities in unexpected ways.

Chapter 4 traces socioeconomic and ethnic inequities as they intersected with local gender dynamics and politics, especially highlighting the viral frictions produced between global health discourses or services and gendered categories of people (e.g., sex workers, wives, and husbands). Financial hardships during and since postelection violence (PEV) increased these frictions and resulted in social changes as men and women struggled to uphold and maintain their gendered ideals and roles. In this chapter, I further demonstrate how HIV became incorporated into these local, regional, and national gender and sexual identity politics to (re)produce already existing inequalities and processes of HIV-related stigma to impact AIDS eradication efforts. In chapter 5, I contextualize the anti-stigma campaigns developed by global health programs and circulated through the community to characterize the shifting nature of stigma in Mahali. Viral frictions in this chapter are framed as anti-stigma campaigns—imported to Mahali and conceptualized using a very individualistic and social-psychological understanding of stigma—colliding with already existing socioeconomic inequalities and knowledge about mental health status. This, alongside the scale-up of HIV testing and ART, helped redraw the boundaries around who was normal and who was not, which in turn impacted interpersonal and intrapersonal forms of self-stigma. The chapter then outlines the moral obligations and ethical dilemmas associated with money and the resources required to live positively (that is, to restore and maintain the health of an ill person), thus exposing what was most at stake (Yang et al. 2007) for all people in this part of the world. In the context of a community marked by extreme poverty, inequitably distributed wealth and resources, and a health care system that (outside of treatment and care for HIV) was inadequate and compromised, those living with HIV or AIDS were perceived to have had access to monies being channeled into the country by global and international donors. Therefore, they were also believed to be benefiting from access to good health care and other material items, such as food and school fees for their children, more than those who did not have the virus or disease. This alleged special treatment was perceived by many people to be unfair. Thus, globalization contributed to new, particular forms of HIV- and AIDS-related stigmas in Mahali. In chapter 6, I center on notions of moral personhood, specifically the interweaving of HIV, generational conflicts and politics, global health efforts, and stigmatization with caregiving.

I explore the way the requirements of living positively and discourses related to HIV as a chronic disease kept people feeling that they were outside the bounds of what was considered a normal person. The chapter then examines the way people living with the virus felt about themselves and how they refashioned the possibilities of their social relationships through forms of therapeutic citizenship and in efforts to restore a sense of normal personhood.

In the conclusion, I reflect on the social tensions and structural inequalities brought about by globalization colliding with HIV knowledges and national services to perpetuate processes of stigmatization and changing everyday social life. I emphasize how stories and social and biological experiences—created and maintained by the viral frictions produced at the intersections of local, national, and global actions—are mutually constitutive. I also offer a practical suggestion for global health policy makers, researchers, practitioners, and activists interested in ending AIDS, which will require ending stigma at individual, community, structural, and ultimately local, national, and global levels.

1 · UNEVEN ANTHROPOLOGICAL AND EPIDEMIOLOGICAL STORIES IN HISTORICAL HIV CONTEXT

I was preparing to conduct another life-history interview with Jane, a key interlocutor, who sat down across from me for our third formal session (we usually met socially). The audio recorder was on a desk in a consultation office, ready to capture her words as the soft voices from a CD of an interethnic, intercommunity peace choir of local women flowed in from the waiting room. We had turned it on to give us added privacy. We were sitting in the truck-container wellness clinic (hereafter, the container clinic) that provided health services to truck drivers and sex workers in the evenings. I had been given permission to use the space for interviews during the days, and Jane and I had agreed to meet very early that cold and rainy August morning.

The room we were in had three metal chairs and a desk on which were scattered supplies: the remains of HIV rapid-test kits, a nearly empty box of rubber gloves, a large bottle of hand sanitizer, a roll of cotton, and a small yellow cardboard box labeled "Biohazard." A few brochures, some blank volunteer counseling and testing (VCT) cards (used for recording the official results of an HIV rapid test), and a dark brown rubber penis and vagina (used for individual and group condom demonstrations) were also in the office. The walls were covered by posters with various pictures, condom advertisements, and HIV-related messages using catchy phrases such as "Be a Trusted Partner" (promoting the Trust brand of condoms), "Responsible Parents Protect the Children from HIV Infections Before, During, and After Birth," and "*Nimekata shauri* [I have decided]: Getting Tested for HIV Is a First Step in Protecting a Baby from HIV." The darkish cream tiles on the floor were smeared with globs of mud from dried footprints, reflective not only of the incessant rain but also of the hustle and bustle of the previous evening's activities. In the corners, also on the floor, were large cardboard boxes of HIV supplies (testing kits and condoms) labeled with lists of contents and the words "Not for Sale" and "Ministry of Public Health and Sanitation and Ministry of Medical Services." Listening to Jane during the interview, it was striking, but perhaps not surprising, how central the HIV epidemic had been across her life story. Jane was not unique in this regard. It was common to hear people repeating the phrase, "Everyone is infected or affected by HIV," which was an attempt to normalize and destigmatize an exceptional disease.

In this chapter, I provide an anthropological story of HIV in Kenya, covering how, why, and where it emerged; the changing responses to it; and the shifting epidemiological profile of the infection since its first diagnosis. To begin telling this story, I share some of what I learned from Jane as she recalled memories from her life during the first two decades of the AIDS epidemic. Building on the oral and anthropological histories and using them as a temporal frame of reference, the last section of the chapter presents an overview of the international funding, policies, guidelines, and programs that have been implemented to expose a contradiction at the heart of HIV-related global and national health efforts since I started doing the research for this book. In practice, HIV was treated as exceptional simply because funding and treatment were available, and the global community prioritized it over other health conditions and local concerns (see Bor 2007; Hardon and Moyer 2014; Dionne 2017; Kenworthy 2017). At the same time, national discourses about HIV and biomedical practices associated with its normalization produced social tensions and helped stigma persist, as people struggled to resolve and make sense of the dissonances. A research assistant merged these two sentiments when she half-jokingly updated me on life in Mahali when we were reunited in 2019: "The only healthy people these days are those with HIV."

JANE'S TELLING OF THE HISTORY OF HIV IN MAHALI

Jane, a self-identified member of the Kikuyu ethnic group and the owner of a small business when we met, agreed to share her story about the first time she heard about HIV. Almost as soon as she began talking about her earliest memories of the epidemic in Kenya, she interrupted herself to offer a broad context that she felt was central to my understanding of the ethnic tensions that were occurring around the same time that she became aware of HIV. She explained that she was married and had moved into a predominantly Kalenjin rural community in the Rift Valley in the early 1980s, only a few years before the emergence of *upungufu wa kinga mwilini* (UKIMWI; immune deficiency) or *slim*, as the disease was originally named by physicians working in this part of the world because patients lost weight rapidly (Knight 2008). She recalled hearing about

HIV soon after she was forced to move to Mahali because of political and ethnic violence:

> In 1992, we had the skirmishes [ethnic clashes and political violence related to the first Kenyan democratic election], and [my] husband was from a different tribe. So after the skirmishes, I was forced to come out of the [rural] area because people were saying that I was stealing a Kalenjin. And it was like I was fighting two wars: one was being a Kikuyu, and the second one was being a husband snatcher from the Kalenjin women. . . . [The rural] community was against me. So I came to the urban Mahali center because of the skirmishes. During the skirmishes, I lost everything that I treasured in this world, like my photos, which I keep on remembering. I lost them. Like the things from my schooling. I don't remember the other things because I can buy them again. I can make another house. I can buy new clothes. But there were things that I could not replace [with money].

In chapter 2, I discuss the history of Kenya and the Rift Valley region in more detail, but what Jane made immediately clear as she presented her oral history of HIV in Mahali was that while the virus was a major crisis, it was not the only one with which people had to contend. Nor was a person's HIV identity (having a positive or negative status) the only one that mattered or that she navigated. Instead, she recalled negotiating and simultaneously balancing a wide range of overlapping and sometimes conflicting identities and relationships—such as gender, sexual, class, marital, ethnic, and rural-urban divides—that mediated her experiences with and perceptions of HIV. Furthermore, Jane took the time to emphasize the grief she felt after losing meaningful and irreplaceable items, such as photographs that had served as reminders of her childhood and personal history. It was only after clarifying these details about how she ended up in Mahali that Jane went on to narrow the focus of her story to when she had first learned about HIV. She described hearing about it through local talk, gossip, and media representations of sex workers who were suffering from a mysterious disease that caused them to lose weight, cough, and have diarrhea. Eventually, the rumors in Mahali about UKIMWI became uncomfortably personal for Jane. It was through gossip that she learned that her husband's lover was suffering from the disease. This news propelled Jane into action and led her to make the following observations and conclusions:

> I very much wanted to go and see this disease that I had been hearing about. . . . [In] 1995, I got the chance to see [my husband's lover]. . . . Because I wanted to see. How does a person look when she has HIV? . . . I saw how slim she was and how she had changed. Before, she was so beautiful—she could have won the beauty of Mahali award—and then I could see that now she has changed to be

black [very sick and close to death].... After she died, many others died also. And I think even they did not die because they were sick, but because of knowing how they had been sharing [sexual partners].... So from that time on ... there was a lot of dying.... By 1999, we were hearing reports that [the rate of] HIV was so high in Mahali. So the [newspaper] articles announced to the entire country, "Take care in that place." It was [because we were located along] the highway. [There were] so many sex workers [and their truck-driving clients].

Through the collision of circulating stories about AIDS and local observations of and experiences with devastatingly high rates of AIDS-related deaths, people living in Mahali came to think about, respond to, and experience the AIDS epidemic and notions of risk in very particular ways (Diane Goldstein 2004). HIV was understood as being heterosexually transmitted and a sex worker disease. Because of Mahali's position along a busy highway and the vulnerability of its inhabitants, HIV was said to be dangerously rampant there, and the town was viewed as a place where people needed to be careful. At the same time, people could experience symptoms or even die of UKIMWI simply by knowing they had had sexual relations with an allegedly infected person. Consequently, people learned to pay very careful attention to sexual networks, which served as an informal yet widely embraced public health prevention strategy in the absence of affordable biomedical care and treatments. This practice and a local form of expertise were present throughout the decade of my research.

The potency of the combination of these stories and experiences led Jane (like other people) to misinterpret her persistent cough caused by allergies as an HIV infection, which prompted her to refuse and avoid HIV testing. She said:

I did not know [my chronic cough] was allergies, so I kept on going to the hospital [in hope of a cure]. So people started talking about me.... Then one day [another lover of her husband] came ... to me and said, "Hey! What is happening to you? It seems you are coughing so much [suggesting that Jane might be infected with HIV]." ... I was feeling I was part and parcel of those who were sick [with HIV] because my husband was reckless with sex.... So I was feeling that the only reason I did not have HIV was just because I had not been tested yet.... By this time, there is still no treatment! ... Some [research was] being done. The Europeans [were] doing research here because the government [could not] help us. At that time, the drugs for HIV were 65,000 shillings, so they were not affordable to anyone in Mahali.... So by that time people were being tested, but they weren't being told [their HIV status] because there was nothing that could be done in the public hospitals. Even the [doctors] did not like to test them.... [Those who were] diagnosed just asked the doctors to inject them with an injection that would kill them. So they could die earlier, ... quickly [without suffering].

During the fifteen years following Kenya's first official case of AIDS in 1984, the epidemic was experienced and perceived as an exceptional disease, which mirrored the broad conditions of uncertainty and violence in the lives of people. AIDS dominated the way people thought and worried about, interpreted, and acted in response to the potential signs and symptoms of disease in their own and others' bodies. As Jane's narrative demonstrates, tensions grew between people and groups as they struggled to control the narrative of who had engaged in "reckless" sex (and who had not) and thus were responsible for potentially infecting others. Since there was no access to life-saving medications and people were physically isolated and socially avoided if they were known to be infected, few people, including physicians, saw value in formal testing for HIV or disclosing an HIV+ serostatus to a patient. Among those who were tested and/or began to exhibit obvious signs of disease, according to Jane, suicide served as one legitimate and compassionate way to bypass the inevitable social isolation, as well as the emotional and relentless physical suffering caused by untreated AIDS. Thus, people like Jane acted reasonably by avoiding testing as a strategy to keep the disease out of their sense of self and as a technique of preserving their mental well-being and keeping future possibilities open (Whyte 1997; Eaton 2008).

At first, Jane spoke of the local sex workers who had died and their orphaned children. She then recalled the tremendous horror of learning that fetuses could contract HIV from their mothers and be born with the infection, and even die from AIDS. She went on to highlight the stories of colleagues, friends, and finally family members. Jane shared stories of brothers who had become infected and died, and she linked these details to the eventual death of their mother: "And so, two weeks after [the] burial of [my brother], my mom passed on after having a stroke. So by that time I knew my mom had died [from] the stigma of HIV. She did not like to be called 'the mother of HIV people.'" Stigma was described by Jane as powerful enough to extend beyond the infected person to affect family members as "courtesy stigma" (stigma by association: see Goffman 1963) and even explain the cause of death.

Jane also spoke of a close cousin who had married into a prominent and wealthy family, been infected with the virus before medication was accessible, and, as a result, attempted suicide. Jane offered the following words to describe her experiences with this relative and to further underscore both the potency of spoken words—their significant role in the activation of HIV-related stigma—and how people living in Mahali sometimes used them to spontaneously "attack" one another:

> The [cousin's] husband became seriously sick. He had tuberculosis . . . and that is
> the time I came to realize he was HIV+. My cousin had [attempted suicide]
> because of HIV. . . . Then it happened. The husband died . . . and . . . I told her,
> "No—don't go [to the funeral]. They are talking ill about you!" But she [would]

not hear. So I went with her. . . . When we went to the burial and [the family of the husband] realized we were [there, his] brother attacked us [with words]. Attacked us! In front of all the mourners. He [said to those in attendance], "You people who are here. . . . This one is danger. This was my brother, and my brother died of HIV. And I want to tell all the young men there. You know the wife—the girl he was moving with! Don't greet [the girl or any of her relatives]. Don't talk to them!" Oh—I felt like fainting . . . my cousin became so stressed.

As Jane made clear through her story, words in Mahali were at least as powerful as the virus. At the time, people living, dying, or associated with HIV and AIDS were construed as dangerous—having the potential to threaten what mattered most to everyone (both the people who were stigmatized and those doing the stigmatizing), such as life chances, reputations, money, health, security, relationships, and a sense of belonging (Yang et al. 2007). To temper the threats he felt, the brother attacked Jane's whole extended family with loud words to communicate that Jane's cousin was dangerous (infected with a virus) and thus was a person and member of a family to be feared and avoided by others. From the start of the epidemic, mirroring experiences with AIDS and responses to it in the Global North, AIDS was a crisis and construed as a disease of the immoral "Other," a term that in most parts of sub-Saharan Africa applied to foreigners, sex workers, long-distance truck drivers, migrants, and city dwellers (Knight 2008, 9). Therefore, processes of stigma and blame were immediately set in motion as people grappled to make sense of a mysterious and fatal disease and protect themselves and others from it in the contexts of limited and ineffective health care, a lack of treatment, and insecurity. This history is important for understanding more contemporary ideas about and experiences with HIV and stigma in Mahali.

Toward the end of our interview, Jane explained that it was the death of her sister in 2003 that had pushed her into the global fight to end AIDS. Maintaining a stoic face, she told a moving story about this painful experience:

One day, she [her sister] called me and said that we were to go see a certain doctor. When she was done [having numerous tests done], we were told to go in [to get the lab results back] together. But on reaching the door, she told me, "No, you should not know [the results]." I don't know what she was told by the doctors. She never told me. She died without telling me. On the first of January, she was very sick. But the best thing is that we had [a peaceful] election in December 2002, and . . . the [elected] favorite was [Mwai] Kibaki. So she told me, "Since I have seen that the man I have voted for has won, now I am ready to die." After telling me that, . . . she had to be admitted in the hospital [where] they tried many things [to improve her health] without success.

Then, after some days [in the hospital], it was like, "Can't you take me home?," and I said, "Let me check the [hospital] bill" [which had to be paid before a patient could be discharged]. She just look[ed] at me and said, "Don't go. Just take care of my kids. I love my kids." She loved her kids dearly. . . . She told me, "Now it is the last day. I'm going to leave my kids. I'm feeling it. Although you are telling me that I am getting better, I'll not be getting better." I told her, "No, Mama." I went to get the hospital bill, but I didn't have money for paying her bill. So I had to go to the National Hospital [Insurance] Fund—I wanted them to assist me. But I overstayed until 4:00! [When I returned to] the gate just near the [hospital] ward where she was admitted, I met [only] her belongings. I met her jacket. I met the basin she was using. I met her sweater. . . . I asked the watchmen at the gate: "There is a person [who owns] these things, where have they [taken her]?" He told me they had gone to the morgue. "Oh, ah—no!" I ran to the ward, but my [sister] was not there. [So] I just slept where she [had been] sleeping. I didn't cry. I just slept there. I covered myself with her things. That is the time when I saw AIDS as a disaster. Not a disaster, but a monster. And then I said, "I'll fight AIDS."

Jane continued to link the intersecting epidemics of AIDS and ethnic conflict in Kenya when she explained that her sister had stayed alive just long enough to see her favored political candidate voted into office. At the same time, it was out of respect and the local value placed on speaking discreetly about this virus that Jane refused to directly state out loud and denied possessing any official knowledge that her sister had AIDS, even years after her death. To further preserve her sister's moral reputation and personhood, Jane refused to let HIV overwhelm the woman's identity. Instead, Jane emphasized her role as a devoted and loving mother, a highly revered position that can help elevate the social status of many women living in this part of the world. Still, Jane credits this loss to the realization that the disease was a "monster." Not long after the death of Jane's sister, ART finally became available in Kenya. When I met Jane in 2010, she was a volunteer at an orphanage and an HIV-related NGO in Eldoret.

A BRIEF HISTORY OF THE ANTHROPOLOGY OF HIV IN KENYA

AIDS became one of the most devastating and threatening global pandemics to confront the human species (Schoepf 2001, 2010). From its first official diagnosis in 1981 in the United States until the end of 2019, this disease claimed more than 32.0 million lives and infected 75.7 million individuals (UNAIDS 2020a). Yet the distributions of HIV and AIDS and of the necessary treatments for them have been hardly even. AIDS is disproportionately responsible for taking lives in countries and communities where social, education, and public health infrastructures have either never been fully established (Prince and Marsland 2013) or were inadequate as a result of historical legacies of inequalities and further weakened by years of economic crisis and the dismantling of social safety nets (Schoepf 2001). The impacts of HIV and AIDS have been especially brutal in sub-Saharan Africa, which has only 10 percent of the people on earth but more than two-thirds of the world's population living with HIV (WHO 2021a). Globally, most HIV infections are found in eastern and southern Africa, which is where 44 percent of all new HIV infections in 2016 occurred. Likewise, while the overall death rate associated with AIDS has declined in this region, 310,000 people died of complications from the disease in 2018 (UNAIDS 2019). HIV and AIDS have become two of the most continually discussed and researched topics in academic, medical, and development circles, and therefore a vast body of literature exists that ranges across multiple disciplines, including anthropology, sociology, political science, education, psychology, medicine, public health, and health systems research.

As the world began discussing the origins of AIDS in the early 1980s, stories circulated globally that it had come out of Africa (L. Thomas 2003). Early reports of cases of HIV and AIDS in eastern and central Africa declared that the nature of transmission of the epidemic in Africa was different from transmission patterns found in North America (White 1990)—where, in 1981, the Centers for Disease Control and Prevention (CDC) published findings in *Morbidity and Mortality Weekly Report* of rare pneumonias among five men who identified themselves as gay (CDC 1981). In response, physicians recalled similar, previous cases among members of the gay community in New York and California (Knight 2008). This impacted initial understandings of the disease, as shown by the disease first being named Gay-Related Immunodeficiency Syndrome, or GRID, in the United States (Mann, Tarantola, and Netter 1992). However, by 1982, the disease had appeared in women, PWIDs, and a child, which prompted the CDC to change the name to AIDS. Also in 1982, researchers working in Europe reported that they, too, had treated similar symptoms among patients who were either from or had traveled to equatorial Africa (Knight 2008).[1] In relation to this, the Ugandan Ministry of Health concluded in 1983 that a disease it had identified in patients from the Lake Victoria region, referred to as slim, was also AIDS. Even more scientists from the United States and Europe who were studying Ebola in the Democratic Republic of Congo (formerly Zaire), including Belgian microbiologist Peter Piot (who was then executive director of UNAIDS) and colleagues, found dozens of patients dying of AIDS in a single hospital in the capital city Kinshasa (Knight 2008). Of particular significance in this latter observation was the fact (controversial at the time) that many women were infected and suffering, which made it clear that transmission was possible through both heterosexual and homosexual contacts. The researchers eventually published their data in the prestigious medical journal *The Lancet* (P. Piot et al. 1984). Piot's colleagues Joseph McCormick and Susan Fisher-Hoch (1996, 173) later described the graphic scenes they witnessed in Kinshasa: "Some [patients] developed such exquisitely sore mouths and tongues that they were unable to eat. ... Their skin would break out in massive, generalized eruptions. Infected fungating masses would appear inside and outside their bodies. . . . [T]here were many other parasites ready to eat the brain alive. None of the victims could comprehend in any way what was happening to them or why. And we? All we could do was watch in horror, our roles as physicians reduced to scrupulous observers and accurate recorders of documentation." As was the case during the first two decades of the epidemic in Kenya, when Jane remembered witnessing her friends, colleagues, and family members dying, doctors from North America and Europe to Africa could do little to ease the suffering and deaths from AIDS.

The earliest years of the pandemic in both the Global North and South have since been characterized as a period of discrimination, failure of leadership, lack of political will (Bor 2007), and wasted time and opportunities, when "only a trickle of funding was made available for research into AIDS, let alone for care and support for those people living with the condition" (Knight 2008, 9). Yet as growing numbers of AIDS cases were consistently reported across every continent, scientists came to understand that AIDS was caused by an agent (identified as HIV) that could be acquired by men, women, and children and transmitted through a variety of routes, including sexual or blood contact, needle sharing, the consumption of breast milk, and the birthing process. In response, WHO leaders coordinated a global network that emphasized the need for international cooperation to tackle the global crisis and, in 1986, established the ACP. Employees of the program held a meeting for potential donors to review its plan of action and establish a budget. Later that year, WHO replaced the ACP with the SPA, which soon became known as the GPA under the leadership of Jonathan Mann, an American physician. Experts from the Global North thus mobilized resources and drafted the *Global Strategy for the Prevention and Control of AIDS* (WHO 1989), the official national, standardized guidelines to be used across countries to tackle the epidemic. This global strategy emphasized medical and behavioral research, information exchange, the rollout of HIV antibody test kits, and the creation and distribution of universalized guidelines, manuals, and educational materials for researchers and the general public (Merson and Inrig 2018). Mann (and later Piot) also framed AIDS not only as a health concern, but as an epidemic that required a comprehensive strategy to protect human rights, social equality, and development. Mann thus warned of the potential impact of stigma in the fight against AIDS when he claimed early on that the third phase of the AIDS epidemic—the social, cultural, and political responses to AIDS, characterized by exceedingly high levels of stigma and discrimination and public denial—would likely be "as central to the global AIDS challenge as the disease itself" (quoted in Parker and Aggleton 2003, 13).

It is worth mentioning that AIDS exceptionalism came to refer to the disease-specific response that has mobilized unprecedented resources around the world (see the introduction), but had its origins in the Global North's response to the epidemic during the 1980s (Julia Smith and Whiteside 2010). That period was marked by a notable departure from standard public health prevention practices in favor of approaches that prioritized societal issues and individual rights over the broad protections of the public health of citizens (Fisher, Kohut, and Fisher 2009). After working in the AIDS industry for more than twenty years, researchers in Uganda recalled the mid-1980s rivalries within and among global health actors and agencies about how best to handle and address the disease, thus exposing some of the earliest roots of viral frictions that I documented in Mahali. Specifically, some international experts wanted to treat the disease as a normal communicable disease, while others argued that exceptional measures were required to take into account local social issues, inequalities, sexual practices, and cultural contexts. Tensions erupted among the global actors and played out on the ground in African countries (Knight 2008).

Global health experts have long expressed concern about the impact of stigma in populations' resistance to HIV testing, prevention, and care across the Global North and South. At the same time, recognizing the uneven impact of HIV on women and their children in Africa and the Caribbean, the GPA and UNICEF united to support and establish early prevention efforts among teachers and students in countries that expressed the need for such efforts, such as Uganda, Tanzania, Burundi, and Rwanda (UNICEF-WHO Joint Committee on Health Policy 1989). Kenya was conspicuously absent from these projects. While its Ministry of Health received a modest amount of funding from donor countries to support a year-long education and prevention program in 1987, the country's government contributed very little of its own attention and resources to preventing the spread of the virus during this early period (Lorch 1993).

Perhaps as a consequence, Kenya experienced one of the world's harshest AIDS epidemics, as clearly recalled by Jane. Given the complex interplay of factors at work when the disease first emerged during Daniel arap Moi's presidency (see chapter 2)—an overburdened health care system, a shrinking health care budget, mounting foreign debt, a dysfunctional government, inflation, corruption, rising numbers of NGOs, growing poverty rates, ethnic conflict, and political unrest—the national HIV prevalence rate grew steadily until it reached its peak in the late 1990s (Raviola et al. 2002). Underscoring the denial and lack of political will in the fight against AIDS in Kenya, Great Britain's Department of International Development (now called the Foreign, Commonwealth and Development Office) characterized the response of Kenya's government during the first two decades of the epidemic as "notoriously slow to admit to its HIV/AIDS problem, to see it without an ethnic focus and to demonstrate high-level political commitment" (quoted in HRW 2001). Jane's mentions of the intertwined timing of ethnic conflict, political violence, and the emergence of AIDS echoed that statement.

Scholars have since documented how the U.S. government, in efforts to shift attention away from the United States being the epicenter of AIDS, traced the routes of transmission from Haiti, the country blamed as the single source of U.S. infections that were brought in by the homosexual population (Kim 2015). Haiti, the story continued, had close connections to Africa—where, by 1986, WHO had epidemiological evidence of even larger numbers of AIDS patients than in the United States, which had allegedly hosted 80 percent of the world's AIDS population in the previous year (Moore and LeBron 1986; Farmer 1992; Knight 2008). In 1985, during the first International AIDS Conference in Atlanta, Georgia, tensions were high among researchers. Mann and Piot recalled the researchers' simultaneously aggressive prioritization of focusing on AIDS in the Global North and refusal to acknowledge that AIDS could be transmitted through heterosexual contact in the Global South. They also described the racist claims about African sexuality and outrageously wild overestimates of incidence in African countries made by journalists and some of the world's most respected and prominent scientists (Knight 2008). As Cindy Patton (1990) noted, through-out the 1980s and 1990s, much of the invention of the African AIDS problem took place outside Africa and was orchestrated predominantly by biomedical researchers and practitioners, social scientists, epidemiologists, journalists, and politicians from donor countries (see also Booth 2004). Consequently, and per-haps somewhat justifiably, early reports about AIDS in Africa were dismissed by Kenyan government officials and politicians, who claimed that journalists were drawing on deep-rooted Western stereotypes about Africans and thus were being racist, as well as exaggerating prevalence rates and frightening the average Kenyan (White 1990; L. Thomas 2003).

While the Kenyan government ignored the rising number of its infected citi-zens, the minimal amount of work being done to control the spread of HIV in Kenya initially was targeted at and focused on changing the behaviors of at-risk groups, especially female sex workers in Nairobi. These workers were described by international medical researchers as "a major reservoir of infection" (D'Costa et al. 1985; see also Booth 2004) and "may have significantly contributed to the spread of the virus" (P. Piot et al. 1987, 1108). These international responses to the disease, which explicitly and directly placed blame on a single population for the spread of infection, likely produced friction and exacerbated the processes of stigma from the beginning. The strategy of targeting sex workers failed to acknowledge and understand how gender and sexual relations in Kenya worked (see chapter 4). It collided with existing gender and ethnic identity politics, inequalities, and beliefs that economically independent and single women were "wicked" (Hodgson and McCurdy 2001) and diseased, and it rebuked women for being autonomous, mobile, and unattended by men (White 1990; Robertson 1996). Meanwhile, a rapidly rising number of Kenyan citizens were infected, including Jane's brother, cousin, and sister, none of whom were identified as sex workers. By the 1990s, cohort studies among high-risk women living along the Kenyan coast pointed to new epidemiological risk groups that included transport workers and truck drivers who engaged with sex workers along truck routes, including the one running through Mahali (Bwayo et al. 1991, 1994; Mbugua et al. 1995; D. Jackson et al. 1997). By the late 1990s, when Jane heard the "creep and seep" (Benton 2015, 7) of national media stories highlighting the exceptionally high rates of AIDS-related deaths in highway towns, the message was spreading that Mahali was dangerous and filled with people whom others needed to avoid or be especially vigilant and careful around. These stories helped position the inhabitants of Mahali as early targets for global health interventions and later made the town an obvious location for a freestanding HIV clinic.

Throughout the 1990s, the denial of the Kenyan government, coupled with the inadequate ability of the country's medical community to deal with the burden of AIDS, further stripped biomedicine of its perceived worth and its cultural influence in Kenya (L. Thomas 2003). As Jane recollected, in the face of the AIDS epidemic and without access to lifesaving medications, physicians were unable to assist their patients or lessen the trauma of so many AIDS deaths during this period. This led Kenyan nationals to abandon or avoid the medical profession (Raviola et al. 2002). At the same time, political and government officials under the leadership of President Moi feared that if too much public attention were focused on AIDS, the international tourism industry would suffer significantly, further damaging the Kenyan economy (Bor 2007). International researchers during the 1980s later explained the great lengths to which the Kenyan state went to hide the magnitude of its AIDS problem from the rest of the world, including when the Kenyan minister of health strongly considered the idea of banishing researchers for speaking to journalists about AIDS in Africa and government officials confiscated news articles about the subject (Altman 1999; Knight 2008). HIV infection rates continued to rise across the general population and soared to an estimated 14 percent among adults, being disproportionately high among women (L. Thomas 2003), and it was not until 1999 that Moi publicly acknowledged AIDS as a national disaster. He reprimanded churches for both neglecting the problem and condemning those who were suffering. Also in 1999, the first National AIDS Control Council (NACC) was established, as an agency independent of the Ministry of Health (NACC 2010), and the country went on to launch one of the most intense, multisectoral, and comprehensive national responses to the disease in sub-Saharan Africa (Knight 2008).

It took several more years of robust activism before members of the general population had access to affordable ART (see the introduction). When I arrived in 2010, residents of Mahali had vivid memories of, intimate and personal experiences with, and knowledge about HIV and AIDS, including the suffering this infection and disease caused and the ongoing possibilities and challenges for people living in their community and country. They also had cultural logics and understandings about how the world and relationships worked and how to use them to navigate the prevention and spread of the disease and stigma related to it, as well as their lives and reputations in a resource-poor place.

While Jane was immersed in the overlapping epicenters of political violence and the early years of the AIDS epidemic in Kenya, a handful of anthropologists were studying and writing about HIV in eastern Africa (Schoepf 1992a, 1992b; Farmer, Connors, and Simmons 1996; Whyte 1997, 2014). Paul Farmer, a medical anthropologist and physician working in Haiti, was a major influence on this early work and published the first full-length ethnography on the topic, *AIDS and Accusation* (1992). He also cofounded Partners in Health, one of the first and most famous global health organizations, which became highly influential and respected. Partners in Health promotes health as a human right and a measure of social justice by ensuring that the most economically vulnerable people around the world have access to quality health care (Kidder 2003). Central to the work of critical medical anthropologists, including all of Farmer's work—from his activism to writings about and medical practices in Boston, Haiti, Russia, and Rwanda—was the idea that while HIV infection is viral, it is fueled by structural violence: physical and/or emotional harm arises from tacit social arrangements and broader socioeconomic forces and inequalities (Farmer 2004). In various texts, Farmer defines structural violence:

The term "structural violence" is one way of describing social arrangements that put individuals and populations in harm's way. . . . The arrangements are *structural* because they are embedded in the political and economic organization of our social world; they are *violent* because they cause injury to people. (Farmer et al. 2006, 1686)

Structural violence is structured and *structuring*. It constricts the agency of its victims. It tightens a physical noose around their necks, and this garroting determines the way in which resources—food, medicine, even affection—are allocated and experienced. (Farmer 2004, 315)

Their sickness is a result of structural violence: neither culture nor pure individual will is at fault; rather, historically given (and often economically driven) processes and forces conspire to constrain individual agency. Structural violence is visited upon all those whose social status denies them access to the fruits of scientific and social progress. (Farmer 2001, 79)

The narrative of structural violence has been a vital contribution of medical anthropology over the past two decades and extremely influential in terms of understanding HIV—how and why it spread where it did, and the inequitable suffering it has caused among the world's most vulnerable people and populations. It was a driver behind successful AIDS activism efforts that exceptionalized the disease internationally, leading to political measures to ensure that ART became available in sub-Saharan Africa (Julia Smith and Whiteside 2010; Crane 2013; Moyer 2015). The narrative also gave rise to the discourse of HIV as a disease of poverty. This has since shaped and limited global and national responses to it.

The concept of structural violence was important because it helped (re)orient theoretical attention away from risky cultural practices and individual behaviors as culprits for bodily affliction and demanded that we pay attention to the larger, socioeconomic inequities fueling the virus and vulnerability to it. From the view of many critical medical anthropologists, as well as others analyzing health through a political-economic lens, carefully constructed global health policies and programs that work to break the cycle of poverty and provide equal access to health care will be the solution to eradicating stigma (Castro and Farmer 2005; Brewis and Wutich 2019). This has become a popular story in medical anthropology and still has purchase in global health through development initiatives. Yet medical anthropology's single story (Adichie 2009), which I have used as a lens to see and recount the history of HIV in Kenya, also has the potential to cause trouble because it is incomplete (Mkhwanazi 2016). An understanding of structural violence is vital for explaining various phenomena and understanding some of the processes of and experiences with stigma that I discuss in this book. But if it is used exclusively, that understanding also limits what we see, hear, and understand. Like the stigma narratives described and critiqued in the introduction, the structural violence narrative is likely to erase details as it attempts to explain the human suffering caused by HIV and the consequent processes of stigma. While contemporary humans everywhere suffer and live inequitable lives (Fassin 2018), the framework of structural violence presupposes a universal kind of suffering that transcends culture (Hannig 2017). Using structural violence as the dominant concept can rob people of their agency as it glosses over the cultural minutiae that help give form to the efforts, desires, and complexities of the lives and identities of people as they struggle with, derive meaning from, act upon, resist, and sometimes find redemption through ill health, misfortune, and even death in a chronically inequitable world.

We need to go beyond structural violence to understand and appreciate the diversity of human meaning making and health-related experiences in the twenty-first century (Hannig 2017, 5). Drawing on various stories of HIV from Mahali and following the work of Anita Hannig (2017), I aim to uncover the larger structural inequalities and global and national forces that help sustain HIV stigma. At the same time, I offer "a grammar of social worlds" (Fassin 2012, 245) produced at the intersection of globally, nationally, and locally constructed stories about and practices related to HIV in Mahali. All people—living with HIV or not—had to work to make sense of and negotiate the complexities of their lives, relationships, and identities within the contexts of multiple ongoing epidemics, violence, and uncertainty. Such insights from people, their lives, and their environments shed new light on how and why stigma persists even as it mutates.

CONTEMPORARY EFFORTS TO ERADICATE AIDS IN KENYA

In 2000, Kenya was selected as one of the first countries to receive $50 million to implement a five-year, multisector response to HIV through the World Bank–supported Multi-Country HIV/AIDS Programme for Africa (MAP). That year marked a turning point in the development of Kenya's national strategy and response to the disease (Knight 2008). To coordinate engagement across the government, civil society, development partners, faith-based organizations, and networks of PLWHIV through MAP, a national coordinating authority was established in the Office of the President. The Kenyan government collaborated with organizations like UNICEF to support, for example, the development and implementation of HIV education in the curriculum for people studying to become schoolteachers. The country benefited from a partnership with UNAIDS that provided start-up funds to bolster and scale up mother-to-child transmission prevention programs and helped with surveillance efforts to collect sound epidemiological data from across the country that were used to mathematically model and predict the impact of the epidemic (Knight 2008). The international community worked to help Kenya harmonize its efforts in support of a national plan, and the country received large grants from the Global Fund to Fight AIDS, Tuberculosis and Malaria (Global Fund) and PEPFAR. These efforts inspired additional contributions from other world leaders, like British Prime Minister Tony Blair, who pledged $3 billion to address AIDS in countries like Kenya between 2003 and 2006. The Kenyan government had difficulty absorbing so much funding, and NACC suffered from early internal corruption. But with the support of UNAIDS, the country worked to repair the image of NACC, and in 2007 Kenya became one of the first countries to initiate a joint AIDS program review: all stakeholders across sectors reviewed the national response. Researchers from UNAIDS credited this move with positioning NACC as the single national coordinating authority with oversight in the review, monitoring, and evaluation of the program (Knight 2008).

With increased money available to address HIV and AIDS in Kenya (much of it from PEPFAR), 5,000 NGOs were registered in the country between 1999 and 2007. While these NGOs addressed HIV in various capacities, most of their efforts were uncoordinated. Therefore, as numerous studies had already argued, structural adjustment programs and neoliberalism had not produced the equalizing outcomes originally promised by globalization (Apter 1999; Ferguson 2006; Watts 2006). Rather, they promoted the privatization of health care in

Kenya, contributed to the proliferation of NGOs that created uneasy relationships with the states in sub-Saharan African countries (Bratton 1989; Chege 1999; Brass 2016), and exacerbated the initial AIDS crisis (Turshen 1999; Schoepf 2001, 2010). Political and economic policies and practices that were first established during the colonial period and continued through structural adjustment and neoliberalism further reconfigured social and political relations (Jean Comaroff and Comaroff 2006; Edelman and Haugerud 2007). These policies created conflict within and between the rich and poor, generations (Buggenhagen 2004; Bornstein 2005; Cooper and Packard 2007), genders (Schroeder 1999; Blunt 2004), and ethnic groups and identities (Hodgson and McCurdy 2001). These broad and exceptional conditions, as they later collided with global health efforts that depoliticized HIV interventions, messaging, and the state with the goal of ending AIDS, helped to give further rise to these national tensions and regional conflicts that were maintained, in part, through the cultivation of new forms and processes of HIV-related stigma. I explore these changes in subsequent chapters.

At the beginning of the twenty-first century, churches began to formally engage with the epidemic. Prior to this time, churches had largely condemned people who were infected, but PEPFAR I (the program's first phase) specifically set aside 20 percent of all funds for organizations willing to promote the ABC model (to practice Abstinence, Be faithful, or use Condoms). By 2005, two-thirds of all PEPFAR I funds were made contingent on their use to promote the "A" and "B" aspects of this model. Likewise, rules governing how the funds could be used explicitly prohibited needle exchange programs for PWIDs (Knight 2008). In these ways, the moralities and politics of the United States and the conservative nature of its Congress merged with already conservative and evangelical Christian churches and ideologies in Kenya, the result of decades of work in the country by missionaries from the Global North. For churches across Kenya, PEPFAR funds offered a new way to both take on HIV and promote their own moral teachings (Parsitau 2009). This complex history of globalization played a role in shaping the moral responses to HIV and AIDS and the persistence of HIV-related stigma in Kenya.

Global health programs targeting HIV and working very closely with Kenyan government officials, civil society, and communities of faith also continued to significantly scale up prevention services to reduce mother-to-child transmissions and increased volunteer male circumcision programs, after male circumcision was clinically proven to reduce HIV transmission. Kenya's Ministry of Education standardized the curriculum and incorporated very basic information about HIV and AIDS into every subject beginning in standard 4 (roughly the equivalent of fourth grade in the United States). Since 2004, UNAIDS and USAID, among other global entities, have supported and encouraged the use of media campaigns to expand public knowledge and understanding about HIV.

Across the Kenyan landscape, mass media advertisements on billboards, walls, and *matatus* (fourteen-seat public transportation minibuses) and other vehicles; popular television dramas; and radio and newspaper advertisements highlighted the latest HIV campaigns and slogans, such as "Kick out HIV Stigma" and "Spread Gospel, Not Virus."

Thus, over the past fifteen to twenty years in Kenya, dramatic improvements have been made in understanding HIV and AIDS, with overwhelming global and national responses to the epidemic. These developments have mobilized exceptional resources and an entire social movement unified in the pursuit of justice and equity in the distribution of and access to medications in Africa and beyond (Hirsch, Parker, and Aggleton 2007; UNAIDS 2020b). What was once considered a global AIDS crisis has since spurred a dramatic scale-up in HIV testing and ART to improve lives worldwide. By the end of 2017, approximately 66 percent of PLWHIV in eastern and southern Africa were in treatment in Kenya (UNAIDS 2018), and by the end of 2019, global ART coverage reached approximately 67 percent (UNAIDS 2020a).

In Kenya, 1.6 million adults were estimated to be infected with HIV in 2012 (Kimanga et al. 2014). While women had a prevalence rate of infection nearly twice that for men, at 8.0 percent and 4.3 percent, respectively (NACC 2010), men had worse AIDS-related health outcomes (Mills et al. 2012; Druyts et al. 2013). Yet men were rarely targeted for specific HIV interventions, except for programs that promoted male circumcision or targeted transport workers and economically insecure individuals within the MSM population (Moyer and Igonya 2018). By 2018, approximately 69 percent of infected adults and 61 percent of infected children were on ART in Kenya (Avert 2020). Throughout my research, people—usually the mothers of boys—occasionally expressed their thoughts and opinions about changing practices related to male circumcision because of HIV. However, in Mahali's urban center and surrounding rural communities, the people I encountered (intentionally or not) were less forthcoming with information on the topic of MSM, and my questions always fell flat or were followed by awkward silences or fleeting comments that lacked substance (e.g., "That does happen."). I also encountered dead ends while trying to explore the subject of PWID: I could not identify people who could offer insights into such practices or people engaged in them in Mahali, even though they have been documented in other parts of Kenya, such as Nairobi, Mombasa, and Kisumu (Kurth et al. 2015; Syvertsen et al. 2015). Consequently, this book does not offer insights into or focus on these topics, although they are important in understanding global health and the persistence of HIV-related stigma in Kenya and beyond.

While it is difficult to determine HIV prevalence rates for any single community, global health professionals estimated that rates in Mahali, given its location along a highway and the considerable size of the sex work industry there, hovered at around 10 percent and was as high as 25 percent among women who identified themselves as sex workers (personal correspondence). Both percentages are considerably higher than the national average, which has continued to hold steady at around 4.7 percent of adults (UNAIDS 2019).

At the time of this writing (2020–2021), HIV in Kenya is still predominantly acquired through heterosexual sex, and approximately half of all people who know they are infected with HIV are involved in a discordant relationship (Gitahi et al. 2020). Since 2004, clinical trials have been exploring and monitoring discordancy across multiple sites in eastern and southern Africa, including Kenya (Lingappa et al. 2009). By 2011, national programs had been established to address issues of discordancy, such as the Prevention with Positives initiative. This program emerged as an element of Kenya's national approach to the epidemic and focused on three main aspects: couple-based HIV testing, encouraging partner disclosure, and regular condom use ("Putting HIV-Positive People at the Centre of Prevention" 2010; NASCOP 2013; Avert 2020). The program was criticized for its exclusive focus on changing the behaviors of PLWHIV and neglecting their social needs and human rights (NEPHAK 2012).

In 2015, epidemiological research revealed that Kenyan adolescents and youth, who make up approximately 24 percent of the country's population, accounted for 51 percent of new HIV infections (Avert 2020). They are now a new priority population for HIV interventions, policies, and funding (UNAIDS 2020b). This shift in priority and focus was evident in some of the HIV infrastructural and social changes I observed in 2019, which included newly constructed buildings labeled as "youth friendly" HIV centers for adolescents. During my fieldwork, I witnessed global health researchers engaged in fierce competitions for limited funding and struggles to stake their claims as experts in adolescent health. If global health prevention messaging and programming are not handled very carefully, they could inadvertently help to increase the already growing tensions between generations (see chapter 6 for a discussion of generational tension and beliefs in curses). The focus on adolescent HIV will be a key area of future anthropological research in sub-Saharan Africa.

HIV in Kenya has been categorized as both generalized and concentrated. It affects all segments of society, but some of the highest rates of infection are found in certain counties (NASCOP 2012; Kenyan Ministry of Health 2014). Although more recent efforts target adolescents and youth, messaging continues to focus heavily on other key populations, including sex workers, prisoners, MSMs, and PWIDs—groups representing approximately one-third of all new HIV infections in Kenya (NASCOP 2013) and 28 percent of new infections in eastern and southern Africa (UNAIDS 2020a). These vulnerable populations are targeted for two reasons: they are deemed more likely to engage in high-risk sexual behaviors; and the activities and behaviors of people within these populations are still criminalized and stigmatized in Kenya, thereby marginalizing them and making them both difficult to identify and hard to reach (NASCOP 2013).

Because Mahali is located on a highway, over my decade of research, HIV-related outreach by NGOs there focused heavily on sex workers and their truck-driving clients (see chapter 4).

Funding to combat HIV across Kenya was impressive and greatly contributed to the biomedicalization of the condition. It also brought together a wide assortment of local, national, and international players from various sectors. Between 2010 and 2019, approximately three-quarters of all funds available for HIV and AIDS came into the country from abroad (Avert 2020). In 2010, for example, the country received $726 million from donors around the world, with HIV funding from donor governments provided through bilateral and multilateral channels. Donations peaked in 2013 and then declined steadily (PEPFAR 2017) until 2019 (Global Fund 2019). After 2001, most multilateral donations were channeled through Global Fund, and starting in 2003, the majority of bilateral ones came through PEPFAR. Private philanthropic organizations, such as the Bill and Melinda Gates Foundation, also contributed significant funding for HIV and AIDS, especially in Kenya and other countries in eastern and southern Africa. After the decline in international donor funding, while philanthropic and in-country funding increased, nations and private donors came together at Global Fund's Sixth Replenishment Conference in October 2019 to donate the largest amount ever raised for a multilateral health organization (Global Fund 2019). PEPFAR has continued to serve as the largest health initiative to focus exclusively on one disease to date (PEPFAR 2019), and it contributed considerably to the funds available for HIV- and AIDS-related services in Kenya while I conducted the bulk of the research for this book.

By 2010, when I started my research, Kenya had already received and used one round of PEPFAR funding (consisting of more than $235.4 million) and was nearing the middle of a second five-year cycle of funding. PEPFAR I (2004–2008) began when President George W. Bush and the U.S. Congress dedicated millions of dollars to the cause. This first phase focused heavily on the global AIDS crisis and aimed to quickly establish and scale up programs in resource-poor countries. The program expanded AIDS-related information and technologies (e.g., ART and HIV rapid tests) in Kenya, drawing heavily on the use of HIV prevention, intervention, and treatment messaging that stressed individual responsibility.

In all PEPFAR-supported countries, PEPFAR I was criticized for the lack of coordination of its programs and a lack of national government involvement. Beginning in 2008, success was not defined by locally identified needs (Hershey 2019) or by entities like PEPFAR in terms of "dollars spent" but rather was "measured in services provided and lives saved" (PEPFAR 2008, 8). PEPFAR II (2009–2013), in the administration of President Barack Obama, shifted focus. The initiative transitioned from being an emergency response to sharing the global burden of the pandemic by making funds available to help strengthen the capacities of partner governments and to help individual countries lead their own responses. However, PEPFAR II grants were still provisional. PEPFAR funding required the "Anti-Prostitution Pledge" and was awarded only to organizations willing to explicitly oppose sex work and sex trafficking. PEPFAR II required reports to the U.S. Congress if a partner country did not spend at least half of its prevention grants on the promotion of abstinence, reduction of partners, monogamy, and fidelity (Gostin 2013). In these ways, while PEPFAR II grants endeavored to promote country-driven and country-owned HIV- and AIDS-related programs, moralities rooted in the United States and the politics of its Congress continued to be embedded within the national health responses. Since Kenya had participated in both phases of PEPFAR funding, people living in or passing through Mahali experienced the shift and the contingencies that accompanied it—and therefore talked about it. As I illustrate in subsequent chapters, these broad shifts and contingencies amplified feelings of uncertainty about the disease and thus impacted the subjective, lived experiences of people in Mahali, a community notorious for high rates of ethnic and political violence, HIV, and AIDS, as well as a large number of sex workers.

Since the early twenty-first century, Mahali has hosted one of Kenya's Comprehensive Care Centers, referred to as an HIV clinic throughout this book. The centers are sponsored by more than a dozen public, private, national, and international partners working in collaboration with the Kenyan government (NASCOP NACC 2013), and the aim of the centers across Kenya has been to offer low-cost interventions to help prevent illness, prolong life, and prevent HIV transmission using evidence-based practices. Despite a decline in the national HIV prevalence rate (NASCOP 2012; Kenyan Ministry of Health 2014), which has been attributed to a combination of increased HIV education and awareness and high rates of AIDS-related deaths (NACC 2008; Avert 2020), the number of new HIV infections remained high in 2011, with 104,137 new infections (NACC/NASCOP 2012). Alongside the implementation of VCT, beginning in 2007 the Kenyan government (in collaboration with numerous international organizations [NASCOP/NACC 2013]) followed WHO's recommendations and launched provider-initiated HIV testing and counseling (PIT) (WHO 2007), especially among pregnant women receiving antenatal care. Also in 2007, one academic global health partnership working in western Kenya implemented a rigorous clinical program of home counseling and testing (HCT) throughout the region (CSIS 2009; Ndege et al. 2016). The goal of this program was to periodically go door-to-door to offer free and confidential rapid HIV tests to individuals, couples, and families living in selected areas across the country.

People who tested positive and were counseled during PIT, VCT, or HCT were immediately referred to an HIV clinic, where they would be registered as patients and provided with low-cost health care, including what was called an HIV Basic Care Package and a variety of other services. By 2012, the packages consisted of a variety of supplies aimed at prolonging the lives of PLWHIV, with such items as mosquito bed nets; condoms; water drinking vessels; Waterguard, a chlorine solution used to treat water to make it safe for drinking; Cotrimoxazole prophylaxis or Septrin, broad-spectrum antibiotics to help prevent secondary infections; and a wide range of material that provided information about HIV, AIDS, malaria, water safety, hand washing, tuberculosis, discordant couples, and nutritional needs, as well as suggestions for living with HIV. People were also given additional blood screenings to determine, for example, their counts of CD4+ T cells and HIV viral load. CD4+ T cells, often referred to as CD4 or T-helper cells, are white blood cells that are an essential part of the human immune system. HIV attacks and kills CD4+ T cells, leaving the body vulnerable to a wide range of infections. The CD4 count was used to determine the degree of weakness of a person's immune system from HIV infection and historically has also been used to determine the need for ART (NASCOP 2012).

From a biomedical perspective, VCT, HCT, PIT, and self-administered HIV testing are believed to be important first steps in the HIV cascade programming and the most effective way to curb the AIDS pandemic in sub-Saharan Africa, especially in locations where ART is readily available. These programs allow individuals who test positive for HIV to learn their status early in the progression of the disease, which is when ART is most effective (CSIS 2009). Clinical evidence reveals that PLWHIV under good viremic control do not transmit the virus (M. Das et al. 2010), which makes it especially imperative that people know their serostatus. If they test positive, they can start taking medication immediately so that the virus becomes undetectable and thus untransmittable—a status referred to as "U=U," which is an anti-stigma campaign that was initiated in 2016 in the Global North ("U=U Taking Off in 2017" 2017) but has been described as less impactful in resource-poor settings because viral-load monitoring there is more difficult (Avert 2020).

While I was conducting research between 2010 and 2014, people diagnosed with HIV were treated only if they were eligible and met certain criteria (e.g., a particular immune status and stage of infection), but in 2015, WHO (2015) adopted a "treat all" policy, which meant that anyone infected with HIV was to be put on ART immediately after diagnosis. By 2019, I was told that health care workers were concerned that patients were still adjusting to this "treat all" policy change, which was described as a viral friction, confusing to people who had no symptoms and felt that they should not be required to take medication (personal correspondence). Previously, health professionals had claimed the opposite, and people then were described as confused that they had tested positive but were not given treatment. Between 2016 and 2017, Kenya had become one of the first countries in sub-Saharan Africa to approve and eventually roll out a national public-sector PrEP program that included guidelines on the use of a one-pill-a-day regimen as a way to prevent those who did not have HIV from becoming infected (NASCOP 2017; Masyuko et al. 2018; Pebody 2019). In 2019, when I visited Mahali, I learned that only a few people had been prescribed PrEP because they had discordant marital partners registered as patients at the HIV clinic (personal correspondence). It was standard operating procedure to require having such a partner for gaining access to the prevention drug. I also found that my research assistants were unaware of the existence and availability of PrEP. They were, however, familiar with postexposure prophylaxis (PEP), a medication that must be taken within seventy-two hours of potential exposure to HIV to prevent infection, and my research assistants said that it was more commonly known and used, perhaps because it was easier to access and people seemed more aware of its availability. Anecdotally, I was at a very well-attended grand opening of a Mahali nightclub with several friends in 2019, and the day after, my research assistants made jokes about the likelihood of a higher-than-usual number of people reporting to clinics to request PEP.

The third round of PEPFAR funding (2014–2018) stressed and prioritized using funds to support TasP to control, normalize, and contain HIV to end AIDS (PEPFAR 2014). During the administration of President Donald Trump, PEPFAR funding for preventing HIV among sex workers decreased (Moyer and Igonya 2018). Likewise, in 2017, the United States reintroduced the global gag rule, which denies funding to organizations that provide abortion services, counseling, or referrals and which has the unintended consequence of decreasing services for contraception, maternal health, HIV, tuberculosis, and nutrition programs in Kenya (Ushie et al. 2020). Internationally, the United Nations—through the SDGs—has placed pressure on the Kenyan government to invest its own resources in HIV care and a national insurance fund, and to expand its approach to incorporate universal health coverage as a people-centered and rights-based approach to primary health care. Worldwide, the United Nations continues to work with national governments toward the ultimate goal of all people having access to the basic health services they need, regardless of their economic, sexual, and HIV statuses (UN 2015; WHO 2022b). Continuing research will show if and how these efforts change the nature of HIV stigma.

In these ways, Kenya has been a pioneering country in major HIV-related efforts over the past two decades. While I was conducting research for this book in 2011–2012 and 2014, testing for HIV and linking the results to treatment and retention in care were heavily stressed through VCT, PIT, and HCT. Global health researchers and employees of HIV programs and campaigns regularly made their way into homes to offer free and confidential testing and counseling, follow up with people who had tested positive for HIV but had not yet reported to a clinic, and even to track and check up on those who were lost to follow-up (that is, they had started ART but stopped going to the clinic). People were constantly trained in ways to practice safe sex, as well as in the lifestyle changes necessary for and nutritional requirements of engaging in self-care and maintaining healthy living with an HIV+ status. People were thinking and making decisions about global health HIV testing, treatment, and services. They were telling stories to each other (and me) about these services that revealed viral frictions.

Some residents of Mahali had experienced, were quite aware of, and spoke about the power that the Kenyan state and its corruption exerted over their lives, especially as the boundaries between NGOs and the state were blurred and the government became more involved in the governance of HIV-related prevention, care, and treatment service delivery (Brass 2016; Hershey 2019). In 2019, for example, a research assistant made a connection between the election of President Trump and her observation of the complete eradication of community-based HIV programming in Mahali, which had historically centered heavily on outreach to sex workers (see chapter 4). She also linked the connection to the end of her involvement and work in the AIDS industry. On several occasions over the years, Peter, a farmer who also worked temporarily as an HIV counselor during the HCT campaigns, expressed anxiety about and bemoaned the shift toward government-led global health initiatives, claiming that lower-skilled, community-based jobs had been cut. He also articulated concerns about corruption and the fact that HIV programs mirrored the ethnic, class, and political divisions and agendas of those in charge in the region. Early one cold evening in July 2012, I met with Moses, a teacher in his late thirties, in the single room he rented in the middle of a large cement apartment building. Moses lived alone (his wife and children had relocated to Nairobi due to security concerns), and a bedsheet served as a curtain to divide the living and sleeping areas. I was sitting next to a research assistant on a wooden couch with velvety red cushions, and there was a small charcoal stove burning to add warmth. Moses explained his perception that people living in Mahali were neglected and excluded by the Kenyan state when it came to HIV. Moses underscored the ideas that people expected HIV care from the state and that they were aware when they were being deprived of it. Moses also pointed out that a community like Mahali needed more than HIV education and medication, such as poverty alleviation. His attitude toward the Kenyan government was based on his own experiences as an educator:

Despite the fact that the government has integrated [HIV into all] the lessons or in the topics [that we teach], that is not enough. For example, in our school, we have a certain [high] percentage of pupils who are infected [with HIV]. But we have not seen [anyone from the] government coming in . . . to see [the impact of their programs in Mahali]. Yet [government officials] are all aware of the community around us [and that we] are vulnerable to HIV because of poverty and violence. [The] government has not come out openly [to] try to find out how [we are] living as a community having a lot of children with HIV. [The government] has left our school to struggle . . . on its own and [only with the support of] well-wishers [international donors who offer temporary support]. Although the well-wishers are no longer there these days, they came. They did something, and then they disappeared. For . . . [the past] three years . . . we have not seen any . . . community-based NGO. [No one] is coming back and trying to find out what the problem is [in Mahali]. . . . So a lot has to be done. So [if I could speak to the government about what they need to do, I'd say], government—we must actually feel the impact [of your HIV programs and policies] here. We must feel the impact of the government coming to find out: How do you live? How do you care for [people living with HIV]? Yet we in [Mahali] still soldier on, claiming to be trying to fight poverty and improve the education of the children.

While Moses noted the positive impact of integrating HIV and AIDS education into the national curriculum, he also spoke of the limitations of this approach on the lives of people living, working, and going to school in Mahali. HIV awareness, the HIV clinic, and access to biomedicine did not appear to him to be lifting people—including schoolchildren—out of poverty, as global and national discourses had claimed they would. Moses thus highlights what it felt like for people living in a community where the measures of success in terms of HIV outcomes are determined by international agencies and donors as opposed to those identified by and rooted in local priorities, concerns, and needs (Dionne 2017; Hershey 2019) that included a desire for the government to focus on the economy (see Bor 2007). He also articulated an awareness of the local impact of the shift in focus from the PEPFAR phases that complicated and confused the boundaries between NGO and state-run HIV initiatives and the governance of service delivery (see Brass 2016; Hershey 2019). Moses believed that the government, which played a powerful role in the AIDS industry, dismissed and ignored the social needs and economic and political realities of residents living, working, and going to school in Mahali. As a result, he felt like a hypocrite as an educator—unable to lift his students out of poverty to become upwardly mobile, empowered, productive, progressive, and healthy citizens.

2 · "THE POSTELECTION VIOLENCE HAS BROUGHT SHAME ON US ALL"

HIV and Legacies of Racism, Political Violence, and Ethnic Conflict

Anthropologists argued early in the HIV pandemic that individuals and groups assessed their vulnerability to and risk of HIV predominantly through the lens of socioeconomic inequalities (Farmer 1992, 2001; Feldman 1994; Parker 2001). Notions of risk, as they related to conceptions of race and ethnicity, were therefore filtered through the socioeconomic positioning of individuals (Gilley and Pfeiffer 2017). Yet Paul Farmer (1992, 2001) noted long ago that rural Haitians theorized AIDS as a tool of white political and social domination used by Haitian elites working in collaboration with those in the Global North. Likewise, early researchers in Kenya and Tanzania pointed to the stigmatizing discourses that circulated about AIDS coming from vilified "Others," including ethnic outsiders (Talle 1995) and those living in modern urban spaces (Setel 1999). To date, however, considerably less emphasis has been placed on how some populations viewed HIV not only as a marker of socioeconomic positioning, but also as related to socially and politically constructed categories of ethnicity in the Global South during the age of treatment. In this chapter, I develop the argument that both views were at play, as well as the politics of gender and sexuality in Mahali.[1]

To make this argument, the chapter gains momentum through a careful, critical tracing of local gossip circulating about the names written in a long list of women (referred to in the community as the List) that were alleged to have been purposefully infected with HIV by one local resident. Using this story, I follow the early ethnographic research from eastern Africa as well as that of Didier Fassin (2007), who argued that the epidemiological profile of AIDS in South

Africa requires an understanding of the social history of the country, in which racial inequalities were institutionalized. To more fully account for the List and the persistence of HIV stigma in Kenya, I consider how individuals and groups conflated notions of ethnicity in their conceptions of disease susceptibility and their explanations of why HIV infection rates were high and so many people died of AIDS. Therefore, in this chapter, I link the individual (or microlevel), intrapersonal, and interpersonal happenings associated with gossip and rumors about the List to broader (or structural) historical, political, and economic contexts. I explain how long-standing legacies of racism and ethnic animosities impacted tensions and levels of trust between people to shape understandings of and experiences with health, health care, and HIV to produce viral frictions and keep processes of stigma in motion. After highlighting stories of the List, the chapter offers a necessarily abbreviated social and political history of the area, beginning with the colonial period and ending abruptly in 2008—after Mahali had become an epicenter of postelection ethnic and political violence—which is also the year I began preparing for the beginning of my anthropological fieldwork in Kenya as a doctoral student. Following the lead of people like Jane (see chapter 1), I continue in the last two sections of the chapter to pay particular attention to the national politics that have contributed to and fueled the animosities and conflict between and within ethnic groups living in Mahali and the land disputes that continue to plague the region and sometimes get worked out, using HIV stigmatization as a tool, between individuals at the community level.

CIRCULATING STORIES ABOUT THE LIST

During my last weeks of a long stretch of fieldwork in 2012, word was spreading within the community that "the fourth woman had died." It was late August, the afternoon and evening rains were heavy, and the maize (corn) was tall again. People were simultaneously excited because the harvest was coming and worried because, in their experience, this meant that cases of seasonal (cerebral) malaria might begin to increase. By this point, unlike in my first days in the field, I better understood how they felt and what everyone was talking about. My time abroad not only had increased my knowledge of the circumstances people faced on a daily basis in Mahali, but it also had positioned me within local social networks of gossip that I, as an outsider, could not fully participate in (Ashforth 2005) but had learned to follow and understand.

All four women's sudden and tragic deaths were connected in the minds of those living in Mahali. Their names were in the List of women who, it was alleged, had been intentionally infected with HIV by a former part-time humanitarian worker and *boda boda* (motorbike taxi) driver. The women on the List were described as "very well-known mothers"—well-respected individuals who died prematurely, "before their days were near." This troubled Mahali residents because "the Mahali community believes that HIV is a sex worker disease. So everyone is wondering how it could be that a married, church-going woman could get HIV." Furthermore, the women were not believed to have died directly from the virus, although they were believed to have been secretly infected, but rather because of the stigma and shame associated with the disease and having contracted it in ways described as corrupt and scandalous. Naomi, a young nurse who lived in Mahali and worked in a maternity ward in another town, spent part of her day off with me at the HIV clinic, and while she was explaining that HIV "spreading sprees" were imagined as typically enacted by sex workers, the topic of the List crept in as an exceptional example. She explained the deaths of local women from her perspective: "People [in Mahali] go on these spreading sprees. . . . Mostly it is the commercial sex workers. . . . But there was recently this motorbike driver. . . . He left a list of over a hundred. He was doing it [sex] purposefully! And he left a list. And that list has taken effect. Imagine [that] a list of names has already killed [four] women! This man did not want to die alone with his AIDS. The women here are being consumed by stress and embarrass-ment." The List had been discussed before my arrival in Mahali. One of my inter-locutors explained that immediately after news of the List had leaked out following the man's burial, "Everyone just thought it was a myth." But then "the first name on the list" died (see the introduction). Residents of Mahali knew the details of this story very well, and being able to participate in conversations about it—and leaking the secrets that it contained—was of value to people as they defined identities, as well as a sense of group belonging and exclusion (Manderson et al. 2015).

I noted slight differences in how the story about the List was told and what parts were emphasized, but the underlying sentiments and messages remained relatively constant. Some people focused on the man's role as a transport worker and emphasized that the women had willingly accepted free rides from him in exchange for sex. In other renditions, the man was alleged to have abused his position as a worker for an international relief organization after the 2007–2008 PEV by requiring women to have sex with him in exchange for his recording them as people who should receive compensation for their losses. Rehema, a widow with five children who did odd jobs like washing clothes by hand for people and cleaning shops, recalled: "This man left a list. . . . He was a young man . . . who used his position in the IDP [internally displaced person] camp to misuse and infect so many women who felt they could get extra favors from him—like sugar or cash handouts—after the PEV." As we talked, we sat in the run-down wooden room she rented at the end of a row of similar living spaces occupied by single women, which had a tattered piece of cloth hung over the open door to provide privacy.

In both versions, the consistent theme and accusation were that women in Mahali had been involved in exchanging sex for money, gifts, or favors, a practice that has been referred to as transactional sex by social science scholars (e.g., Hunter 2002, 2010; Poulin 2007). The term was used to emphasize the everyday norm of economic exchanges for sex in sub-Saharan Africa and to eliminate the stigma associated with notions of sex work (Thomas and Cole 2009, 9). The focus on transactional sex emerged as a critique of the initial HIV prevention efforts that directed outreach toward core groups, especially sex workers (as discussed in chapter 1). More recently, social scientists have argued that the concept of transactional sex continues to be conflated with sex work by HIV-related agenda-setting organizations, especially in sub-Saharan Africa (Stoebenau et al. 2016; Wamoyi et al. 2016). While transactional sex has various nuanced forms, scholars suggest that an overarching, unified definition of the term is necessary for improving global health HIV interventions. One proposed definition is that transactional sexual relations are "noncommercial, non-marital sexual relationships, motivated by the implicit assumption that sex will be exchanged for material support or other benefits" (Stoebenau et al. 2016, 187). Transactional sex has become a central part of sexual development and practices among youth in sub-Saharan Africa (Kaufman and Stavrou 2004), and while scholars have argued that the exchange of sex for money is often a survival strategy, it equally serves as an expression of love and intimacy that provides women with agency in their lives (Poulin 2007; Hunter 2010). Such practices have helped transform notions of masculinity (D. Smith 2017) and what it means to be a woman in sub-Saharan Africa (Mojola 2014).

But as the story of the List suggested to me, exposing the married women's involvement in transactional sex in Mahali cast them publicly in a very negative light. Locals ultimately construed this as being humiliating enough to kill people who internalized the broad, circulating public messages about HIV and argued that the judgment had enough merit to warrant suicide, which is an extreme form of self-stigma. The purpose behind the gossip and the scandal of the List was, in part, an attempt to make sense of and manage the social tensions, uncertainties, and contradictions produced by HIV. At the same time, stories about the List regulated morality (G. Reid 2010), reinforced social values and roles, and stigmatized people with the goal of keeping community members in line (White 2000).

I was never able to track down the List, not from a lack of trying. I very much wanted to see it and hold the object in my hands. At one point I was told that it had been destroyed so the scandal would not escalate into physical violence. I wanted empirical evidence, as there was also the possibility that it might never have existed. Josphat, an employee at the HIV clinic, shared my skepticism because he too had never seen it and knew no one who had. As we sat in a private consultation room at the clinic and enjoyed the chai and *mandazi* (fried bread) delivered to us by a staff member during the midmorning tea break, he made it clear that he had heard the stories and dismissed them:

Even I have never seen an actual list. . . . Just recently there was a lady who died, and we were told that there is a very big list of people and that she was the first name on it. But we never got a list. This [sort of] thing has been happening for a long time. I remember before we even started doing ARTs—it was about fifteen years ago—there was a man here, and we were told that he was going through centers [small towns along the highway] and . . . sleeping with people. [But] I don't think these stories are real. Every person has their own rumor and they want to spread rumors differently, and you can get the same story from different people differently.

In contrast, the List was not generally doubted by others living in Mahali. Even if the specific details varied, the overall story was believable and sounded probable to those who were hearing and sharing stories about it. Therefore, it was real: it adequately summarized the public opinions, tensions, and anxieties of the majority of those embedded within a very particular shared social world (White 2000). But because I remained skeptical, one day, as I walked slowly with two research assistants through one of several crisscrossing dirt alleys that ran along the back of the urban center, I asked them if they thought that such lists were "really real." We were being careful to avoid the swampy puddles and scattered piles of trash that lined our path. A large unattended pig was grazing in a narrow space between two buildings as we passed behind a pool hall and then a local bar spray-painted with the words "Do not urinate." It was early morning, and as we moved past a string of metal and wooden kiosks that offered a variety of prod-ucts and services (such as cards to "top up airtime" for a variety of cell phone providers and mobile phone repair and charging services) and were just begin-ning to open, one of my research assistants replied without hesitation and with confidence, "[The lists] are very real! I have heard of three. One in 2002. I saw that one with my own eyes in [a rural community adjacent to Mahali]—a woman had left it. There was one in 2008. It was December, or maybe it was January 2009? I did not see that one, but I heard people talking about it who had seen it. And then there is this most recent one—have you heard? There was a motorbike driver who was employed by [a relief organization]." I heard the story about the List during semistructured interviews and through local gossip and casual conversations with other people in and around the community. I even read about it in my interlocutors' conversational journals.

The story had very real effects on local bodies—harming people if not physi-cally, then certainly socially and psychologically. It terrorized people, women in particular. I also found that the local story about the List bumped up against the logics of the global and national responses to AIDS to produce unexpected out-comes. A story relating to the List came up in a late-night casual comment made by Judy, a VCT worker, while we sat in a blue camping tent set up as a makeshift HIV testing station in front of a line of pubs and nightclubs. We were waiting for the next person to enter and be tested for HIV. We later scheduled an interview in the container clinic, where I inquired more formally about the story. Judy's answer provided evidence of viral frictions:

> There was one woman who was so worried that she came to me and insisted that I test her [for HIV]. She said she knew she was positive because she was on the list. So the first time we tested her at home, she was negative. And she said, "No! I know I am positive!" . . . So I told her that if she refuses to believe, she should come to the [VCT clinic building] when they are testing. She came to the center and had [a different VCT counselor] test her. Again the test was negative. But she still could not accept the results. So I told her, "Go now and don't test again until after three months. Then if you are still negative, you will know that you are negative." She came back to me in three months. She tested at the [district hospital] and . . . told me, "No, it is just negative again. But I know that I am HIV+." And now I don't know how to help her, because she was on that list! And she told me that she did not use a condom, so she cannot believe that test. It was like, she told me, she didn't have money and so this man who was working on the motorbike . . . would give her [rides for free in exchange for sex]. . . . She was very worried.

Living in a community inundated with various global and national HIV-related programs, prevention messages, campaigns, and testing programs, this woman, like others, had learned well that having sex without a condom could lead to an HIV infection. She also had clearly received the message that practices associated with transactional sex were risky from a public health angle. Consequently, she had carefully kept her personal engagement in both of these behaviors— globally deviant, yet locally practical—a secret. This was especially important because she also had been taught that as a married woman, she should remain faithful to her husband, even if they lacked the financial means and stability to maintain such a practice. But the List exposed her reckless behavior and threatened to destroy her social reputation and potentially her marriage. Given the clarity and certainty with which these HIV prevention messages (be faithful and use a condom) had been presented to and received by the woman and the fact that she had clearly violated them, she could not believe that she was HIV negative. In these ways, the words, trainings, and technologies brought into the community through global and national health responses produced friction in the lives of people as they pressed against local knowledge, expertise, politics, and distinct ways of knowing HIV.

The scandal of the List was an extraordinary event in Mahali's urban center. It reflected instances when enacted stigmatization erupted and power dynamics were perceived as threatened. While the case can be interpreted in many ways, including as a form of community building and providing a temporary sense of justice (by uncovering corruption and who might be secretly living with HIV), it served to perpetuate national and regional ethnic, class, gender, and sexuality politics, as well as HIV-related public stigma related to the possibility that people were maliciously spreading the disease. Stories about the List reflect fierce struggles for power over what was most at stake—social values and roles, moral standards, ethical principles, and a secure sense of belonging in the community—during a contentious period of upheaval and social change. While global public health professionals might have dismissed gossip and rumors about the List, it provided an opportunity to understand the lived social, historical, and political realities of the people they sought to assist and highlighted the ways broader structural inequalities and discourses help sustain HIV stigma.

A BRIEF HISTORY OF MAHALI

Colonialism (1895–1963)

White settlement during the colonial period had a profound impact across present-day Kenya, and specifically in the Rift Valley (where Mahali is located). The effects have been long-lasting (R. Reid 2009). In the first decades following the establishment of the East African Protectorate in 1895 (it was renamed the Kenya Colony and Protectorate in 1920) (L. Thomas 2003), the early colonial administrators identified two major problems they felt they needed to address before they could create a viable economy in the area (R. Reid 2009). The first problem was the indigenous populations who inhabited the territory. Confronted by people such as the Maasai, who lived in pastoral and stateless societies with no apparent leaders, the colonial administrators were unable to easily identify and rely on local chiefs to serve as instruments of colonial change and to implement new policies on behalf of the colonial regime (R. Reid 2009). The second problem was geography. Most of Kenya is arid savanna that gets little rainfall. Only 24 percent of the country is arable land (Kamungi 2009), and that is mostly in the western zone—the Rift Valley and surrounding areas. This area eventually became known as the White Highlands (R. Reid 2009).

As a result of these two problems, early colonial administrators opted to turn away from their initial plan of implementing a peasant agricultural system in the territory (R. Reid 2009). Instead, at the beginning of colonial rule in Kenya, the Rift Valley became one of the most popular places for whites to settle. At the beginning of the twentieth century, after the railway system was completed in Kenya, the colonial regime began to implement policies and offer financial incentives to encourage other Europeans to settle in the area and take responsibility for overseeing intensive agricultural initiatives. By 1926, approximately 12,000 white settlers were living in the region (L. Thomas 2003). This part of Kenya was thus an early space of migration, displacement, and, consequently, ethnic and political conflicts, tensions, and violence (Ashforth 2009; Kamungi 2009).

In order to accommodate white population growth and support new agricultural patterns, Europeans engaged in two activities. First, they pushed the original inhabitants, including Maasai, Nandi, and other Kalenjin communities, onto less fertile lands. The Maasai were the first to experience this marginalization, as groups were pushed south into the driest regions of the country. Second, using land ordinances to establish native reserve policies beginning in 1915, the Europeans forcibly removed Africans from fertile lands to accommodate the development of plantations for the economic benefit of white settlers and the British Empire (Kamungi 2009). The rapid population growth of Europeans increased the need for more Africans to provide labor on large, white-owned plantations of tea, coffee, and tobacco. This led some early settlers to want to clarify racial boundaries to prohibit social and sexual relations between the groups (L. Thomas 2003). Using a native reserve system, colonists divided Africans according to ethnic groups and restricted their movements within and between particular geographic regions (R. Reid 2009). In this way, the colonial administrators sharpened the distinctions between cultural groups (Ashforth 2009): they implemented a divide-and-rule strategy that served to separate and polarize groups of people based on ethnic identities. As we shall see, postcolonial politicians continued to maintain their positions of power by building on this tactic in ways that helped create HIV stigmatization along ethnic lines from the beginning of the HIV epidemic.

Throughout the colonial era, Africans were politically, socially, and economically marginalized, despite the fact that they were essential to white settlers for the (often forced) labor they provided. As colonists steadily increased in numbers, more Africans were squeezed into smaller reserves, putting pressure on land that was already of poor quality. During the 1940s, there was an increased international demand for African cash crops such as cotton, tobacco, coffee, and sugar, which once again resulted in a further expansion of white settlers (R. Reid 2009). By 1960, over 7.5 million acres of land in the White Highlands (approximately 75 percent of the area) were owned and farmed by only 4,000 Europeans. This forced the original inhabitants of the area to become reliant on small-scale subsistence farming practices in reserves or to move into major cities like Nairobi and Mombasa in search of work. This fundamentally altered and fragmented family, marital, gender, and sexual roles and relations (see White 1990; Hodgson and McCurdy 2001; L. Jackson 2002). It also resulted in a "social crisis" (R. Reid 2009, 206).

Early in the colonial period, while African labor was being exploited to improve the living standards of white Europeans (Cooper 1996), settlers felt a sentiment (which they considered a "burden") that Africans were incomplete and needed to be assisted economically, morally, politically, physically, and psychologically by more "adult persons" (James Smith 2008, 26; see also Karp 2002). Missionaries in particular endeavored to improve the health status and change the beliefs and behaviors of Africans (Burke 1996; James Smith 2008). Later in the colonial period, development initiatives emerged as a colonial state-centered practice, with the primary aim of moving Africans back to the country-side and away from the cities. Thus, massive labor-intensive rural agricultural projects expanded during the 1940s and 1950s and were used to control Africans' use of land and movement. This control was prompted in part by growing fears among colonists that Africans were modernizing too quickly between epochs, a process that many whites believed would inevitably lead to chaos (James Smith 2008). Migrant laborers moving between rural and urban areas were construed as being the most dangerous, because they shifted rapidly and regularly between the traditional areas associated with rural communities and the modern spaces of cities, a pattern that colonists felt would result in a variety of perverse behaviors and/or a form of schizophrenia (James Smith 2008). Europeans reasoned that Africans, especially those imagined as not being fully traditional or modern, could have no morals or values and thus could not be held accountable to any custom or system of belief (Lonsdale 1992).

Colonial and agricultural practices, policies, and early development initiatives sparked social problems in Kenya, including major disputes over land and ethnicity. Land alienation resulted in growing discontent among rural Africans and hostility toward white settlers, particularly among the Kikuyu. These land issues and the colonists' control of Africans' movement are often cited as some of the factors leading to the Mau Mau uprisings and violence in 1951 and 1952 (Kamungi 2009), with the uprisings and their popular support contributing to the British granting Kenya independence in 1963 (R. Reid 2009). Although the British military defeated the Mau Mau insurgents, the uprisings reinforced questions about whether the colony should be maintained.

Independence and Jomo Kenyatta (1963–1978)

At independence, the postcolonial government of Kenya inherited the land problems that had been produced during the colonial period and had, in part, motivated the British to get out of the area. In the final months of colonial rule, the British developed land-purchasing schemes, designed to assist an independent Kenya to resettle the landless poor that the colonial administration had created. At the same time, individual British colonists started selling the lands they owned to any buyer with resources and financial, social, or cultural capital. This meant that land areas in the Rift Valley and White Highlands were purchased by individuals from various ethnic groups, but only by those wealthy enough to afford to do so (R. Reid 2009). Therefore, some people in Kenya began moving about the landscape, making formerly white farms considerably more cosmopolitan. The majority of Kenyans, without capital, were left scattered about the country and remained landless, unsettled, and frustrated.

Jomo Kenyatta had been sentenced to prison for being a Mau Mau rebel. After being released, he was made president of the Kenya African National Union (KANU), the political party that formed the first government and led the new country to independence in 1963 (R. Reid 2009). An anthropologist and Kikuyu, Kenyatta placed many other Kikuyus in leadership roles and positions of power. He also focused on resettling thousands of angry Kikuyus on farms in both the central region (where Kikuyus are said to have originated) and the Rift Valley. People from the Kikuyu, Meru, and Embu ethnic groups also formed cooperatives and created alliances so they could purchase large tracts of land. This left many other original inhabitants, including Maasai and Kalenjin, living on reserves nearby but unable to acquire land in their former territories (Kamungi 2009).

President Kenyatta offered Daniel arap Moi, a man of Kalenjin ancestry and the deputy chair of the opposing political party, the Kenya African Democratic Union, the position of vice president of KANU in 1964. Kenyatta selected Moi because he had helped ensure Kalenjin support for a one-party political system and had worked to diffuse land problems as the government implemented resettlement policies. The government endeavored to resettle over one million Africans by giving preference to farmers, who would produce food for the country and products for export, over pastoralists (Kamungi 2009). Some scholars have argued that through Kenyatta's resettlement schemes, classes became even more divided in Kenya. This was in part because the original occupants of the Rift Valley and areas of the White Highlands could not afford to resettle there. Prisca Kamungi (2009, 350) writes, "Kenyatta gagged the articulation of ethnic grievances over land by rewarding individual leaders rather than addressing the matter at the community level." In this way, instead of solving the land problems and ethnic tensions of the colonial past, he complicated them. During Kenyatta's presidency, the state became Kenya's primary employer, and development programs were dependent on government funds and initiatives to build infrastructures such as roads, schools, and health facilities, as well as dams to generate electricity, provide flood control, and store sufficient water supplies in arid regions. This meant that government-led development initiatives became the dominant mechanisms for securing power over populations (James Smith 2008; see also Haugerud 1995). Under the leadership of Kenyatta, Kikuyus were perceived to have easier access to land and other economic, social, and political advantages and were able to enjoy better infrastructure and other amenities.

By the late 1970s, global prices for Kenyan exports such as tea and coffee had fallen. At the same time, world prices for oil escalated, and as the Kenyan government's debt increased, the income earned by Kenyans began to steadily decrease (L. Thomas 2003). Former colonies, like Kenya, became dependent upon countries in the Global North (James Smith 2008).

The Moi Era (1978–2002) and Beyond

Jomo Kenyatta died in 1978, and Daniel arap Moi moved into the central position of leadership in Kenya. By this time, individuals from the Kikuyu ethnic group and those from the Kisii, Luo, and Luyha communities had purchased land not only in their traditional homelands, but also in the Rift Valley, including in and around Mahali. Many other ethnic groups felt that this was unfair and considered it the result of Kenyatta's having favored Kikuyus. During Moi's presidency, the Kalenjin community was perceived to benefit more than other ethnic groups, as Moi worked to reverse Kenyatta's efforts by shifting resources and development initiatives to Kalenjin communities. By this time, land problems had become an issue between and within ethnic groups and were related to socioeconomic class divisions. Kenyatta's initial failure to resolve land issues that had emerged during the colonial period was used by Moi to incite ethnic violence, with the goal of maintaining his political power. Moi's leadership has since been characterized as repressive, as he used arbitrary arrests; detentions without trials; intimidation; the disappearance of people; torture; police brutality; and the state control of the media, judiciary, and parliament as primary methods to maintain his power and leadership (Kamungi 2009). State-led development initiatives (*maendeleo* in Kiswahili) were equated with modernity and science by Moi, and Kenyans' access to those initiatives was based on their loyalty to the state (James Smith 2008; see also Wipper 1975). Critics of the Moi regime were branded as disloyal, detained, and/or silenced.

During the 1980s and 1990s, three significant things happened that fundamentally altered Kenyan society under Moi's leadership. First, in the early 1980s Kenya began taking out structural adjustment loans from the World Bank and the International Monetary Fund that were accompanied by tight regulations, restrictions, and conditions set by the lenders. By 1992, the annual debt repayment was equal to 40 percent of the country's export earnings (James Smith 2008). Second, the end of the Cold War and the collapse of communism in Eastern Europe in 1989 led to the creation of movements centered on democratization and respect for human rights. Aid flowing from the Global North to the Global South became contingent on good governance and democratic reform (Haugerud 1995; Mkandawire 2002). Kenya's foreign aid funding was significantly cut as a method of pressuring Moi to transition the country toward a democracy (Haugerud 1995). Moi was eventually forced by Western donors to change a constitutional amendment enacted in 1965 that outlawed opposition political parties and to hold a multiparty democratic election for the first time since independence (James Smith 2008). During this period, there was also a shift in international development funding to channel money to NGOs rather than governments, in part due to assertions that governments were corrupt. While scholars have pointed out that NGOs are not immune to corruption and often must cooperate with and operate within the bounds of the nation-state (Bratton 1989), Moi warned that any NGO that dabbled in politics would be deregistered and construed as threats to the government (Chege 1999). Third, during the Moi era and against this political and economic backdrop, HIV tragically emerged in Kenya and began to spread rapidly across the general population to completely transform social life for all citizens.

As HIV infection and AIDS death rates were rising, and as Kenya moved toward the 1992 democratic presidential election, Moi drew on colonial and racial legacies and historical animosities related to land and ethnic tribalism in efforts to thwart and limit any success of a multiparty election (Lynch 2011). His goal was to stay in power as long as possible. In repetitive campaign speeches, he emphasized that Kenya lacked the national cohesion required for democratic practices. He also suggested that the majority of Kenyans, who were poor, were "backward" and had "witchlike natures" that made them a jealous, resentful, contentious people and thus unable to participate in democratic processes (James Smith 2008, 32). During political rallies, Moi and other politicians vilified "outside ethnic Others" and called for the removal of *madoadoa* (spots), *kwekwe* (blemishes), or *chui* (leopards) from historically Kalenjin territories (Lynch 2011). Through his words, Moi promoted ethnic and class rivalries and hatred across the general population.

The result of these political tactics was an eruption of violence in October 1991 in the Nandi Hills, located in the Rift Valley. Violence spread systematically across the country in the name of the removal of the so-called tribal outsiders from various areas, causing people like Jane to flee their homes for safety. By December 1992, Maasai and Pokot (a Kalenjin group) "warriors"—dressed in uniform T-shirts, with their faces painted with white clay, and armed with traditional weapons—instigated fighting against the Kikuyu living in areas like rural and urban Mahali (Lynch 2011). Some scholars (e.g., Lynch 2011) have argued that the clashes were initiated with the full support of the government under Moi's leadership, using the same divide-and-rule tactic that the colonists had employed. Another interpretation of this violence was that the clashes served to vindicate Moi's earlier predictions that multiparty elections would end in ethnic conflict and to bolster the belief that Kenyans could not handle democracy (Morton 1998). The consensus has been that the violence associated with the 1992 election was politically motivated and coordinated, with ethnicity as a central political strategy (Schmidt and Kibara 2002). Later reports revealed that government officials had not only supplied weapons to skilled attackers from outside areas but also trained, paid, and transported them to cause chaos by burning houses, destroying farms, and killing people in communities like Mahali (Lynch 2011).

During the 1992 election, the Moi government also siphoned off more than half a billion dollars from the treasury and illegally printed and distributed millions of Kenyan shilling notes that were never registered with the Central Bank of Kenya (James Smith 2008). This led to a fiscal crisis the following year, as inflation hit 100 percent (Barkan 1993; James Smith 2008). The Moi regime became equated with theft, counterfeiting, and corruption, which led to the rapid and total deregulation of the Kenyan economy (James Smith 2008). At the same time, HIV infection and AIDS death rates were rising, and the government faced pressure from key development partners such as WHO and the World Bank to finally admit the presence of HIV in the country and make AIDS control a priority. Some international donors refused to disperse development funds, citing bad governance, with entities such as the International Monetary Fund and World Bank imposing additional austerity measures that further eroded social programs, including those related to health and education (Okuro 2009). Moi was forced to accept donor countries' demands and began to shift his position on the growing epidemic. However, he started sending contradictory messages about HIV and AIDS to citizens through the Kenya Broadcasting Corporation (the state-owned radio station formerly called the Voice of Kenya). Moi's misguided position on HIV was particularly damaging to those living in rural areas, where people relied on the radio for their information (Okuro 2009).

The experiences of the 1992 election were duplicated in 1997, when Moi again successfully preserved his presidency. Violence was once more directed against the Kikuyus in the Rift Valley, where Jane was living when she and her family were declared dangerous because they were associated with a rapidly spreading infectious disease. At the same time, the International Monetary Fund withheld a $220 million aid package to Kenya, claiming pervasive corruption. Aid was not resumed until 2000 and was withheld again in 2001 (James Smith 2008), when the country was experiencing a high number of deaths from AIDS. By the first years of the twenty-first century, Kenyan citizens began to lose faith in their country and its leaders. Robert Blunt (2004, 295) contended that citizens had come to view the state as an oxymoron—both "excessively empowered" and "impotent" because it could not provide services for its citizens, especially in relation to health. A widespread belief emerged that the decline in national sovereignty was a global conspiracy and that international development institutions, such as the International Monetary Fund and World Bank, were evil and "false fronts for the transnational corporation known as the Satanic Church, which many Kenyans held was a global organization dedicated to undermining national economies through the incorporation of drugs, condoms, used clothing, and the exportation of human organs and children" (James Smith 2008, 35; see also Blunt 2004). The number of NGO programs continued to grow, including those newly designed to tackle HIV (L. Thomas 2003). Thus, many Kenyans became suspicious of the intentions behind Westerners' offering money to change their society (James Smith 2008).

As Jane noted when she spoke of the death of her sister, in 2002 Kenya experienced peace for the first time since independence during a democratic election. Citizens were unified around the notion of removing Moi and his repressive regime from office and ending his twenty-four years of patrimonial, ethnic politics (Ashforth 2009; Kamungi 2009). In December, KANU, which had ruled the country since independence in 1963, was defeated, and Mwai Kibaki, leader of the Democratic Party and the National Alliance Rainbow Coalition, was elected as Kenya's third president (Throup 2003). Despite the unity felt among Kenyans during the election process, soon after being sworn in, Kibaki and a handful of other influential politicians from the central region (later known as the Mount Kenya Mafia) began to advantage certain individuals on the basis of ethnicity. The Kibaki government favored Kikuyus and kept non-Kikuyus from positions of power, further fracturing the nation across lines of ethnicity and difference. The country was divided, and public distrust and tensions began to rise again (Kamungi 2009).

As in the democratic elections under Moi's leadership, the 2007 pre-election campaigns were marked by politicians giving hate speeches, thus exacerbating tensions between ethnic groups and resurrecting historical animosities over land (Kamungi 2009). While peace was maintained throughout the pre-election period, the general message conveyed by Kalenjin politicians during political rallies and conversations, and through the use of media stories was that it would be possible to rid all "Others" from the Rift Valley once and for all (Kamungi 2009). When Kibaki was suspiciously and suddenly declared the winner over his opponent, Raila Odinga, the results were quickly contested. Again, violence and lawlessness erupted, occurring for several months in various places across Kenya, with most destruction and aggression in the Rift Valley (Ashforth 2009; Kamungi 2009; Lynch 2011). While Kenya was generally viewed as "a bastion of peace in an otherwise volatile region" (Lynch 2011, 2), given the mood before the election and previous interethnic community violence, the 2007–2008 clashes were neither new nor spontaneous (Kamungi 2009). Scholars described Kenya during this period as having "imploded from continued structural weaknesses" (Kamungi 2009, 345).

Between January and February 2008, over 1,300 people were killed, more than 600,000 were displaced, and 12,000 were left as refugees who fled to neighboring countries (Ashforth 2009; Kamungi 2009). These numbers, combined with the number of people who had been displaced and never resettled during the 1992 and 1997 elections and their aftermath, meant that by 2008, Kenya had over a million IDPs (Kamungi 2009). While the media frequently portrayed the 2007–2008 conflict as being between Kenya's two main tribes represented by the presidential candidates—the Kikuyu and the Luo—the epicenter of this violence was the Rift Valley, where neither Kikuyus nor Luos were the majority (Lynch 2011). According to Adam Ashforth (2009), the fighting that occurred in the months after the 2007 presidential election presented itself in five ways: police violence and brutality against civilians; targeted attacks on Kikuyus; the forming of vigilante gangs by individual Luos and Kikuyus in response to the violence; opportunistic crimes, in which individuals took advantage of the chaos and looted shops, homes, and businesses and/or raped women and girls; and Kalenjins engaged in the ethnic cleansing of Kikuyus in the Rift Valley. Ashforth claims that it was the fifth form of violence that contributed to the highest rates of deaths and displacements.

Displaced people (the majority of them Kikuyus) lived in IDP camps until May 2008, when the government initiated Operation Rudi Nyumbani (Operation Return Home). But according to Kamungi (2009), most Kenyans refused to leave IDP camps, fearing to return to their homes or farms. In response, in December 2008, the government cut off water, food supplies, and protection to the camps and announced that Operation Rudi Nyumbani was over. With this declaration, echoing the kinds of stories circulating about the List in Mahali, the government compiled detailed lists of how much monetary assistance each former IDP resident would receive from various aid and humanitarian organizations, to make sure that compensation for losses was fair and accounted for. Because most people living in IDP camps were Kikuyu and corruption was rampant, no one believed that the amounts in the lists were correct, which enhanced the perception that Kikuyus were once again the favored ethnic group (Kamungi 2009). It was just as people were contentiously negotiating "fair" compensation for losses sustained during PEV that I started my PhD program in anthropology and decided to focus my studies on HIV in Kenya. I began making arrangements for my first trip to Mahali—four months of preliminary dissertation research in 2010—where the scars of PEV, as well as the fragility of interethnic harmony, remained visible in the landscape, and anxieties at each election cycle were still audible in the stories people told in my subsequent research trips in 2011–2012, 2014, and 2019.

Local knowledge about and intimate experiences with these global and colonial legacies of racism, national issues, and ethnic and class politics impacted and mediated how people experienced, engaged with, and made sense of the HIV epidemic and processes of stigma. For example, Samuel, a health worker, described the impact of PEV on the care and treatment of PLWHIV in IDP camps and how it produced viral frictions:

[The PEV], that one was very bad for HIV [in this area]. Those who were on medication, their drugs were burned. Their [health] documents were burned. They ran away, and they [didn't] know where they [were going] when they [were] running away. Okay, [for] those whose medicines were not burned, [everyone was] grouped in tents [in the IDP camps], so there is that confidentiality [issue]. They were not taking their drugs. You see? A lot of our clients died [during the PEV]. Those people who were dying were [experiencing] the highest stigmas. They could not come out and take the ARTs publicly.

The constant threat of violence, which sometimes occurred, meant that people living in Mahali might suddenly be cut off from access to ART, even if the medication were free and had the potential to transform their disease from fatal to chronic and nontransferable. As a result, even though HIV was technically no longer a fatal disease, the epidemic continued to evoke fear, insecurity, and social anxieties. It also had become a marker of some of the corruption and atrocities committed and/or experienced by people during and since PEV. HIV was described as one tool that could be used to perpetuate local inequalities, tensions and conflicts, and stigmatization. The stories that circulated about the List illustrated this point.

ETHNIC VIOLENCE AND CONFLICT IN MAHALI, A STIGMATIZED PLACE

As stories about the List were circulating, I also heard a handful of statements by locals suggesting that I was studying HIV stigma in a place perceived and experienced as being stigmatized, discriminated against, and abused by the Kenyan state. This perception did not sink into my mind until one day when I was visiting Nduta at her three-room home—the front two rooms had rickety wooden floors, and the back area served as a dirt-floored kitchen—which doubled as a den serving chang'aa (a strong, traditional, illegally home-brewed spirit). Nduta had a warm smile and contagious laugh, her place was cozy though crammed with furniture, and I enjoyed visiting her. One morning I was seated on a couch in Nduta's house when Mwangi, one of her regular customers and one of my close companions, sat down in the chair across from me. He visited this den nearly every morning before heading out in search of work in the informal economy, making his daily attempt to "break the lock" (take a shot of hard alcohol as a way to reduce a hangover). This morning, as Nduta used a small white plastic cup to carefully measure the strong liquor and pour a shot into a blue-and-white enamel mug, Mwangi made a fleeting, unexpected comment: "Eliza[beth], it is too late for everyone in [Mahali]. We have all heard that gospel [messages about HIV and AIDS], but everyone is already either infected or affected. There is no saving anyone here—the people of this town are all evil. The only ones left who are not infected are those who have not tested themselves, and they are just pretending to be . . . good people." Over time, I heard many people articulate this negative view of the place. They imagined that "all" people living in it were "evil," as evidenced by their (or their loved ones') vulnerability to HIV infections. HIV was not seen as the root of the moral shortcomings per se, but it was the logical, embodied, and warranted outcome of living amid "evil." Furthermore, for Mwangi, the suggestion that everyone was evil reversed the narrative that increased HIV awareness produced morally good citizens and therefore served as a local, leveling move and attempt to destigmatize HIV: if "the people of this town are all evil," no one could legitimately claim moral superiority or point fingers at or blame anyone else.

Mahali was perceived as "evil" due, in part, to the recurrent and chronic violence, death, and chaos that had erupted episodically across ethnic lines every five years, along with nearly every democratic presidential election.[2] Kiprono, a pharmacist who had recently moved to the area, explained his perception: "[Mahali] is known to be one of the most chaotic areas in all of Kenya. Even where I come from, we have heard of [Mahali]. It is just a bad place. I think it is just perception. Even some time back, there were [interethnic] clashes. It was unfortunate that [Mahali] was the worst hit area by the recent [2007–2008] clashes. This was just the one area you would hear about the most. So it made people think even more negatively about [Mahali] [laughs]! It is too much in the media." The town was an "imagined community" (Anderson 2006), reported in the media to be plagued by ethnic and political conflict and unrelenting chaos. Kiprono noted that because the area had been chronically represented negatively in journalists' accounts, Mahali—as "a place"—had experienced very public "discourses of vilification" (Wacquant 2007, 67). While he added that "it is just perception," he circled back to the notion that PEV substantiated what outsiders thought they already knew—Mahali was a "chaotic" and "bad" place—and this served as a self-fulfilling prophecy.

The collective moral experiences of people living in Mahali were shaped in part by such negative media representations of the place, but also by the residents' subjective, lived encounters during and in expectation of the cycles of political and ethnic violence. A *fundi* (mechanic) and long-time Kikuyu resident summed up his view of the place concisely: "Every five years—there must be fire." A Kalenjin man who had been born and raised in the area and worked at the *posho* (cornmeal) mill elaborated on this idea: "People fear [Mahali] because of tribal clashes. That is all. Anything else, they don't see [here]. When you say the word [Mahali], people say, 'Hey, that is [where] fire can arise at any time!' Now, as we are moving toward election year, we [who live here] worry. What might happen? Will it be like the other times?" For outsiders, Mahali conjured up images of fire and destructive clashes. But violence was also a chronic source of worry in the minds of locals. Central to everyday existence, especially when an election loomed on the horizon, was the probable manifestation of violence.

ETHNIC ANIMOSITIES, BLAME, AND THE PERSISTENCE OF HIV STIGMA

People who connected the stigmatization of the area with PEV (and other pre- and postelection disturbances) emphasized the perceived immorality of long-term inhabitants as emanating from two sets of behaviors: having committed horrific acts against rival ethnic group members and having engaged in immoral activities (e.g., sex work and corruption) to rebuild their lives. Conversations about PEV often morphed into discussions of high rates of HIV and memories of untimely deaths of people living in Mahali. Both PEV and the high number of AIDS-related deaths early in the history of the epidemic were perceived and experienced as catastrophes that fueled undesirable social changes and tensions. Thus, the two constantly evoked each other in ways that made it difficult to untangle them.

Most people in Mahali (including some health professionals) either rejected the reported HIV national and regional prevalence rates as too low or imagined that they were substantially higher in the Rift Valley than elsewhere. In 2010, the estimated rate of 10 percent cited by international researchers involved in global health work in the community, while higher than the national average, still meant that most people in Mahali did not have HIV (see Kaler and Watkins 2010). Despite this, when asked, most interlocutors said they suspected that the actual rate was significantly higher, claiming that more accurate estimates would be closer to 50 percent. One interlocutor even imagined that 80 percent of the population was infected. Many people said that they felt the rates had to be higher than the published statistics because of their personal and very vivid memories of PEV, and because social and family life had been (and continued to be) disrupted. For example, Kimaiyo, a farmer and secondary teacher at a private school who lived in a spacious cement-brick house with his wife and children in a rural community a few miles from the urban center, suggested:

I think clashes [after the election in 2007] increased the spread of HIV because the family structures were broken down. And when people have fear and trauma, they tend to look for solace or something to embrace [to] move on in the next life. So . . . all families were separated, and people came to a common village. There were no proper rules, proper moralities . . . that is, no proper families. So those people who had HIV found themselves in an awkward situation, whereby they could access immorality and all manner of vices, which made others who were not even infected with HIV to have HIV. . . . Everyone [during and following the PEV] lived in a small village—and it was a global village [people were from all over and no one knew anyone]. So they had the opportunity [to spread HIV]. Clashes contributed to [higher rates] so much! [The clashes during PEV] impacted the most on the spread of HIV. [PEV made the rates] around 70 percent of the people [living in the area]. The level of HIV has just increased [since the last PEV], because those who came with it spread it around freely. That is one of our major challenges.

PEV contributed to an imagined explosion of HIV cases, and as a result, people living with the virus served as scapegoats for the ongoing chaos associated with the area. However, that chaos stemmed from much larger and more complex social and structural inequalities and global, historical, and national processes that also fueled local tensions and animosities between people living in what Kimaiyo negatively referred to as a "global village" that lacked social cohesion, rules, standards, and norms. HIV was thus perceived by people as a possible device used to further these conflicts.

Links between PEV and HIV were made frequently. Many interlocutors recalled the chaos during PEV: brutal deaths; audacious looting; the burning of fields, houses, and other personal possessions; reliance on sex for survival by women of all ages and groups; and rapes of women and girls. People also remembered being temporarily cut off from global and national health services, including ART. The topic of the atrocious living conditions, especially in IDP camps where even the healthiest individuals could hardly avoid illness, also was raised in interviewees' responses, as was the division and scattering of families. In 2012, some people said that they still were unable to locate loved ones. The disorder evoked by memories of PEV among people I interviewed often served to link the violations of social and cultural norms and moralities to high rates of both HIV transmission and deaths from AIDS, thus disorder became part of local stigmatizing practices and discourses of blame.

On several occasions, I was specifically told that women living in IDP camps, because they lacked arrows and machetes during PEV, had sometimes used their HIV-infected bodies as weapons to strategically infect men of opposing ethnic groups. This was accomplished as they supposedly allowed themselves to be raped by their enemies. These kinds of stories blurred the boundaries between victim and perpetrator and demonstrate a form of symbolic violence (Bourdieu and Wacquant 1992), through which already existing and intersecting ethnic and gender inequalities and sexual identity politics were internalized and made to appear natural and commonsensical. Specifically, these stories reveal a taken-for-granted notion that Kikuyu women, and sex workers in particular, were responsible for being raped during PEV because they were parading themselves and thus ultimately to blame for the ongoing spread of HIV within and between members of different ethnic groups (see chapter 4). These kinds of discourses helped strengthen the links made between the notions of sex work and HIV. For example, Wawiru, a Kikuyu shopkeeper and one of my research assistants, recalled memories about living conditions after PEV. As we sat in the tiny, cluttered room where Wawiru lived behind the shop and she nursed her baby, the two women described events they claimed to have witnessed and overheard being discussed among women living in the IDP camps that unconsciously reinforced the status quo and ideas about the subordinate, political positioning of Kikuyu sex workers and their relationship to HIV in Kenya and especially the Rift Valley. Wawiru recounted from her memory:

The Kalenjin men raped Kikuyu women in such a way that the Kikuyu women decided to use rape as a weapon. They went to the river . . . just to be raped, as a way of spreading HIV. I don't know why the Kalenjin boys were not thinking they were not getting HIV . . . or maybe it was the insecurity that everyone was just doing anything, as if we were all going to die the next day. . . . The boys raped the old grandmothers, the mothers, the daughters, the granddaughters, and . . . they were not choosy. And it is like I have [already] said . . . you cannot tell who is HIV+ . . . but it was like those in the camps knew . . . , "Oh the Kalenjin boys are raping women." So [some of] the sex workers started going to them. . . . They just went to [the Kalenjin males] to be raped, not knowing that HIV would be a circle. These boys would rape these HIV+ women and then . . . the same boys would [later] rape [the daughters of the sex workers who had allowed themselves to be intentionally raped], who were not already HIV+. So . . . you cannot refuse [to be raped] because they are forcing you . . . but [it does not mean] you should go parading yourself! [Or think] "I have a weapon and this is a big weapon. It is a cold weapon!" It was a form of warfare against these people. . . . You know, there is nothing else we can do to these people. So they used [HIV] . . . as a weapon of revenge here in [Mahali].

As a "weapon," HIV also was said to be used to harm and cause suffering among ethnic rivals outside the IDP camps. One man stated, "We do use HIV for our tribal fighting." The sentiment that HIV was used to socially, emotionally, and physically harm others suggested that global health efforts aimed to normalize and destigmatize the disease had taken on new meanings as a double-edged sword in a community where the disease was still perceived and experienced as difficult to manage. I spoke about this with Joseph, a man who took care of a farm on behalf of the nonresident owner. Perched on the edge of a wooden chair inside an otherwise empty house with board walls and a dirt floor that had been constructed by a humanitarian relief organization, I listened to Joseph recall how locals had been using HIV as a tool for revenge since "the war" (as he characterized PEV): "Because people [are still bitter] because of that war, they have grudges and think of revenge through spreading [HIV]. A friend [of the rival ethnicity] could tell a female [who he knew to be living with HIV] to make love with [the man] so . . . he becomes [HIV] positive."

Once again, as in the conversation between Wawiru and a research assistant, Joseph blames the actions of women for new HIV infections as he notes the strategic use of their bodies to fuel the spread of HIV across ethnic lines and throughout the community. In the moments of conflict, chaos, and insecurity that surrounded PEV in Mahali, people had engaged in activities that they would never have performed during times of peace, behaving as though they were "all going to die the next day." This was a time of exception. Residents of Mahali were described as having acted as though there would never be any social or moral consequences for these deeds. Perhaps to the surprise of many, however, people did not all die the next day. Instead, they had to return to life as normal, as soon as the government declared the conflict over. Once peace was being restored, no one was supposed to be angry anymore.[3] Living in the same community, however, meant that people occasionally bumped into perpetrators. This left those who had survived PEV to live with painful memories and constant reminders, and people had to deal with the repercussions of what they (or others) had done to one another.

Gossip about HIV, such as stories about the List, often was less about the actual infection and, reflecting this context, more about how talk of an HIV diagnosis triggered images of the physical war and the so-called cold war—the secret use of HIV as a weapon. The knowledge that someone was living with HIV and the gossip about that sometimes served to fuel existing cultural politics, including ethnic animosities and anxieties, even though things might have seemed peaceful on the surface. Viral frictions were produced when local knowledge about activities during PEV and ongoing ethnic conflict and national politics collided with the distribution of local and global health care and efforts aimed at normalizing the disease to reduce stigma.

Ethnic inequalities were suspected to have worked their way into the general national health care system in Kenya, thus further strengthening a general distrust of the institutionalized structure of the medical establishment. For example, Joseph shared his rationale for distrusting the medical community in the Rift Valley:

JOSEPH: I will speak the truth to you. Our hospitals employ people who have tribalism. So there is negligence. If you are in a certain tribe, you are received [at the hospital or health center] willingly. They favor some [ethnic groups]. . . . You may even be treated and sent to a laboratory, but when it comes to the [pharmacists], they will tell you that there is no [free] medicine here [although it is supposed to be distributed for free], and so you should go and buy it. . . . And if you don't know any doctor at that place, you are not treated well.

ELIZABETH: You have to know someone?

JOSEPH: Yes. You [referring to me as an example] may be prescribed medicine, and we suffer the same disease. You [for example] are a Kalenjin and I am a Kikuyu. I will be told there is no medicine and you will be told there is free medicine.

ELIZABETH: So medicine is given by tribalism?

JOSEPH: Yes!

Likewise, the need to carefully navigate ethnic politics was described as posing a challenge to those seeking employment in the AIDS industry at the national level. For example, Jeptoo, a young and unmarried HIV counselor, described the

dangers, corruption, and politics of her own efforts to find work as a VCT counselor in a nearby town. It was a hot and dry day in early February—the wind was
fierce, and the dust from the dirt road we were walking on swirled around us
and periodically made us cough—when Jeptoo claimed that getting jobs often
demanded certain things from women: (1) "knowing the right people," (2) align-
ing themselves with the parliamentary minister favored by "the boss" (or the
person doing the hiring), (3) having sex with potential employers, and/or (4)
bribing someone in an organization. Later, in the privacy of the spacious living
room at her natal family's rural homestead that Jeptoo wanted me to visit, we ate
ugali (a thick, white, dough-like starch made from maize flour) and drank *mursik*
(a popular Kalenjin milk that is fermented in a calabash gourd) prepared for us
by her mother. Jeptoo spoke of learning from others about how and where to
apply for work as a VCT counselor, claiming there were rumors that people
should avoid certain organizations throughout the region because "everyone
working at [name of an HIV-related organization] is HIV—is known to be
infected." Finding work in the AIDS industry was sometimes described as complicated and competitive and demanded careful navigation of local, regional,
and national ethnic politics as well as potential participation in corrupt practices.
Sometimes finding work required a person to risk contracting HIV. But this was
often construed as less risky than not being able to earn a living. In another setting, Jeptoo offered an intriguing summary of the challenges of earning a living
for young women, in the context of extreme job scarcity and high rates of
HIV: "Sometimes you just have to pretend—for that one night—that the HIV
is not there."

HIV and local ethnic identity politics also blended to shape local discourses
of stigma and blame that I heard either during interviews or when I was spending time in and around the community. I heard members of one ethnic group
placing blame on a person from a different ethnic community for intentionally
spreading the disease. For example, in November 2012, I accompanied Cherop and
her next-door neighbor—both women were married and had several children—
as they delivered milk and eggs to the homes of several customers away from the
urban center. As we walked, I observed large, rolled-out tarps covered with
maize kernels that had been harvested and were being dried by the sun and air.
Occasionally, the air filled with laughter as barefoot children delightedly slid
through the maize, which was described as providing fun and speeding up the
drying process. As we walked on this particular day, some of the children started
running after us, as they often did, happily shouting at me, "*mzungu* (white person)!" The women I was with gossiped about a local Kikuyu husband who had
allegedly died of complications from AIDS. What the two women found especially interesting was that he was a Christian and quite wealthy. There was more,
however. He had supposedly been seducing Kalenjin women because several of
his shops had been destroyed during PEV and he was "bitter." While I regularly

heard ethnic labels used to describe locals in general, they were also used to refer to those who were allegedly spreading HIV on purpose. The logical explanation that often quickly followed was that they were still "bitter" about PEV, thus further cementing local links made between the chronic conflict and this virus. Additionally, moralizing discourses of blame about the spread of HIV were sometimes mediated by ethnic identity politics and, on occasion, springboarded into and out of already existing national political and ethnic animosities and inequalities.

HIV was construed as a real, albeit invisible, threat suspected of being used by those with malicious intentions to harm ethnic rivals. Such gossip (true or not) was evidence that people continued to harbor feelings of distrust and suspicion toward one another, despite the fact that more overt forms of hostility had receded. Likewise, this kind of casual talk about a disease being used to harm others socially, psychologically, and physically underscored the fact that despite intense efforts to normalize HIV as a chronic condition, it was still widely regarded as exceptional. Gossip provided an outlet through which people expressed concerns and offered commentaries about the abuse of power, most notably the idea that wealthy ethnic rivals were able to infect others with HIV, wreaking havoc on those with limited resources and social networks. Such gossip was as much about a circulating virus as it was about providing a cautionary tale about the dangers of living amid the violent conditions of Mahali, a form of local knowledge and disease management perceived as necessary for people to protect themselves from harm and infection. At the same time, however, this gossip served as a device to further fuel ethnic animosities and public moralizing discourses about the HIV epidemic, and it fed the stigmatizing sentiment that people living with the virus were dangerous, oversexed, and willfully spreading an exceptional disease.

The inequitable distribution of health care and even HIV-related stigma sometimes presented themselves across historical legacies of racialized global structures and ongoing national ethnic animosities, political violence, inequalities, and insecurities in the area, and therefore reverberated loudly in many of the stories about HIV that I collected. Milicent, a vendor in a market stall, described PEV as having completely shamed the community, resulting in the place being cursed. From her perspective, the high rates of HIV in the area were not the cause of the shame or curse directly, but rather, reflecting the sentiments expressed by Mwangi earlier, were the logical consequences of the chronic fighting and conflict among locals and their failure to fulfill their proper roles and social, moral, and ethical responsibilities to one another. Mahali was a bad or stigmatized place. For me, this also suggested symbolic violence, manifested in the form of collective shame through which locals internalized blame for their choreographed actions against each other that brought to their community both the devastating consequences of political violence and the AIDS epidemic.

Milicent made the following comment: "[PEV] affected this place so much. So many women were raped, and many more became associated with sex work [because of poverty]. . . . Some people in Mahali even say that [HIV doesn't exist]—only that the place is cursed [because of all the immoral practices that took place during election violence]—and that is why so many live with HIV and die from AIDS here. [PEV] has brought shame to us all."

PEV and rates of HIV in Mahali made both national and international headlines, attracting much attention to the place from around the world. Relief money, food, and services poured into the area, at least for a while. A school, a new market, and some houses were rebuilt in selected spots by various international donors. Compensation for losses was also distributed, albeit unevenly and corruptly. This was interpreted by many in the community as simultaneously helpful and another source of disgrace, because people living in Mahali were characterized as useless and unable to live up to their proper social and gendered roles and obligations, as well as depending on sex work and/or aid for survival. International aid was described as both felt and enacted sources of stigmatization toward the place and those living in it. (I return to questions of gender and sexuality in chapter 4.)

Mahali became defined, in part, around ethnic conflict and local corruption. People living in the community also knew that it was filled with secrets. According to legal scholar Robin West (1992), conflict sometimes builds community and constitutes a way for people to know and interact with each other. This conflict, in turn, then unifies and motivates members in the pursuit of justice (see also Stoeltje 2009). In the context of Mahali, HIV was incorporated directly and distinctly into already existing forms of conflict and corruption during and following PEV. Locals were united around the task of working to identify (often through gossip and occasionally through scandals) who was and was not living with the virus in their search for justice and security, and for a local sense of belonging in the contexts of tremendous uncertainty and rapid social change. Circulating stories about the List reflected these efforts. Being able to talk about and leak the secrets contained in such stories helped sustain social relationships (Manderson et al. 2015). Viral frictions perpetuated stigma at various levels— individual, community, and structural—even during a period of increased efforts to normalize and end AIDS by the global health community.

3 • STIGMA AND THE CULTURAL POLITICS OF UNCERTAINTY

The article I was reading as I traveled in a *matatu* said that a building in Mahali damaged in PEV had been "resurrected from the ashes," complete with a *hoteli* (restaurant) on the ground floor, two levels of lodging accommodations, and a pub on top. This news piece went on to say that the building served as a "yardstick" or measurable evidence that years "down the line, the town is receiving a new lease on life."[1] I was thrilled that here, unlike in other media stories I had read or heard about, Mahali was finally being cast in an apparently optimistic and hopeful light, so I tucked the article away to share with others later. I had learned early in my trips to Kenya that people from all walks of life kept up with the latest media stories in various ways: listening to radio and watching television, purchasing a newspaper individually or as a group, or gathering around newsstands to memorize the headlines and imagine through talk and debates the contents of the stories inside the paper.

This chapter opens with a more detailed, ethnographic story about commuting into Mahali from Eldoret with an emphasis on the local reactions to and interpretations of the abovementioned news piece that I had not anticipated and that contrasted with my own initial reading of it. The chapter then continues the historical thread started in chapter 2, which I extend by highlighting a series of other media stories over the past decade that chronicle more contemporary circumstances at play and that shaped everyday social life in globalized Kenya. My goal is to describe the relationship—and frictions produced—between Kenya and the global community to center the uncertainties, insecurities, and political realities that characterized the everyday lives of people in Mahali. I develop the concept of local cultural politics of uncertainty, which I argue intersected with global and national health efforts to address HIV to produce viral frictions and keep various forms of institutional, public, and courtesy stigma in place.[2]

"PREPARE YOURSELF FOR ANYTHING"

During my early commute on the day Mahali was featured in the news, I was sitting in the very back row of the *matatu* with my legs propped up by the bags of produce and various parcels of other passengers that took up much of the available floor space. Matching the color of local soils, a reddish-brown cockroach skittered across the top of the seat in front of me. On this October morning, it was drizzling. Maize had been or was being harvested and collected to dry in tepee-shaped bundles across many of the *mashamba* (farms) along the way. The seemingly unending rain, which I had been told should have ended by then, was a matter of unease that everyone was talking about. People were concerned that the maize would rot—leading to food insecurity—or pose a health hazard if not dried and stored properly. They debated whether or not global and local climate patterns were changing and, if so, what this might mean for their subsistence farming and agriculture, the bases of the economy across the Rift Valley. Also on the minds of some people was the fact that their pit latrines (their only toilets) were flooding, which heightened concerns about poor sanitation and the potential for increased transmission of diseases already endemic to the area, like cholera and typhoid. While it was cool and damp outside our vehicle, inside it was warm and stuffy. The windows had fogged up from the heat and humidity emanating from our bodies. And the stale air reeked, combining the smells of car exhaust, sweat, cooking smoke from wood stoves, and a hint of the sweet scent of *chang'aa*. The driver frequently wiped the windshield with a handkerchief. Desiring a view of my own, I mimicked the driver and cleared a small circle so I could peer out across the landscape. The scenery outside was breathtakingly beautiful and fascinating because I never knew what I might see.

As we started to make a steep climb, my eyes focused on the roadside, and I noticed a woman holding a rooster upside down by its feet toward the oncoming traffic, hoping to sell it. Not far from her were three huge metal jugs used for carrying milk, evidently waiting for someone to pick them up and transport them to wherever their contents would eventually be consumed or they would be refilled. Farther along the road, I watched two women with babies tied to their backs (protected from the cold under thick, plaid wool blankets) navigate around several donkeys carrying weighty loads of neatly cut firewood through a large herd of oncoming cattle shepherded by two boys wielding long sticks. I heard the muted rustling of feathers nearby and realized that the passenger in front of me was transporting more than one chicken in a small cardboard box.

When we neared Mahali's urban center, the passengers of the vehicle I was in were jostled as it bounced across a set of speed bumps. Several hands, including mine, reached toward the ceiling as if choreographed to protect our heads from hitting it. The *matatu* conductor[3] flicked the inside of the roof to indicate to the driver that a passenger wanted to be dropped off at the next stop. As we rolled to a stop, a few passengers got out. As I started my tedious climb over people and products to get out too, the driver and conductor verified that I was exiting at the proper place and hadn't intended, as a white woman, to go to another, more secure location. While it was common for white doctors and students from the Global North to visit the HIV clinic in Mahali, it was rare to see them walking around the center and especially unusual for them to travel by public transport. Instead, most of them were in the center for only a few hours at a time and arrived in private SUVs, sometimes with red-and-blue lettering saying "USAID— From the American People" on the side. While there was a gated compound— topped with rolls of barbed wire—where people from China regularly lived in Mahali, I was told that the area had not housed expatriates from other countries (such as India or Holland) for decades because of the history of violence. Instead, it was more common for expatriates to live in larger towns and cities, where the living standards were considerably more comfortable for those with access to resources like stable internet service, electricity, and running water. After successfully convincing everyone that I was where I wanted to be, I stepped out, being careful to avoid the precipitous drop from the edge of the jagged pavement into the mud. While the weather patterns were often distinct in Mahali (when compared to Eldoret), it appeared that today the sun would once again be unable to fight off the clouds or dry the maize. I pulled up my hood, zipped up the maroon fleece I was wearing, and carefully made my way across the slippery and muddy terrain, dodging the oncoming traffic that flowed steadily between a long line of storefronts and the highway. I was headed toward the container clinic, where I would conduct interviews that day.

The clinic, funded by collaborations between the Kenyan state and international entities, sat across a small grazing field from the compound that housed Chinese workers who had come to Kenya to repair the main roads through the country. On many mornings, men in Mahali who relied on *kibarua* (casual labor positions, such as digging ditches) to earn their living arrived early and sat outside this compound, hoping to be the first ones in line and ready when the Chinese bosses emerged, looking for workers to employ for the day. Jobs in Mahali were not only scarce but often short-term and competitive. The container clinic was run by a public-private partnership that, according to a brochure about the organization, offered health services at "major truck stops and border crossings in Africa, India, and Asia." This tiny health center was open to truck drivers and sex workers and provided free medications for a variety of conditions as well as screening for HIV. While the clinic was equipped to treat several sexually transmitted infections, it referred clients who tested positive for HIV to the nearby HIV clinic.

When I arrived at the clinic, I stepped into the main room, which had a desk and watercooler in one corner under a mounted television that frequently aired a documentary highlighting the dangers of AIDS-related stigma and discrimination. Around the perimeter of the room and under a sign with an arrow pointing down that read "Ngojea Hapa" (wait here) were about 6–8 lightweight, white plastic outdoor chairs. Above one of the chairs was a gold cardboard box that served as a condom dispenser and had the following words written on the front: "Sure; Lubricated Condoms; 144 Count; From the Government of Kenya." There were two doors to the left and right of the waiting area that bore wooden signs saying "VCT" in handwritten black letters. Under each of these signs was a sticker showing a Japanese flag and the words "From the People of Japan."

Soon, Rehema appeared to mop the floors, so I went back outside to wait. I wandered past a large pile of fresh sugarcane stalks for sale and a bicycle repair stand to a nearby storefront, where colorful plastic-wrapped mattresses, small propane stoves, large jugs of various sizes and shapes, and washing containers were set out for sale. There I found a small group of familiar individuals who were already socializing. As I greeted them, I pulled out the newspaper, and Henry began reading the article about Mahali aloud to the rest of us. When he concluded his reading, there was an awkward silence that I had not anticipated. This was interrupted by Judy, who offered an alternative interpretation: "That building shouldn't have been rebuilt! I have vowed never to step foot in it because it could fall at any moment. I do not trust it. It was built on a deep crack. Every one of us saw that crack with our eyes!" Jane added: "It is true. That building was for Kalenjins, and during the [2007–2008 PEV], the Kikuyus looted and burned it. The owner was told [by authorities] to tear it down before rebuilding it, [but] I heard that he paid *kitu kidogo* [literally, a "little thing" in Kiswahili, meaning a bribe] so he could build it quickly and without hassle. It was rebuilt on corruption. He only smeared over the cracks. But they are still there. That crack runs deep into the ground. . . . That building is not safe."

After this comment, the group began to discuss the insecurity of the building, its history, and its sudden scandalous, if not mysterious, reconstruction. As I listened, I was once again struck by the intensity and depth of the ethnic animosities that influenced the interpretation of this article and recalled Luise White's (2000, 113) comment that newspapers did not necessarily render the words in their articles "true" but were used by locals as a space to offer contending versions of a story. When the conversation paused, Henry turned to me and in a gentle, yet firm, tone reminded us all of what was required to successfully adapt to the complexities and dangers of living in the modern global world: "Not everything is as it appears to be on the surface in this world. You must learn that anything is possible. From this moment forward, do not be surprised by anything—not anything good that happens nor anything bad that happens. Prepare yourself for anything." People living in Mahali were acutely aware of the precariousness of everyday life, and this uncertainty influenced the ethnographic moments and social mood of my research over the past decade.

In Mahali, almost anything did happen, and life was chronically uncertain and insecure. As is the case everywhere, maintaining health—especially among those suffering from chronic conditions—heaped further complexities on top of the problems of uncertainty (Whyte 2002; McGrath et al. 2014). After the 2008 global economic crisis, rates of poverty had increased, which coincided with PEV and brought about even higher levels of unemployment and concerns about food security. Food prices climbed sharply. The media reported scandals involving corruption among Kenya's wealthy, ruling elite (Prince 2012). And with the corruption that flowed from the top of the social hierarchy to the bottom and back up again (Apter 1999; James Smith 2008), nothing was as it seemed. This left locals to decipher on their own who and what they might or might not trust. Many people emphasized that in Kenya it was not safe to trust anyone, precisely because anything could happen: loyalties might shift without notice. The image of a deep, smeared-over crack created an illusion that all was normal and well. The crack's masking of unseen, uncertain, insecure, corrupt, and dangerous conditions serves as an excellent metaphor for thinking through the broad contexts that are muted when global health efforts bracket individuals out of them. Understanding these uncertain conditions is central for explaining the persistence of HIV stigma and helping make sense of how local perceptions of and experiences with HIV impact AIDS eradication efforts.

THE UNCERTAINTIES OF LIFE IN KENYA (2010–2019)

Issues highlighting events in Kenya in relation to the rest of the world were often reported in the media, which left people in Mahali talking about and remembering just how uncertain, corrupt, and dangerous life was there. Such stories created and sustained anxieties within and between people and groups. For example, in 2011, a number of grenades exploded unexpectedly at various locations in Nairobi and near Kenya's eastern border, with Somalia. After thorough investigations of each incident, reports circulated that the deadly assaults represented a nationwide security risk. The attackers were identified as al-Shabaab rebels, an al Qaeda–linked terrorist group of Somali militants. These kinds of attacks had occurred in eastern Africa since August 1998, when—a consequence of orders from Osama bin Laden—truck bombs exploded just outside the U.S. embassies in downtown Nairobi and Dar es Salaam, Tanzania, killing more than 200 people and injuring more than 5,000 in Nairobi alone (USDOS 2018). In videos broadcast after the terrorist attacks, bin Laden claimed that the bombs were to protest Kenya's alliance with the United States. During my 2011 trip, things became even more unnerving when news stories announced that those responsible for the explosions did not look like people of Somali descent but rather resembled ordinary Kenyan nationals, making it difficult to identify the enemy. In the weeks that followed, I overheard half-joking comments that an al-Shabaab terrorist might even have the face of a *mzungu*.

The grenade attacks prompted the Kenyan military to invade Somalia, and several media articles predicted the grim impact it would have on the tourist industry, the value of the Kenyan shilling, and thus the whole Kenyan economy. The terrorist attack not only discouraged foreign investment in downtown Nairobi for some years, but it also was the first in a series of periodic, random terrorist attacks in Nairobi that continued throughout my decade of research. For example, there was a shooting at Nairobi's popular, high-end Westgate Mall in September 2013. Several months later, while I was doing research in 2014, there were concerns about a terrorist cell operating out of a larger town close to Mahali, and a Somali man passing through Mahali in a *matatu* was temporarily placed in jail while locals inspected the vehicle for explosives out of fear that he was a terrorist. In April 2015, four al-Shabaab gunmen stormed Kenya's Garissa University College and began firing, singling out, shooting, and killing approximately 147 people who were identified as Christians (BBC 2019). And in January 2019, just prior to my trip that year, men armed with guns and explosives attacked and killed dozens of people at an upscale hotel in Nairobi.

In January 2012, the International Criminal Court (ICC) confirmed charges of crimes against humanity against four of the six Kenyan politicians suspected of having played the largest roles in instigating the 2007–2008 PEV (see chapter 2 for details about PEV). The Kenyan government had established the charges but was unable to set up a special local tribunal to prosecute the men, so the cases were taken up by the ICC. Later that year, as the country began to prepare for its next general election, scheduled for March 4, 2013, two of the men facing trial in The Hague emerged as potential presidential candidates. This increased tension in Mahali. When Hillary Rodham Clinton, then the U.S. secretary of state, visited Kenya in August 2012, she warned leaders and citizens not to repeat the deadly violence that had erupted during previous elections and hinted that if William Ruto or Uhuru Kenyatta were elected while still facing charges by the ICC, the United States would consider imposing economic, diplomatic, and even military sanctions against Kenya.

Kenyatta and Ruto were elected president and deputy president, respectively, in 2013 and 2017 with only minor fighting, and at the time of this writing they remain in office. Yet anxieties remained high as the initial results of the election in both years were contested by Kenyatta's opponent, Raila Odinga, who refused to accept the outcomes and, in 2017, contested the results in the Supreme Court, which nullified the results from the original election and ruled that it must be repeated in October of the same year. Still, the threats made by Clinton also pointed to Kenya's connections to and position in relation to the world at large and global politics, as well as highlighting the perceived fragility of international funding. After Clinton's visit, people frequently asked what, if any, implications such sanctions would have on foreign aid, specifically in the distribution of free ART through PEPFAR. People in Mahali wanted to know what economic sanctions would mean for PLWHIV. Funding through PEPFAR had previously been reduced in Kenya due to the country's inefficient spending following PEV (PEPFAR 2008).

My interlocutors recognized that shifts in unequal international and global relations, such as those between the United States and Kenya, could very likely produce real effects on the bodies and experiences of residents of Mahali.

Other incidents and media reports also circulated in relation to the insecurities and uncertainties more directly associated with HIV and health and contributed to sentiments like "nothing is as it seems" and "anything could happen." For several years, newspaper stories and political cartoons highlighted health challenges facing the Kenyan government, as officials worked with international entities to locate and remove batches of counterfeit ART from circulation. In 2012, at one of Kenya's largest public hospitals, services and the distribution of basic drugs such as antibiotics were temporarily interrupted during a cash crisis blamed on an allegedly corrupt hospital administration and the Kenyan treasury. In the months that followed, services at this hospital and numerous other public facilities across Kenya were suspended again during a series of strikes by doctors and/or nurses. People in Mahali had a variety of opinions about the local impacts of these events. Some people considered the actions of health workers to be unprofessional, unethical, and contributing to unnecessary deaths of otherwise innocent people. Others empathized with the public health professionals, citing the poor wages, limited resources, and difficult working conditions provided by the government as legitimate and reasonable motivations for the strikers' actions. Still others did not care about the suspension of health services, claiming that such services were chronically inadequate and erratic for people living in Mahali, with or without a strike. Some public health employees who were involved in the strikes spoke about the tensions that had emerged between government employees and foreign and international employees working for global health institutions and other humanitarian organizations. In particular, public health officials worried that the Kenyan government would not feel the full impact of the strike, since international workers and organizations continued to provide health-related services to patients during the strikes.

In August 2012, a small Ebola outbreak occurred in Uganda, generating an Ebola scare in the Rift Valley. During my 2014 research trip, a major Ebola epidemic was in full swing in western Africa, causing anxiety and stress across the continent and beyond. When I reached Kenya, I and everyone else arriving at the airport had our temperatures taken to screen us for Ebola. When I returned to my home in Indiana a few months later, my next-door neighbor would not come near me for weeks out of fear that I had been infected. During my 2019 trip, there was another outbreak in Uganda and the Democratic Republic of the Congo. The latter was declared by WHO (2020a) to be the second-largest Ebola outbreak ever and a global health emergency, and it lasted through June 2020. During the 2012 and 2014 Ebola scares, rumors circulated around Mahali of patients being quarantined at a nearby public hospital, and media stories offered health updates, lists of the signs and symptoms of Ebola, and strategies to avoid contracting the disease. Kenyans were discouraged from shaking hands, riding in a *matatu*, traveling to Uganda, or interacting with people who were from or had been in Uganda. People living in highway communities, like Mahali, that regularly hosted foreigners, were warned to be especially vigilant. Some residents of Mahali were skeptical of the whole story and doubted either the ability or the willingness of the Kenyan state to protect the people living along the highway. During these Ebola scares, another story was broadcast about a Protestant Kenyan church group whose members had been planning to attend a women's mission retreat in Uganda. The group changed its plans at the last minute and traveled to Tanzania instead, in the hope of avoiding the deadly Ebola virus. But the group, traveling in two buses, never made it to the retreat. Instead, thirteen women were killed and seventy-one injured when both buses were involved in road accidents.

My interlocutors were quick to share the irony of these stories. Maina, who identified herself as a sex worker, linked Ebola, HIV, and road accidents in Kenya to contextualize things for me one afternoon while we sat alone together in a booth at the empty pub where she worked: "You can spend your life trying not to contract a virus, and then you suddenly get struck down during a road accident. This is why I would rather have HIV—at least there are ARTs nowadays, which can keep you alive for over twenty years." I heard similar refrains in 2014 and 2019, which emanated from an escalating cancer epidemic that had followed the AIDS epidemic across sub-Saharan Africa and was in part a result of the fact that more PLWHIV were living longer on ART (see Livingston 2012). People said, "I would rather have HIV than cancer—at least there is ART." More recently, my six-week research trip to Kenya, planned to begin in May 2020, was canceled due to the COVID-19 pandemic, when many countries went on lockdown and banned international travel. Messages from friends and colleagues across Kenya via email, text message, and video chats echoed familiar phrases: "People are saying, 'I would rather die of COVID-19 than hunger. With COVID-19 you can live for fourteen days, but you can only live seven days without food.'" This kind of talk about diseases and the unevenness of access to safety, treatment, and food illustrates the many uncertainties and inequalities facing ordinary people living in Mahali that maintain HIV's exceptional status as a disease (see also Hardon and Moyer 2014). This talk also demonstrates the ways people constantly weighed health conditions, tried to manage and control disease uncertainty, and evaluated which (and when) diseases posed the most threats (and to whom) and caused the greatest potential disruptions to their normal living and the aim of staying alive. These efforts and evaluations influenced interpersonal relationships and power differentials between people, or what I refer to as the cultural politics of uncertainty. As we shall see, the cultural politics of uncertainty intersected with global and national health messaging and technologies to keep processes of public and courtesy stigma in motion.

Uncertain Maladies

"HIV has not come for dogs. It has come for people. If we get HIV, we get it. If we don't, it has not come for us." These words were said by a woman I did not know after our paths had literally crossed on a log footbridge that enabled people to pass over a frequently rushing river that ran between urban Mahali and its more rural community neighbors. The woman was carrying a heavy load of goods and was probably returning to her rural home after having spent the day at the Mahali market. I was with Irene, who translated for me because I did not know KiNandi (the language of the Nandi, a major Kalenjin group in Mahali). We had been following a dirt path that led down a large hill and through a lush green grazing pasture to the river, and we were on our way back to urban Mahali after spending the day in a nearby rural community where we had conducted life-history and semistructured interviews. As this woman made clear, most people in Mahali were not paralyzed by HIV: it was one of many dangers lurking about that they tried to avoid. What was especially striking about this statement was the ambivalence that seemed to increase as the same sentiment was echoed by many others. The ambivalence seemed to emerge not from a place of denial, ignorance, or lack of knowledge about the presence of a dangerous virus or disease (Eaton 2008), but rather from a place of articulated awareness and continued observations of the inconsistencies, contradictions, uncertainties, and dangers associated with the realities of HIV, AIDS, and daily life.

Stacey Langwick's (2011) classification system of maladies in Tanzania is useful for further understanding the uncertainties associated with HIV and the persistence of stigma in Mahali. In her detailed ethnographic study of East African healing and healers, Langwick argues that the Kiswahili word *ugongwa* is best translated as malady, rather than as disease, illness, or sickness, as is usually done. While all these terms imply a lack of physical health and well-being, the English word *malady* also refers to notions of moral defect and corruption, as well as the idea that the person suffering is in a state of "not being held well by the seen and unseen world, by spirits or kin, or neighbors, or in other things in the world" (Langwick 2011, 11). Langwick also writes, "The concept of malady holds biomedical and nonbiomedical discomforts, disabilities, and other undesirable states of being in the same frame" (10).

Langwick (2011) identifies three types of maladies in East Africa: maladies caused by God in the natural order of things; maladies of person, sent by the malicious intentions of others, usually in the form of witchcraft; and maladies caused by run-ins with nonhuman devils (*mashetani*). She notes, however, that "these distinctions are not rigid categories of complaints as much as they are narrative technologies through which stories may be created and experienced, and conditions may be described and engaged" (153). In general, people in Mahali had come to classify HIV as a malady from God, which Langwick argues has to do with a local practical understanding and knowledge that nothing really can be done to avoid or completely remove a particular malady. She contends that some maladies come to be classified as having been sent from God when people come to believe that biomedical practitioners are unable to fully negotiate the threats produced by them. At the same time, there is an implied sentiment that accompanies such maladies. That is, there is no ultimate cure for or prevention against them, as the woman on the log bridge put it. Langwick writes that "the distinguishing characteristic of maladies of God is that there is no protection, no defense, and no way to avoid them if they come your way" (155).

The classification of a malady from God helps us understand the local logics being drawn upon to think about and respond to HIV—a condition that has to be managed and controlled, but is not curable (McGrath et al. 2014). This was especially true in Mahali as the global health community pushed the normalization of HIV, using a chronic disease rhetoric in a place already characterized by uncertainty. The concept of a malady from God is also useful in helping interpret why many people resorted to medical pluralism, exploring various healing options available to them, including paying exorbitant rates for prayers from priests, herbal remedies, and/or treatment by traditional healers. Especially in the domain of health, in the context of uncertainty, people everywhere are willing to consider and often try anything (Kleinman 2006). As Susan Reynolds Whyte (1997, 2002) documented in eastern Uganda and Jane mentioned of the Kenyan experience, early in the crisis and before treatment was available, people embraced the uncertainty of AIDS by avoiding HIV tests and found agency in trying out different healing strategies. In Mahali, people were provided with a sense of hope that perhaps someone else, beyond the medical establishment, might one day be able to negotiate with God and cure them of HIV.

Hope for a cure was certainly in the minds of many patients at the HIV clinic. Interviews often ended with some variant of questions such as, "When will there be a cure for HIV?" and "I heard there is a cure for AIDS in America but that it is too expensive for Africans. When will it be made available to us here?"[4] On one occasion, Moses (introduced in chapter 1) spoke of a cure for stigma. He had recently buried his sister-in-law, who had died from the synergistic complications of her dual diagnoses of HIV and diabetes. Moses linked her death to the fact that she had delayed accessing ART while she focused her efforts on "paying witch doctors [traditional healers] 80,000 [Kenyan shillings, or about $1,000 in 2014] for a cure from stigma."

Numerous people explained that at one time in Mahali, AIDS was considered to be the result of witchcraft, or to use Langwick's (2011) classification, a malady of person. However, most people went on to say that from a combination of their own observations and experiences and the increased education and awareness campaigns of global health initiatives, they now "knew better": AIDS was transmitted by a virus spread predominantly through unprotected sexual intercourse. Many of my interlocutors formally rejected the idea that witchcraft caused HIV[5] (see also Ashforth 2004), the exception being if all members of a single family had become infected. To locals, this seemed like too much misfortune for a single family to endure, and stronger and evil forces were likely at play in these instances. I do not intend to suggest that people in Mahali never resorted to seeking cures and remedies from traditional healers before seeking biomedical treatments. Signs advertising such traditional services were common across the landscape. Many people did consult traditional healers for protection, prevention, and treatment, but they often ended up at the HIV clinic after they had exhausted other possibilities. For example, one early December after the maize had been harvested, I spoke with Mercy, a widow with four daughters. As we sat on the grass in front of her rectangular mud house and chatted, while our children sorted through the residue of picked-over maize cobs and husks to make pinwheels, Mercy said: "People go to the witch doctor [traditional healer] when they start to feel sick. And that is the time that they take their money [in search of healing]. But then if it is [HIV]—will it be cured? No! You just come back and continue to be sick. Because with a disease like [HIV] or cancer— there is no cure. So the person will just be coming back, and he continues being sick. The witch doctor [traditional healer] can give you something that will help, but only for a time."

Ironically, witchcraft claims and most maladies of person allow blame to be shifted away from the individual sufferer and his or her individual behaviors to an outside entity. While local politics certainly lie behind both who can and cannot legitimately claim to have been bewitched and the potential violence that could erupt from formal accusations (F. Thomas 2008; Ashforth 2015; Pfeiffer and Maithya 2018), being able to locate blame outside the individual is useful because it transforms explanations of the causes of suffering from a socially stigmatizing condition to a more socially acceptable one (Rödlach 2006). Furthermore, such healing rituals are sometimes able to address and/or reflect on the interpersonal social issues and human conflicts imagined to be the root origin of maladies and their associated stigmas (Evans-Pritchard 1976).

As people increasingly turned toward classifying HIV as a malady from God, they simultaneously began attributing contraction of the virus to the individual behavior of people who had engaged in behaviors that were described as "immoral" or "reckless" and thus had only themselves to blame, as I explore in greater depth in later chapters. This shift unintentionally exacerbated the processes of structural or institutionalized forms of stigmatization and sometimes influenced the relationships between patients and their health care providers in Mahali. For example, it was common for me to hear remarks from exasperated workers at the HIV clinic such as "You got the disease on your own, so you will have to suffer alone" or "You got the disease alone, you can find a way to get yourself to the clinic every month." But the idea that people living in a resource-limited setting could manage a chronic condition like HIV on their own was a myth, especially for those who struggled to manage stigma beyond the walls of the clinic (McGrath et al. 2014). Social support and emotional care—within and beyond the clinic—was necessary to sustain a person's whole and healthy life on ART (see chapter 6).

While some researchers have argued that the use of the chronic disease paradigm would destigmatize HIV (Swendeman, Ingram, and Rotheram-Borus 2009), my research, like the work of other scholars in sub-Saharan Africa (Russell et al. 2007), suggests that this approach complicated processes of stigma. Consequently, as others have argued, the notion of HIV as a manageable chronic illness needs to be reconsidered in sub-Saharan Africa (Whyte 2012; McGrath et al. 2014), where HIV has been biomedicalized "but not socialized" (Steenberg 2020, 212). While global health programs that prescribed ART and developed anti-stigma interventions (described in chapter 5) aimed at extending and improving the lives and experiences of PLWHIV, they sometimes aggravated rather than resolved the interpersonal tensions created and maintained by this particular malady. These tensions intertwined with the larger social and structural inequalities at the core of stigma. The shift in classifications of the malady reflects a viral friction produced as global health messaging, technologies, and national programming and policies wrestled with local logics, experiences, and the politics of uncertainty to change processes of stigmatization and local socialities.

Managing the Uncertainties of Stigma

Given the uncertainties and inequalities associated with HIV, people's discussions of the malady, people living with it, and subjective experiences with stigma were wide-ranging and even incongruous at times. People across the social spectrum—men and women, young and old, urban and rural dwellers, and individuals from various ethnic groups—were well versed in the basic biomedical aspects of HIV they had access to,[6] but their stories about the virus tended to be extremely varied. The presence of diverse and contradictory responses to HIV and the range of dissimilar discourses seemed to trouble only me, as I was in search of things that were neatly packaged so I could assess public stigma. That is, I wanted to determine whether the general public accepted or rejected people living with or associated with HIV (Pescosolido et al. 2010). What I found was that both were happening at the same time, and it was precisely this kind of uncertainty that made public stigma, like HIV, a potentially chronic condition that demanded careful and skilled social navigation.

In retrospect, it was likely the bias of my own binary thinking and dualistic assumptions that complicated matters for me. Life in Mahali was uncertain, and chronic insecurity plagued everyday existence and health experiences. Consequently, HIV was also perceived and experienced as uncertain: anything could happen, and nothing was as it seemed. Translated into a discussion about stigma, this meant that the effects of stigma might always be considered possible at any moment, but were not a given. Just because no obvious stigma or discrimination was occurring did not necessarily mean that it was not happening quietly, indirectly, in some other nuanced fashion that might leak out at a later moment or in a different location. For example, a person who had not previously been stigmatized overtly because he or she did not look sick (which was usually attributed to the use of ART) could unexpectedly become subject to all sorts of stigmatizing remarks and behaviors the moment the person's HIV (or another illness) began to appear. ART was construed in Mahali as offering (at least temporarily) relief and an overall general perception and hope that all was well. However, ART—as documented by other scholars (e.g., Kalofonos 2010; Wilhelm-Solomon 2013; McGrath et al. 2014; Steenberg 2020)—was not uniformly construed as having completely resolved the problem. Rather, it produced new ones, thereby making stigma even more complex. Therefore, people still felt the strong need to conceal an HIV+ status, which ART made possible (see also chapters 5 and 6).

On any given day, many people worked hard to destigmatize and normalize HIV to diminish its seriousness by making statements like "HIV is a disease like any other," "It's no big deal," "Just normal," "The order of the day," "That's the preferred disease," or "Like a *homa* [common cold]" and in the very next moment, or sometimes in the next sentence, they would say something like:

HIV is a bad omen or a curse—the result of sin and/or negligent living.
[HIV is a] serious disease—feared above the rest.
[It is a] scary disease because if you are infected, you cannot ever be cured. Even with these drugs, you are not being healed, so you will just die. So that is why people are just committing suicide, rather than die that slow and shameful death.
[That is a disease only for the] immoral and promiscuous.
That disease makes me see only death—I can just [get] diarrhea at the mention of the word. I have witnessed so much death and dying because of it.

Some interlocutors offered their interpretations of what these conflicting messages meant. A handful of people said that such incongruous comments reflected the mixing of local logics about and memories of AIDS with global health technologies, words, and knowledge. Justifications supporting this belief took on two different but related forms. First, people said that free biomedical technologies and HIV-related messages offered new glimmers of hope for locals, as they carried the possibility of managing uncertainties and restoring a sense of a normal life and identity. Global health interventions and knowledge had theoretically shifted the malady from being a death sentence to being a chronic condition that could be controlled to extend the future life of a person indefinitely. Local doctors spoke of the great lengths they went to as they tried to normalize HIV as a chronic condition—for example, when they were carefully disclosing the news to an adolescent that he or she was infected. They explained their strategy of slowly educating their teenage clients about a wide range of chronic lifestyle conditions that people managed before proceeding to discuss their patients' seropositive status and equating their lifelong need for ART to the need for medication for people living with "any other disease," like diabetes. Second, global health programming had literally put new words and phrases, such as *HIV is a disease like any other*, into circulation through education and outreach efforts, clinical programs, and globally produced anti-stigma campaigns. Yet this latter, popular type of approach for combating stigma (for a wide variety of health conditions), which has long emphasized education about scientific theories and biological understandings of a disease and the "disease-like-any-other" messaging in the Global North, has become regarded as an ineffective strategy. Social scientists have noted that the combination of scientific information and the "disease-like-any-other" discourse might exacerbate public fears about a disease, reinforcing the idea that a condition is not curable (thereby rendering it as a malady from God) and increasing—rather than decreasing—community rejection of those living or associated with it (see Dingfelder 2009; Pescosolido et al. 2010). This appeared to have happened in Mahali.

On several occasions, while chatting about my research with employees at the HIV clinic, I mentioned my struggle to make sense of the conflicting statements that I was hearing. To my surprise, workers appeared enthusiastic: "A disease like any other? That is what we tell our clients at the clinic!" These individuals were pleased to hear that the words being spoken at the clinic—strategically designed to normalize and destigmatize the disease and those infected or associated with it—had made their way into local discussions, an indication that the knowledge and ideas being distributed through their efforts were effective. Others in the larger, general community said that such expressions as "HIV is a disease like any other" were spoken strategically to encourage and offer hope to people. Sitting in an empty sanctuary on a weekday, a Protestant pastor who had been relocated to a church in Mahali from Kisumu said:

When somebody says, "HIV is a disease like any other," that is only for supporting those with the disease [and giving hope]. You see, saying that . . . can help maintain [the health of] someone for some time. . . . But [it] can also destroy. Because if someone says to you, "After all, it is a disease like any other" . . . then that [statement] makes another person become infected . . . and they will quickly come to find that it is not a disease like any other. But it can be a positive thing—like in a pastoral way to tell [people] that they can continue if they just take the drugs and eat well. So that phrase is just used in a positive kind of pastoral perspective—but sometimes [it] can be used in a destructive way.

The words "HIV is a disease like any other," imported to Mahali, blended with the local knowledge, moralities, and politics of uncertainty. People in Mahali used popular global health phrases as a strategy for offering social encouragement to others in an attempt to help them psychologically. But at the same time, these messages were frequently said to be used to destroy a person, since it was common local knowledge that HIV was a condition that required substantial and exceptional social support so a patient could manage ART. The phrase was therefore imagined as being used to cut both ways.

Like the local talk and discourses about HIV and categories of people living or associated with the disease in Mahali, the subjective experiences with the malady among them were exceedingly varied. The answers to questions about stigma were never a simple "Yes, I have felt/experienced enacted stigma" or "No, I have never felt/experienced enacted stigma." Instead, people presented their experiences as contingent and shifting. Sometimes individuals would feel and/or experience rejection in one context (e.g., in their rural community or at church) and feel and/or be accepted in the next (e.g., at the HIV clinic). Stigma was sometimes a problem, but not a problem at all at other times. Stigma often felt possible, which made it uncertain and dangerous: HIV was a status that could be used against a person in certain situations. As Erving Goffman (1963, 18) noted long ago, those in a position of being potentially stigmatized "have special reason for feeling that mixed social situations make for anxious, unanchored interaction."

Over my years of research, some PLWHIV reported having been or felt stigmatized—usually in the form of a verbal attack, and very rarely in the form of physical abuse. However, verbal attacks were construed as being at least as dangerous, if not more so, than corporeal attacks because words were perceived to be able to kill a body physically and/or socially. Words left little if any proof for locals to complain about or to use as evidence against a person who stigmatized someone else. Josphat, who worked at the HIV clinic, said that this latter belief made it hard for health workers to intervene in a situation where a patient was being stigmatized or discriminated against:

> Stigma, that is still a challenge here in Kenya. It is very difficult to intervene in such cases, apart from when one has been physically assaulted or a child has been thrown out of school or someone has been chased out of employment . . . there are laws on that. . . . But stigma may be very hard to intervene [in] because the laws are not very clear. Proof, proof is difficult. And those patients don't want to expose their families to such ridicule. So even if [our patients have] a problem in the home, they will not tell [us]. [We at the clinic] try to encourage them, counsel them. Sometimes we do home visits and talk with the family.

In general, workers at the HIV clinic felt that there was little they could do to help their clients who were experiencing stigma, apart from offering encouraging words (e.g., "HIV is a disease like any other") and very basic counseling services on how to live with HIV (see chapter 5). Their patients were rarely forthcoming about such matters—they did not want to shame their family members or themselves by reporting or complaining about such abuses—and it was often challenging to find any tangible evidence against those who discriminated against others, especially in the context of unclear and unevenly enforced laws that required tangible proof that was described as difficult to produce. Health workers who were living with HIV themselves were more forthcoming. People who consistently reported never having experienced any stigma were also employed in some capacity by the groups involved in the AIDS industry, where disclosure was encouraged. These interlocutors had also often lived with HIV for a considerable time, and even though they had developed new friends and social networks, and in some instances had moved away to another area, they no longer interpreted past events as being motivated by stigma. Rather, they maintained that since they had been able to financially provide for their families and larger kin networks, they had never had any overt troubles with others. As described in chapter 6, however, these individuals maintained that they still did not feel completely like a normal person at the intrapersonal level and when they compared themselves to others. This suggested that even health workers sometimes internalized both the more uplifting words and the negative and moralizing societal messages about those living with HIV that constantly swirled around them.

While a small number of people said they had never experienced any stigma or stigmatizing sentiment, everyone I interviewed or engaged with in casual conversation on the topic had heard or read about someone else being discriminated against, usually in the form of rumor or gossip and/or from reading or hearing something in the media. Stories about circulating gossip and messages communicated in these instances pointed to two processes that occurred simultaneously. First, gossip helped uncover who was "sick" and taking "all those drugs," a combined set of subtle discourses that denied PLWHIV full status as normal, healthy individuals (see also chapter 6). Second, the notion that spoken words about HIV—especially those uttered to suggest that the disease was still a death sentence in the age of treatment—could escalate quickly into physical violence was often suggested. As Nekesa, a Luhya woman who was the second wife (co-wife) to her Kikuyu husband put it, "I hear people gossiping all the time about people living with HIV. People say quietly, 'Do you see that person? He is very sick—he goes to get all those drugs!' Once I even witnessed my friend having a verbal confrontation with [her] sister. The sister told my friend [who was living with HIV], 'You are not to be proud as a living corpse!' Then [with that comment] the sisters started [physically] fighting in front of everyone!"

Several people at the HIV clinic reflected that they had never experienced any form of stigma or discrimination, but they quickly qualified that they had never told anyone of their status, other than those attending or working at the clinic, because they feared the verbal attacks and judgments of others. One woman who worked at a kiosk made it clear that she had seen others being abused in various parts of Kenya for being HIV+, which is what she claimed continued to motivate her to keep her own seropositive status private: "No one knows that I am HIV+. I have witnessed others of my status being abused with words and physically. I am not special, so I [could] go through the same thing. Once I was at [another market center] where businesswomen were buying potatoes to resell. The victim [one living with HIV] wanted her [share] of the potatoes [to sell] but she was told by another, 'I cannot talk or share with a skeleton like you!'" Sometimes announcing the seropositive status of a "victim"—as people living with HIV were sometimes described, which served as a linguistic strategy to counter stigmatizing forces and moralizing claims that suggested individuals were responsible for contracting HIV—could still be used by others to get ahead and, as the woman quoted above pointed out, as an economic strategy in a fiercely competitive market and resource-poor place.

Despite the varied and sometimes contradictory discourses I heard from research participants, nearly everyone in the general community said that because of the politics of uncertainty, an HIV diagnosis was best kept private and that it was safest not to tell anyone publicly and keep a seropositive status secret in some relationships. As one man put it, "You never know when someone will become angry with you and throw damaging words that could harm you." Others revealed the cultural logics around "proper talk," or the idea that it was considered rude to directly say that they or someone else had HIV. Silence or not talking directly about the disease was actually about being a respectable person (see also Moyer 2012). Consequently, while gossip about HIV was very rampant, it was still considered inappropriate to straightforwardly or publicly mention that someone was using ART outside of a clinic setting. One man stated, "ARTs are never mentioned in this community. We do not speak of them. . . . You cannot tell who is HIV+, unless someone starts [rudely] shouting. You only share [your HIV+] status with your doctor. We do not speak of such things [out loud] in Mahali. We are disciplined [respectful] people!" The continued link made locally between HIV and immoral "Others" demanded that anyone living with HIV must conceal the disease, lest his or her social reputation be potentially tainted. Of course, this required a delicate balancing act between concealing information across the general community and needing to disclose it at the clinic to receive services (see Frank and Rödlach 2013). The need to manage secrets about private information in some public settings but disclose them in others blurred the boundaries between the public and private lives of people and created a contradiction that PLWHIV had to learn to negotiate as they moved between diverse surroundings and social relationships (Manderson et al. 2015). Critical reflection on the complexities of disclosure thus offers a "mechanism to 'rethink' stigma" (Manderson 2014, 14), as well as its persistence in places like Mahali.

Despite the overlapping local moral rules, logics, and knowledge about proper talk and local politics of uncertainty, global public health programs endeavoring to end AIDS generally start with the idea that definitively knowing and disclosing one's HIV status—the earlier the better—is morally good, gives people power over their lives and bodies, and motivates them to behave in healthier ways (Kaler and Watkins 2010; Nguyen 2010; Hardon and Posel 2012). Therefore, disclosure is a central component and imperative of global public health interventions aimed at preventing the spread of infection (Davis and Flowers 2014; Manderson 2014).

Employees working at the HIV clinic regularly spoke of the "problem" of concealment and secrecy, which they described as needing to be "fixed" (see also Hardon and Posel 2012; Pfeiffer and Maithya 2021), especially among men. Socializing people to use the global health technologies of HIV—such as rapid tests, ART, the clinic, and "confessional technologies" (see Nguyen 2010, 35)—to communicate private biological information to others was thus an activity that occurred within the walls of the clinic. For example, when Omar, another employee at the HIV clinic, discussed the "problem" of disclosure, he shared the creative strategy he used to help his patients balance the need to disclose their HIV status to their sex partners while also maintaining their respectability in terms of proper talk and preserving the lives of their intimate, loved ones:

> Mostly this problem [of not disclosing] affects the men. Women tend to be much more open. But with men—they can't [say such things directly]. We just had one [man] here. For ten years he took drugs, but the wife was not aware! Yet he knew [he was HIV+], but he never revealed it to the wife. . . . There is that belief that if they tell [loved ones], they can easily lose them [the person will die]. It is just too hard for them to say, "I am HIV+." So we normally advise them—just pretend that you are not positive. Just take this person [who you want to know your status] to [a VCT center] and test yourselves. And you just pretend. Just look for a way so you can communicate [with that person] in that easy way. That way, you will just avoid a lot of quarrels. After [the person knows], then you can focus on encouraging [him or her]. Otherwise, you will be tricked. But it will not be good. But you cannot just say, "I am HIV+!" No—because people react differently! A person could even be killed [if he or she says such a thing]. So the best thing to do is pretend that you are not using [ART] and insist to your partner, "We [should] test ourselves!" You will then find that you are both positive and you just come to [the HIV] clinic together from there.

As Omar suggested, the way people talk about private information, including revelations of secrets about living with HIV, matters (Manderson et al. 2015).

Disclosure, in this setting, requires careful negotiation to mitigate potentially damaging consequences (Squire 2015) and, accordingly, Omar adapted the practice for his patients that were men, thereby underscoring the ways that "disclosure is complexly performative" (Davis and Flowers 2014, 74). Yet this performance of HIV disclosure rested on the faulty assumption that if one sex partner was HIV+, the other partner must be too. Thus, it discounted global health knowledge about the phenomenon of discordancy to produce viral frictions, a topic to which I return later in this chapter.

During my observations of the support groups held at the HIV clinic, a significant portion of the time was spent preparing clients to disclose their HIV status, or make public confessions, to others (see Nguyen 2010), and the national HIV testing and counseling policies about such disclosures were strict in Kenya (Hardon et al. 2012). As other anthropologists have observed about the rapid spread of modern medicine around the world from the Global North, disclosure or "public testimonials" by those infected with HIV became "indicators of success of governments' national AIDS control programs and a key argument in favor of keeping aid money flowing to these programs" (Nguyen 2010, 31). Thus, secrecy in the domain of public health was increasingly presumed to be bad for individuals, communities, and nation-states. Health care workers, including support group leaders, trained patients to negotiate the "interpersonal and cultural politics of disclosure" (Manderson et al. 2015, S183) and (re)fashion their own identities and sense of self (Davis and Flowers 2014).

For example, the support groups at the HIV clinic usually began like meetings in a U.S.-style twelve-step Alcoholics Anonymous program. First, sitting in chairs arranged in a circle, the group recited "The Serenity Prayer" (AA 2009) in unison, an activity quickly followed by the mandatory practice of each person standing up and confessing boldly, "I am HIV." Surprisingly, people in Mahali were instructed not to say that they were living with the virus, but that they were the virus, and thus their whole identify was absorbed by HIV—at least during their time with the support group. The regular and casual use of this metaphor among PLWHIV in London has been documented by Mark Davis and Paul Flowers (2014). In Mahali, people who refused to make the statement could not participate in the meeting. The logic behind the practice of stating that a person "was HIV" was the notion that by the end of the meeting, each person would have already disclosed his or her status to at least thirty people, which in theory would make it easier for them to do the same with people in other settings. Leaders sometimes poked fun at each person who did not want to publicly announce his or her status, which often resulted in an eruption of laughter among other group participants. The mocking regularly resulted in compliance, and the new group member would eventually say the words, "I am HIV." Disclosure during support groups at the stand-alone HIV clinic was both performative and redundant. However, by participating in such practices, the HIV identities of people were rendered highly visible in ways that made other aspects of their self-identity less visible (Davis and Flowers 2014), which is a topic I return to in chapter 6.

An essential part of recognizing and accepting one's seropositive status is trusting the test results. Biomedical and public health researchers have studied and produced a sizable body of literature on testing initiatives (Cherutich et al. 2012; Dalal et al. 2013), with many studies highlighting the successes of testing and counseling in Africa when the five key components outlined by WHO (2012)—the five C's: Consent, Confidentiality, Counseling, Correct test results, and Connection to prevention, care, and treatment—were respected and practiced (Kyaddondo et al. 2012; Fylkesnes et al. 2013). During an interview at an empty pub, Samuel spent forty-five minutes talking passionately about the importance of disclosure, as well as the notion that global health policies that demanded the confidentiality of patients and local practices of secrecy and concealment were "enemies." He described the conundrum and contradictions he experienced as an employee of the HIV testing and counseling industry, and he continued to equate HIV infection with a death sentence to emphasize his concerns about confidentiality:

> I am HIV+ and you are keeping that confidential. You cannot tell. Not even your own sister. And I go to the extent of infecting your sister—your blood sister! And because of this word—confidentiality—I am hiding a gun here. I am going to kill your sister. And you can't say so? So counselors should eliminate or at least say that it is not a mandatory thing that the HIV status [of our clients] is confidential. You won't even tell my wife before I consent for you to tell her? And I go in the evening and I infect my wife with HIV? Had you disclosed it—could I have infected my wife? Had you disclosed it—could I have infected your sister? And now you are crying, "I wanted it to be confidential, so I didn't tell my sister!" That confidentiality is what makes HIV spread. That one is an enemy to [preventing or stopping the spread of] HIV. Why are we testing all these people? To help the community? To make me access these drugs? But all alone? The word *confidentiality*—that one is killing us here [in Mahali]. At the end of the day, you have only put a cover over a fire that is burning. But you have not yet stopped that fire from burning. . . . But suppose you unveil the fire and you expose the smoke [a sign of danger]. Would somebody go there? HIV is a disease like any other. But people don't want to talk about it? [Confidentiality] is our barrier.

The contradictions and tensions facing HIV counselors have been documented by other social scientists in sub-Saharan Africa (e.g., Angotti 2012), where global health HIV testing norms of the five C's conflicted with local, ethical, and moral concerns for the health and well-being of the people, and thus maintaining confidentiality was perceived as harming communities and was not always prioritized in practice (see also Dionne 2017). Because of this tension, during my 2014 research trip, numerous people spoke of the uncertainties surrounding confidentiality during the HCT campaign that passed through Mahali on several occasions and made them ambivalent about being tested (Pfeiffer and Maithya 2021).

The Uncertainties of Discordancy

Previous anthropological scholarship has centered on the challenges of managing ART under the chronic disease paradigm (McGrath et al. 2014, 303) and living with HIV under conditions described as continuous uncertainty (Moyer and Hardon 2014). In this section, I expand this focus to examine the impact of these conditions on general discourses and public forms of stigma and discrimination as community members grappled with and negotiated the uncertainties of HIV by creating an informal public health prevention management system that maintained a form of courtesy stigma. Forces of stigma were powerful and uncertain to the extent that such processes, at times, could extend beyond the HIV-infected individual to family members who would experience courtesy stigma—especially sex partners, including those who were HIV−. The uncertainties surrounding the management of HIV became especially clear to me as people struggled to make sense of and attach meaning to discordant couples (in which one sexual partner is HIV+ and the other is HIV−). Throughout much of the research for this book, as I discuss in chapter 1, clinical trials were enrolling and closely following thousands of discordant couples across Kenya. Discordant couple studies are the primary way that global health experts have been able (and continue) to monitor the effectiveness of TasP programs. Likewise, programs targeting discordant couples strongly emphasized the value of marital and sexual counseling, monogamy, and the importance of couples staying together (Moyer 2015). While locals were familiar with the term *discordant couple* and could correctly define it, they were less clear about why some people got HIV while others did not: "If we get HIV, we get it. If we don't, it has not come for us."

However, over the years, HIV prevention messaging across the community made it very clear and stated with certainty that unprotected sexual encounters, especially adulterous ones, result in infection. But this did not always happen, as we learned from the woman who had unprotected sex with the man who allegedly wrote the List and therefore would not believe her test results that repeatedly indicated she was not infected. Another incident at the HIV clinic also related directly to the general uncertainties and assumptions related to the possibility of discordant couples. A man whose wife had tested positive for HIV during the HCT campaign had been sharing the ART that his wife brought home from the clinic each month, though he had never been tested. For reasons that were never fully disclosed, the man started having physical complications and reported, for the first time, to the HIV clinic in Mahali. Because he was not yet registered in the medical system at the clinic, he had to start the process from the beginning, which always included a series of biomedical tests. When he was tested, he was found to be HIV–. Thus, global health technologies of HIV—tests, ART, and prevention messages—intersected with local politics of uncertainty to produce a rather unexpected outcome not only for the man (and presumably for his wife, who must have been taking only half of her prescribed medication), but also for the clinic's staff.

People came up with their own explanations that made sense in context but also served to marginalize both HIV+ and HIV– partners. Terms such as *AIDS carriers* and *slow progressors* emerged to describe some people who locals knew were having sex with people already infected with HIV but who never seemed to suffer any overt symptoms. These terms were defined inconsistently by locals, which I interpret as a generalized uncertainty about the topic. Still, locals had learned early in the epidemic—long before global health initiatives were offering consistent HIV testing and ART—to pay careful attention to the sexual networks of people as a local strategy of managing HIV and protecting oneself from potential infection (see chapter 1). This practice of monitoring sexual networks informed local interpretations of discordant couples. Regardless of their varying definitions, the words *AIDS carriers* and *slow progressors* were consistently used disapprovingly and to demarcate especially dangerous people living in the community who were potentially and perhaps even purposefully spreading the virus. For example, even Naomi, a health professional, defined the local logics behind and the overlap between the two terms. The "carrier," she claimed, was an HIV–person involved in a discordant relationship, while a "slow progressor" was an especially negative term used to describe an individual who outlived a series of sexual partners who allegedly died of AIDS. According to the logic, although someone is not infected with HIV, no one believes his or her HIV– status if the person's sexual partners keep dying, and the person becomes characterized as dangerous and a "slow progressor." Another community member defined *AIDS carrier* in the following way: "The person who is a carrier is very strong, and his blood is very strong. He is HIV+ but very healthy, and he never changes [in appearance] even if he takes the ART or not. He always looks healthy and, [even if he is taking ART, he is spreading] the disease to others in this community."

Even in the age of treatment, HIV was still perceived and experienced by members of the general public as an extremely uncertain malady without a cure, which mirrored the insecurities of everyday life in global Mahali. Some people got the disease. Some did not. Still others were imagined to be able to mysteriously spread it, even if they had tested negative or claimed to be negative. ART worked exceptionally well for some bodies, but not for all. Usually ART was available, but sometimes people could be cut off from it (as occurred during PEV) or cut themselves off to avoid revealing their HIV status to others while living in IDP camps (see Wilhelm-Solomon 2013).[7] Additionally, the prevention and awareness messages about the disease—which were presented with certainty—did not seem to completely match what people were observing and experiencing, so they created terms such as *slow progressors* and *carriers* as a way to obtain a sense of security and safety and to manage the uncertainty and protect themselves from people who were imagined to be potentially dangerous. The cultural politics of uncertainty produced viral frictions to reinforce processes of public stigma, which in some cases offered people at least a temporary sense of control over their lives, health, and bodies.

These kinds of viral frictions slowly transformed local relationships. For example, in 2010, I volunteered at an NGO that focused on peace-building and youth empowerment initiatives in a nearby town. I became friends with several of the employees, including Mary and Ndegwa, who also lived in Mahali. It was not until I returned in 2011–2012 for a year of ethnographic research and became more familiar with local community dynamics and the lives of people that I realized Mary and Ndegwa had two children. As we spent time together, I observed that the two seemed to enjoy their companionship, a sentiment confirmed during a series of life-history interviews with them and as my friendship with Mary grew over the years. One day over a cup of chai and my favorite Kenyan dish, *mukimo* (made from potatoes, maize, and green vegetables), which she graciously prepared for me whenever I visited her home, Mary told me that she had decided after a series of HIV tests not to continue her relationship with Ndegwa because his wife was HIV+. Mary said that she did not want to constantly battle a reputation as a carrier.[8]

Mary was a widow with several children, and by the end of my 2014 research trip, she was involved in a stable relationship with a truck driver who regularly passed through and spent time in Mahali. Mary prided herself on being a lifelong, hard-working, and respected member of the community who was able to educate her children, and she identified herself as a skilled farmer who, above all else, loved to cultivate the land. She cultivated a larger plot of land in a nearby reserve, where she grew things like pumpkins, tomatoes, maize, onions, cabbage, and carrots. She needed to supplement this work with other side "hustles," as people often referred to their need to participate in various income-generating activities. Fortunately for Mary, one of the ways she supplemented her farm work was by occasionally working at the NGO in a neighboring community. Mary spoke of her continued feelings for Ndegwa and said that at one point she had desired to become his co-wife. But she went on to explain that things became complicated when Ndegwa and his first wife tested for HIV together, and that the wife, but not Ndewga, turned out to be infected with HIV: thus, they were discordant. The results of these rapid HIV tests triggered a series of gendered responses and social challenges that this triad had to negotiate. Mary and Ndegwa felt strongly that it would be wrong to discriminate against the woman, and thus they determined that Ndegwa should remain committed to his first marriage and wife, who he loved dearly and who Mary respected. At the same time,

Mary and Ndegwa reasoned that, given Ndegwa's love for alcohol and his propensity toward drunkenness during the late evening hours in bars with his friends, it would be risky for Mary to remain within this sexual network. Mary imagined aloud that Ndegwa, while drunk, might forget to use a condom with the first wife, contract the virus, and in turn inadvertently infect her. Furthermore, Ndegwa and his wife did not actively conceal their HIV discordancy. Mary went on to articulate her experience of having already been at the center of false local gossip about being a carrier and explained how difficult it was to overturn such gossip. She worried that if she remained in this relationship, others in the community would assume that she, too, regardless of her actual serostatus, was living with HIV, leaving her with a tainted reputation that she made clear would ultimately be impossible for her to reverse.

While the details of this case were exceptional in several ways, it was striking to witness how carefully people paid attention to other people's sexual networks to know or at least assume their serostatus, as well as the local logics used to understand discordant partners and make sense of their relationships, which seemed to marginalize them (see Rispel, Cloete, and Metcalf 2015). The cultural politics of uncertainties related to the complexities of living in a community with high rates of HIV infection, including forces of HIV-related courtesy stigma—whether accepting them, as Ndegwa did, or resisting and seeking to avoid them, as Mary did—was powerful. It impacted the way people made decisions about how to navigate their sexual relations and social reputations, even as they cared deeply for people living with HIV and those living without it.

4 · "WE CALL HIV A SEX WORKER DISEASE"

Economic Inequalities, Social Change, and the Politics of Gender and Sexuality

Since at least the colonial period, processes of transnationalism and globalization have been shifting manifestations of gender and sexuality on the African continent in ways that have intensified gender inequalities (Davison 1989, 1996; Grosz-Ngaté and Kokole 1997; Weisner, Bradley, and Kilbride 1997; Cole and Thomas 2009). In more recent years, anthropologists have noted the impacts of changing consumer markets and the monetization of daily life on gender, marital relations, and ideas about and practices of intimacy in sub-Saharan Africa (Cole and Thomas 2009; Hirsch et al. 2009; D. Smith 2017). Such changes have had profound impacts on the spread of HIV (Hunter 2007; Parikh 2009), including its stigmatization. In turn, this epidemic continues to reconfigure sexual, gender, and marital interactions and transform ideas about the meanings of masculinity (Wyrod 2016; D. Smith 2017) and what it is to be a modern woman (Mojola 2014) in globalized Africa. After critically reflecting on and contextualizing a story about a major scandal and intense conflict that erupted between two women living in Mahali, this chapter considers the impact of living in a community with limited resources on gendered relationships. The chapter then moves on to explore the intersections of local and national gender and sexual identity politics and power struggles with HIV, the global health infrastructure, and national programming to produce viral frictions.[1]

A SEX WORKER BEWITCHED

"I did not hear people discussing HIV today. People think my friend [Maggie] is a witch and tried to kill [Wambūi]. I did not go into the [urban] center all day" (Pfeiffer and Maithya 2018, 239). These were handwritten words in a conversational journal belonging to Njeri, who worked in a Catholic church dispensary. In the days leading up to Njeri's refusal to go into the town center, Wambūi, an unmarried woman, had become ill. Her symptoms were described by Mary, who had witnessed the suffering firsthand: "The stomach became big, like a woman about to deliver [a baby], and all of a sudden, it disappears. . . . And then the legs became big. She was in great pain. She screamed!"

Gossip about Wambūi's illness spread throughout the community, as did the belief that she had been bewitched. Everyone knew Maggie was jealous of her. Wambūi was known to be a lover of Maggie's husband, Paul, and witnesses had previously spotted the two women in a hostile confrontation. Kamau, a friend of Paul, explained the logic behind the jealousy: "[Paul] loves a lot of ladies, and those women are the prostitutes of this area. . . . [Wambūi] is a carrier [of HIV]. You know, most of the women [in this area] are carriers because they sleep with men from all over Africa and with locals. So [Maggie] came to envy [Wambūi], so she bewitched her. It was like [Wambūi] was about to take over [Maggie's] family. So [Maggie] put a snake in [Wambūi's] stomach." As Kamau demonstrated, the concepts of HIV and sex workers as "carriers" constantly evoked each other, and he attributed Maggie's retaliation to both her envy and blame for spreading HIV. While HIV was a relatively new disease, the notion that unmarried or independent women were evil and therefore responsible for spreading diseases in sub-Saharan Africa was not.

When asked how people knew that Maggie was responsible for Wambūi's illness, some of those I spoke to cited mounting evidence, which included details such as the fact that two public hospitals had denied Wambūi treatment and officially declared her condition to be the result of witchcraft. Mary, who had escorted her to the hospital, recalled: "[At] the hospital, the nurses refuse[d] to treat her. They said, 'There is nothing we can do about this because this is witchcraft.' . . . They could not understand what was happening, so they said, 'Go and solve [the problem] in your home!'" Wambūi also named Maggie as the person assaulting her as she pleaded for the pain to cease. Mary went on, "[Wambūi] was saying, 'No, stop, [Maggie]. Stop harming me! I'll leave your husband alone.'"

A group of single women, outraged at the harm being directed toward Wambūi, united in a violent and frenzied witch hunt. Kamau recalled, "The fellow prostitutes demonstrated—they wanted to kill [Maggie]." As the gossip was legitimated, a contagious sense of panic involved an even wider diaspora of residents. Maggie initially found refuge at a nearby police station and later in a distant city, while the crowd of women grew in size. When the police exerted force and used tear gas, the multitude thinned. When people learned that Wambūi was still ailing the next morning, a new mob gathered to issue a stern, verbal threat to local authorities: "If you are not going to take any action, then we will take the law into our hands." As community leaders deliberated the case, the heightened sense of panic was described by eyewitnesses as miraculously calmed by a Pentecostal pastor when he prayed for Wambũi and successfully rid her of her suffering. Soon after, Wambũi was commanded by the police to leave the area, and provided with money to do so: being bewitched had threatened the peace. The message was clear that Wambũi's continued presence might provoke new violence in an already volatile region.

Though peace was restored before Maggie was physically assaulted, the accusations of witchcraft were socially destructive to her. She temporarily moved, but the time she spent away from Mahali did not repair her blemished reputation. Instead, the story solidified that Maggie was a witch and devil worshipper and a person to be feared and avoided. Several of my interlocutors said they were leery of socializing with her and supporting her business. A gendered variant of social death befell Paul, described by Kamau as "an embarrassment [to Paul]. People are saying, 'Ah, your wife is a witch.' Even [their] kids don't interact with other[s]. You see, he was a Christian, although he was evil. He is the cause of all of this, being a prostitute! He [is] now a hard drinker. . . . [After the ordeal] they [Wambũi and Paul] fought directly in daylight! Then the fellow prostitutes came and were shouting at [Paul] like a child, embarrassing him in public! I told him, 'You have a wife, land, money, and your kids are educated. What else do you want?'" Kamau held Paul responsible for his shameful inability to maintain control of the women in his life and used the derogatory term *prostitute* here to underscore the greedy behaviors of Paul and to convey a sense of his status loss in the community because of his involvement in this public scandal. As Mary reflected on this event, she suggested that a shared moral lesson had emerged: "It has made the sex workers fear having relationships with men who are from within this center. So now they just stick with the truck drivers . . . because the married women have been saying, 'Now we know what we will be doing to them [the sex workers] if they snatch our husbands!'" Residents interpreted the effects of this ordeal as challenging yet ultimately reinforcing local power dynamics and gender conflicts between categories of people (e.g., husbands and wives, wives and sex workers, and husbands and truck drivers) in the urban center of Mahali.

Maggie, a wealthy, Christian wife, was publicly accused—and attacked—for allegedly being a witch and devil worshipper around the same time that residents were also circulating stories about the List. Like Maggie, the women on the List were characterized as wealthy, Christian, and married. These scandals appeared to be working to reinforce larger social values and rules and keep people (married women in particular) in line when gossip alone could not (White 2000). Like processes of stigma and discrimination, discourses about witchcraft and devil worship have been conceptualized by anthropologists as a form of power (Geschiere 1997) and as a way of explaining misfortune (Evans-Pritchard 1976), as well as the existence of malcontents brought about by modernity, including its economic crises, spiraling inequalities, rapid social change (Jean Comaroff and Comaroff 1993), and historical legacies of colonial and postcolonial state formations and transformations (James Smith 2011, 56). Formal witchcraft accusations—while rare (Ashforth 2015)—represent one way in which broader, globalizing forces and uneven structural arrangements play out between people (often those most intimately connected; see Geschiere 2013) interpersonally and at the community level.

Scholars have argued that in Kenya, accusations of witchcraft and devil worship are related to the particular circumstances afflicting a community at a given moment in time but that have roots in a larger process associated with a "history of traumatic state betrayal and violence" (James Smith 2011, 77). This case—of witchcraft and devil-worshipping accusations—reflects local anxieties about shifting gender roles and tensions between men and women and between various categories of people (e.g., wives and sex workers, husbands and truck drivers, and those who were HIV+ and those who were HIV−) that were associated with the destructive and chaotic consequences of ethnic and political violence, poverty, and the moral failings of state-imposed order and peace (see James Smith 2011, 56) in Mahali. It also shows people fiercely competing over the meanings of those changes to reveal what was most at stake: the scarce financial and emotional resources of men, status, power, and reputation. Furthermore, local, circulating discourses about Maggie being a witch and devil worshipper helped to legitimate and reproduce state violence. Specifically, Maggie emerged as a visual representation of the collective fears (see James Smith 2008) within Mahali and became a "personified scapegoat for complex social problems, including the growth of illegal economies and spiraling inequalities" (James Smith 2011, 77) that were fueled by failed development in the community. In part, HIV was to blame, but PEV, the global recession, and Kenya's political history all worked together to aggravate problems related to gender roles, relations, and inequalities.

The gender politics playing out in Mahali mirrored those circulating across the country that were shaped by the state through a series of media stories that "poached images from a troubled past" (James Smith 2011, 77). During 2011–2012, a persistent refrain related to changing gender roles and relations "creep[ed] and seep[ed]" (Benton 2015, 7) through a series of media reports and political cartoons claiming that violence against men was on the rise. News coverage included images of assaulted men, touted as victims, who sought care in public hospitals, and headlines such as "Battered Men Silent for Fear of Being Rebuked" (*Daily Nation*, February 14, 2012) and "Male Edifice Crumbles as Women Rise" (*Daily Nation*, February 18, 2012). These and other articles linked the source of "dangerous trends" to men shirking their conjugal duties and frustrated women who were challenging African men's traditional dominance. One political cartoon had the caption "*Tunaomba serikali ije itusaidie na tatizohili*" (We beg the government to come and rescue us from this problem) over a drawing of wounded men carrying signs with messages like "Stop violens [violence] against men" and "Maendeleo ya Wanaume" (Men's progress) ("*Tunaomba serikali ije itusaidie na tatizohili"* 2012). Ironically, the latter message harkened back to the historical, countrywide membership group Maendeleo ya Wanawake (Women's Progress) that originally promoted the advancement of African women and sought to raise the living standards of rural women during the colonial period (see Wipper 1975). Many of the articles emphasized that Kikuyu husbands were battered by their wives in Kenya's central region, where allegedly women were aggressively independent and in the habit of beating up their men. Economic, ethnic, and political sentimentalities and animosities thus intersected with and crept into country-wide media reports under the guise of national gender conflicts that had complex histories. These national discourses, I believe, are reflective of the tensions and frictions produced as overlapping gender, economic, and ethnic politics across Kenya bump into global knowledge. The UN's Millennium Development Goals[2] and SDGs focus heavily on promoting gender equity through programs to empower women economically, educationally, and in terms of health through targeted interventions (UN 2020).

PEV, ECONOMIC INEQUALITIES, SHIFTING GENDER RELATIONS, AND HIV TESTING

In chapter 2, I developed the idea that Mahali was perceived and experienced by insiders and outsiders as a bad or stigmatized place due to its chronic legacies of racism and ethnic and political conflict. But racial and ethnic discriminations rarely exist as a single axis of power through which people are differentially treated. Instead, these discriminations intersect with other systems of social stratification, such as those related to socioeconomic class, gender and sexuality, or what Kimberle Crenshaw (1989) has termed "intersectionality." PEV resulted in failed development, which people described as having had a profound impact on their economic possibilities in ways that exacerbated social inequalities and tensions. For example, James (introduced in the introduction) described the political violence and the impact it had on the image of the place and, by extension, those living in it:

> The people here don't have income-generating activities.... There is absolutely nothing. The people here are farmers. We don't have any entrepreneur. Because of the history of this area, no one will put a business in right here. They will put it somewhere else because they don't know what will happen in the next election. You see the fear now? Outsiders fear this place. [Mahali] is not stable. People are not united. And because this place has no income-generating activities, outsiders think that all the people are infected with HIV because the women here depend on the truck drivers [for financial support]. [The rate of] prostitution is very high.

Because of the history of the area, the name *Mahali* had been tainted, and people were divided and devalued (their dignity was assaulted) in ways that seemed natural and that continually located blame and responsibility in the bodies and behaviors of local women who were described as financially "dependent on the truck drivers." PEV was characterized as having pushed people into poverty and women toward practices of sex work and pathogen exposure (which disrupted normal gender relations) to make outsiders and insiders leap to the conclusion that everyone in Mahali was infected with HIV, a disease and situation that continued to evoke the sense of ethical failures. As Brent Steenberg (2020, 212) convincingly argues of stigma in South Africa, it is frequently attached to location "because of the avenues through which location is tied to social networks." The national portrayal of and local experiences of living in Mahali—as a chaotic and violent place with a substantial sex worker industry—was described as negatively marking the location and the relationships of those connected to it.

After PEV, many residents participated, at least temporarily, in corrupt and illegal practices. Some felt criminalized by the Kenyan state for being poor. This was ironic: local experiences with and manifestations of poverty worsened as political violence erupted alongside a supposedly democratic presidential election. People had felt firsthand the power of the Kenyan state in their daily lives. Those who engaged in illicit activities, which they hoped would eventually springboard them out of poverty, sometimes lamented that they had few alternatives, though they never complained about their actual work. During one of our many lengthy conversations in the living area of the house where Beatrice had graciously given me a bedroom while I worked in Mahali, Mwangi spoke of his lack of employment options, which made him need to maintain a position in the illegal sector. The walls in this particular room were lined with old brown cardboard boxes, marked occasionally with the labels "Relief Food" and "Not for Sale." Exposed wooden studs that composed the inside walls were decorated with Christmas wrapping paper and garland. And like many of the other homes I visited, old and outdated calendars served as wall decorations, as did framed pictures of the president and the patriarch or matriarch of the house—in this instance, Beatrice with her children. While I was living at this house during one research trip, Beatrice was taking care of her daughter-in-law, who had just given birth to a daughter named Beatrice.[3] It was delightful to have the added company of a baby and her mother, who was now referred to as "Mama Beatrice"[4] around the house in the evenings. Not only did I get to observe and participate in a variety of ceremonies for infants—to provide names and when people from different ethnic groups came and sang songs (in various languages), danced, and welcomed the new baby by showering her (and the mother) with gifts—but I also enjoyed being in a household where ugi (a sweet, fermented porridge made from maize, millet, and/or sorghum flours) was served daily because of its nutritional value for breast-feeding and postpartum mothers. It was in this setting, as we drank ugi together, that Mwangi told me: "You know, there is no employment in Kenya. Please, let me tell you one thing. You can tarmack [look for jobs or work]. You can *tarmack*! You can go anywhere, but there are no jobs. . . . And ah, when you join that [illegal] sector, you have to fight. So that you can fit. You have to fight so you can get that job there. Ah, it is very difficult. And there are no jobs in [Mahali]. There are no investors here. The veterans [long-term residents of Mahali] can just do any business." Mwangi reviewed his own employment options as I naively kept making futile suggestions, given that he had a license to drive a truck but lacked a university degree and, most importantly, that he did not have social networks including people with political power: "Drive a tractor? I am a Kikuyu—that is Kalenjin work. Who would hire me? Drive for someone with a private car? I don't know anyone wealthy enough to employ me. Cut down timber from the [nearby] forest? Hey—that forest work is only for the government nowadays. If you get caught, you are jailed. Forest is for government. When they get you in the forest . . . you see fire [the wrath of the government]!" Mwangi went on to talk about police harassment, the hideous conditions of Kenyan jails, and the toll all of this took on his physical health and well-being:

> [In my position] you can't spend a month without entering a [jail] cell or meeting a judge! You get thrown in a cell monthly for [the job]. Eh! And for drinking. Both, anyways. If a police officer sees you drinking . . . the charge sheet will be "Drinking without eating!" . . . You are fined 3,000 [Kenyan shillings, and he made only 300 on average per day]. [And] you don't have [the money], so you just have to serve the [jail] term. . . . That is where you contract cholera or TB [tuberculosis]. There was a time I was jailed . . . ; when I was released I had chronic TB. . . . Hey—you can just pity [those detained there]. It is very dangerous! [So] you just pay that police bribe.

For many Mahali residents, especially the landless, combining employment opportunities from the formal and informal economies was a reasonable way to carve out a living. This usually translated into a person spending the day engaged in *kibarua* and earning approximately 200–300 shillings a day, which over the past decade has held steady at roughly the equivalent of about $2–3. While this could easily put enough food on the table for a day, it was hardly enough to pay for rent, firewood or gas, clean water, or school fees for children. People creatively carved out additional income-generating activities, like starting a fruit stand or selling secondhand clothes in the market. Some women used small businesses as a front for attracting men, with whom they could develop relationships and eventually exchange sex for money or favors. But small businesses required some capital. For those lacking such assets, selling *bhangi* (marijuana); brewing, selling, or distributing *chang'aa*; or even selling sex at night (by walking the streets) required very little and thus were realistic alternatives. Such work sometimes meant having to offer free sexual favors to men or spending the occasional night, week, or month in jail, if they were unable to pay local police bribes, which at the time of my research were about 500 shillings ($6.25) to be paid twice per month. I once spent a day sitting in the kitchen (made of mud and covered by a grass-thatched roof) of a Kalenjin woman who people referred to as Mama Chebet, while I observed her. Mama Chebet was showing me how she brewed *chang'aa* (which is how she earned a living and provided for the eight children in her care) when she explained that a police officer had passed through to collect his monthly payment the previous day.

Women engaged in the sex trade had shared accounts similar to that of Mwangi. Again, no one ever complained about the actual work they were required to perform. While selling sex had been initially difficult, they explained that it got easier and that they were ultimately grateful for the work, because it enabled them to provide food and education for their children, and this made them feel proud as women and mothers. To further emphasize their material successes, several wealthier sex workers invited me to their apartments to show me their living conditions—they had rooms in concrete (not mud or wood-slat) structures with electricity—and requested that I take pictures of them posing next to their television sets and among the stuffed toys they were able to purchase. In the case of less wealthy sex workers, who described having to walk outside urban shops at night rather than wait in their homes to be called on by clients or sit inside bars, the problems they shared with me included long, cold nights spent alone and unable to get clients, a customer refusing to pay for the services they had provided, or a night when they had been raped by one or more people. In the latter case, women explained that it was fruitless to report a rape or endeavor to obtain justice: they would likely be ignored or even blamed by the police for having brought the problem on themselves, as sex workers. Like Mwangi, they spoke about the challenges of being caught soliciting sex or simply being a woman out past the 11:00 P.M. curfew that had been imposed as a government strategy to increase security in the area. They explained that their choices were paying a police bribe, offering the police free sex, or being incarcerated in one of the small, cold, cement cells at the police station.

Many of the women who spoke of their sex work offered personal stories of having been sexually abused by men. But rather than focusing on recounting these horrific acts, they emphasized the days of work they had missed as a result of them and the money they had lost as their bodies healed and recovered from the violence. Once in a while, women described abuses they believed were far worse than sexual assaults as even more socially and morally degrading. For example, Ester experienced the most humiliating and demoralizing encounter a sex worker had ever endured. While I never met or spoke with Ester, she crept into the stories of a few other women who identified themselves as sex workers and tried to derive meaning from the upsetting story. As the story went, once Ester and her client were alone in a room, the man undressed and exposed a body covered with oozing sores. The man did not request sex but rather demanded that Ester "lick his wounds all night, like a dog." Since Ester had been involved in an illegal act of sex work and because she had "no proof" of the man's abuses, she could not seek the protection of the state or redemption for this abuse. Ester was consistently described as having told as many women about the man as possible so he could be avoided in the future. While I anticipated stories that centered on gender and structural violence against women, I was not prepared for the details of Ester's story. They have bothered me ever since I first heard it.

As I conducted research for this book, the possibility of legalizing sex work was constantly (and contentiously) being debated in Nairobi. Articles on the topic often filled newspapers. Those in favor of the new legislation cited the positive impact it might have on reducing the spread of HIV. Politicians who rejected the idea emphasized moral and social concerns. To my surprise, when I asked local women who identified themselves as sex workers to share their views, most were completely against the idea. The main reasons they cited included (1) suspicions that this would be a strategy employed by the government to take large portions of their earnings through taxation, and (2) fear that it would inadvertently send the message to their daughters that being a sex worker was a reasonable occupation for which to strive. To date, government leaders have always voted against such legalization. The requirements of international funding agencies combating HIV, some of which demand formal opposition to sex work and abortion as part of the criteria for funding, likely influenced this debate and its outcome.

The insecurity and dangers associated with election cycles frequently led to an increase in the number of military and police officers across the community and, in turn, to considerable ambivalence about their presence. While most people appreciated the increased protection, they simultaneously felt harassed (and, as just described, criminalized) in ways that disrupted and complicated gender dynamics. The case of Simon, a civil servant stationed in Mahali with a first wife and children who lived in Nairobi and a younger, second wife in Mahali who was pregnant, illustrated this sentiment:

PEV affected our people so much. So much. So much. . . . I would say that PEV brought [higher rates of HIV into Mahali]. It was when the soldiers were there. [They were] brought [into the area] because of the skirmishes. They could arrest each and every lady [and make them] have sex. And the women agreed. For protection! Just protection. By then, if a soldier wants to hold your hand, [you can't say no]. He'll take you where he wants. . . . So the skirmishes had a very big impact on the community. And a lot of *askaris* [police guards] were brought around. Even today [they are still here]. The work of the *askaris* right now [is] just to look around, move [have sex] with women—move with people's wives! [The police] have nothing else to do. We are not at war [now]. . . . [But the extra security officials] have not been taken back [to where they came from]. [There are] very many police. Some new police stations were [even recently] opened [here]. They are still here. So what are they doing? Just [harassing locals].... [And] nobody can hold them accountable...because you cannot question a police officer.

Citing economic reasons, people described gender roles and relationships as disturbed in ways that were imagined as unsettling and disruptive to the moral and social order. An increasing number of women—single or married, young or old—had to sell or offer their bodies to truck drivers and police officers to protect themselves and their families economically and physically and thus were construed as changing normal gender roles and responsibilities. Men were described as unable to perform their proper male duties, especially serving as protector and provider for the family. Therefore, some local men had also come to be characterized as powerless and/or useless. For example, as Kipruto, a casual laborer, and I sat in the container clinic, he said that the soured economy and his inability to find consistent employment made him "powerless" to provide the global products that his wife had come to desire: "One of the challenges [in marriage nowadays] is that I am the provider, and my wife depends on me. But I don't have a stable job, and you know how women are. A woman wants to make her hair pretty and to buy clothes, and I don't have the power.... I want to make her happy, but I don't have the power."

Other men made fleeting and sardonic remarks about local wives no longer being married to their husbands but rather to national and international aid organizations better equipped to support them and provide their families with food. In so doing, the men described themselves and other men living in the community as "useless." The reliance on international aid, like PEV, was further described as upsetting and transforming local norms and roles and was perceived as fracturing gender relations in ways that were destructive to everyone. The demoralization of men was described as extremely troubling, as Eunice, a rural shop owner, put it: "So that time in the [IDP] camp, husbands became useless because the one who was feeding everybody was the [humanitarian organization]. So women could be saying, 'My husband is [name of a humanitarian organization], not you—we are all being fed by [them].'" We were sitting in her cramped house, made from local clays, with a small group of her neighbors during an impromptu gathering that turned into a small-group discussion. As the conversation continued, the women built on one another's comments to vent about the "uselessness" of men, until one woman linked their "uselessness" to the ease of contracting HIV, thereby concluding our discussion in a way that perpetuated moralizing and stigmatizing sentiments about people living with the disease: "It is easy for a person to get HIV when he become[s] useless. [He] start[s] playing unprotected sex, plays sex with different people, [he] doesn't care about his life anymore. For those reasons, a [useless] person must get HIV." Perhaps this demoralization of men offers a context for understanding the moments during my research when vividly (and understandably) upset women and health workers at the HIV clinic reported troubling accounts or suspicions of their own or their clients' infections as being purposely transmitted by their husbands. Men feared abandonment and stigmatization by their wives or feared that one "might leave if she feels superior because she is not infected," as one employee tearfully recalled one of the patients saying bluntly to her. As Nancy Scheper-Hughes and Philippe Bourgois (2004, 1) observed, "structural violence— the violence of poverty, hunger, social exclusion and humiliation—inevitably translates into intimate and domestic violence."

The potential for this kind of marital violence produced viral frictions and (re)shaped people's lives in unexpected ways. For example, I sometimes spent time in the home of Lydia, who brewed chang'aa. Like several women I met, Lydia had been forced to move out of her matrimonial home because she gave birth to only girls and did not provide her husband's family with a son. While divorce was not permitted in the Kalenjin community, the failure to have sons can be a ground for men to take a co-wife. It was when I was in Lydia's rectangular, two-roomed, wooden house that I met Sharon, who identified herself as Kisii and had been living in a rural community with her Kalenjin husband. Sharon was convinced that her husband, after being diagnosed with HIV, was purposefully trying to infect her so that he and her in-laws could "shift that blame to me for bringing it into the family." In tears as we sat in the privacy of the container clinic in 2012, she offered several pieces of evidence for why she had these suspicions. Sharon explained that she had fled to the home of a friend who lived just outside Mahali's urban center—with her three children, one of whom always cried and hid from me when she saw me because the color of my eyes, hair, and skin appeared so strange—and eventually moved in with Lydia and helped brew and sometimes deliver the chang'aa to dens. When we reunited in 2014, Sharon was visibly pregnant—the father was a truck driver—and Lydia had insisted that she return to her husband because Lydia could not "feed any extra mouths."

Before leaving Kenya that year, I looked for Sharon. I found her at the roadside, where she was packing up her things after having spent a short day selling charcoal. She was distraught, so I helped gather her things and carry them home. It was a market day, and we purchased some food staples along the way. As we slowly wound our way through the market we passed herbalists, rickety wooden booths lined with dozens of pairs of used shoes, tarps piled high with used clothing, and market stalls out of which women were selling fruits, vegetables, honey, buckets of potatoes, and large baskets of grains, until we came to an alley that led us toward the slum area where Sharon lived (she still refused to return to her husband). Sharon unlocked the padlock on the door and led me into a dark and dank room, where we sat and chatted while she used a small cooker to prepare the *sukuma wiki* (a vitamin-packed collard green), onions, and tomatoes we had just bought. Before I left, we exchanged phone numbers. From abroad I received a few text messages from Sharon, which is how I learned that the baby did not survive beyond its first year. But I have not seen or heard from her since receiving that news. I still wonder how Sharon and her children are doing.

Limited access to material resources—and its ensuing effects on gender roles and relations—was characterized as simultaneously burdening women with new forms of responsibilities and fueling competition between gendered categories of people. For example, in 2014, Rose, a tailor, echoed the idea that men had become "useless" in recent years before she offered a critique of development efforts that promoted equality between the genders, which she identified as further complicating the lives of women: "Women are depended on for everything . . . [caring for] cows, fetching water, firewood, food, taking care of children, educating them, cleaning the house. . . . When we [women] got an ID [a government-issued identification card], it generalized the work, so we are equal. . . . Men don't support their wives; . . . the husband depends on the wife to look for food—[so] nowadays, both the children and the husband depend on you." Cherop mentioned the increased dangers of being a married woman in Mahali because [that status] increased the conflict between various categories of women: "It used to be that you only had to worry about the single women being husband snatchers. But today, young school girls, or even someone like you—a married woman—might even steal my husband to get money!" Leah, another young woman, reflected on her experiences of what life was like after she married:

> When you are married you start trying to compete with every woman in the plot [over who has more possessions]. This one has this, and you don't have. This one is living a better life and you are not . . . [and] living in those renting places, you are facing one another's house [living in close proximity to one another]. It's like so many houses together. So if your neighbor has a TV and you don't have one . . . you are feeling bad. You go and watch the program at that house. [But] in time you feel you don't want [others' possessions], you want yours! So life becomes competitive because you are trying to get this and this. That is why they try to even get your husband! Even if your husband is next door and he has money— that is when everyone is trying to get him! [laughing] And so there are always fights.

In line with conversations about the fierce competition between women—in the globalized world, or where "Westernization" made people "increasingly brainwashed to look for money," as Mwangi framed it—my interlocutors spoke about suspecting that others were using love potions, a form of witchcraft to keep sex partners faithful (Rödlach 2006; Wilson 2012). Mercy summed up the frequent use of potions and the perceived root of the problem: "We have so many women, and [wealthy] men are few." Love potions were thus deployed not only to control sexuality and scarce resources, but as a strategy of women to keep a limited number of men—who were employed and thus did not have to rely on their wives—available exclusively to themselves.

These kinds of shifting gender and power dynamics led to added tensions and struggles between men and women in relation to HIV testing, specifically over who was more adversely impacted by a positive result. This was clear in the ways people spoke about the HCT program that passed through the community during my two research trips in 2011–2012 and 2014 (see Pfeiffer and Maithya 2021). One consistent theme across these narratives was the perception that very few men were actually tested or counseled in their homes. This matched the results of epidemiological research in sub-Saharan Africa demonstrating that men have higher rates of AIDS-related morbidity and mortality because they are less likely to accept HIV testing and thus delay entering into HIV care (Mills et al. 2012; Druyts et al. 2013). My interlocutors seemed uniformly amused as they recalled men running away, "hiding in the maize," and "chasing away counselors with machetes." I also learned that men sometimes relied on the HIV test results of their sexual partners to determine their own. For example, Mwangi, who could not afford to pay the (expensive) bridewealth (or sometimes referred to as brideprice) to formally marry the woman he loved and therefore was involved in what he (and others) referred to as a "we come, we stay" (or informal, cohabiting) relationship, seemed eager to tell me that he was HIV– when we reunited in 2014. Since he had previously asserted that he feared and avoided HIV testing, I immediately pushed him on the topic, asking what had changed while I was gone. He clarified that he had not been tested, but his "wife" had agreed to be tested during HCT because she had grown suspicious of his having "*mpango wa kando*" (literally "a side plate," which meant a secret love affair). He seemed relieved to report that "when she told me, 'I'm HIV–,' I knew I was HIV–." Discourses about, responses to, and experiences with this regional HCT program were portrayed as intersecting with power dynamics, norms, and performances of masculinity and femininity.

While people acknowledged that "everybody is afraid of a positive [HIV] result," most expressed the sentiment that it was easier for women to get tested because "women are confident about their HIV statuses." By 2014, many people were remarking that "stigma nowadays is only for men." Yet these remarks sharply contrasted with many of the stigmatizing stories I collected, including the practices associated with the List that unevenly disadvantaged and discriminated against women. When asked why it was easier for women to get tested, people mentioned several factors, including classic stereotypes about women being perceived as faithful and men as polygamous. As Zephaniah, an unemployed man in his late thirties explained, "It is obvious. If my wife was tested and found to be positive, there was no need for me to be tested because it was me who contract[ed] the HIV." Others claimed that women's confidence in themselves and their willingness to be tested for HIV emerged from a sense of responsibility shared by women to produce children for the family and then care and provide for them. Kioko, a *fundi* and self-described Kamba, stated that women get tested and seek treatment "immediately [because] it is the only option to uphold the family values and to continue the family." Likewise, nearly everyone credited the ease with which women were tested as a direct result of national programs to prevent mother-to-child transmission. Nyambura, a woman in her early thirties who identified herself as a sex worker, explained, "When you are [pregnant], you have to be tested. So it is mandatory." A young mother, Alice, who had a fruit stand behind Mahali's urban center, added that if expectant mothers were not tested, medical professionals would not help them deliver their babies. Testing was a good thing, even if it was coercive; pregnant mothers could opt out of being tested, but they had to consider the consequences.

Gender ideals—norms of being good women as faithful wives and/or responsible mothers—were depicted as facilitating women's participation in the HCT program. Testing symbolized that women were upholding ideal gender norms and duties. This mapped onto the realities that women increasingly carried an uneven proportion of the familial responsibilities, including HIV testing. Men had few programs to prepare them psychologically for testing and bore the brunt of the blame for infecting others, and thus were characterized as being more at risk of the negative effects of HIV testing because of uncertainty about how they might react. Makori, a casual laborer in his forties, admitted: "I would rather stay that way [without knowing test results] because if I . . . am positive, stress will kill me. . . . Stress kills men, and that is why we don't test. Knowing is much worse, better to stay without knowing." A farmer, Kimutai, articulated the view of others about the imagined impact of being "officially diagnosed" with HIV on the reputation of a respected man:

> HIV has a very negative impact on a man—he loses dignity and social value—the moral value of being a father or the man of that house. . . . Economically, that family will go down, and the upbringing and the social life of that family will be low because the stigmatization [is there] that [the] father is HIV+. He will no longer be recognized or appreciated by others. . . . The marriage will not be stable as before because the mother will be the only one now who will be looked upon. Socially, he will be rejected.

Some men therefore avoided getting tested during the HCT campaigns to protect their reputation, status, family, and power, as well as to manage the social and psychological uncertainties of HIV, as documented early in the HIV epidemic before there was access to ART (Whyte 1997; Eaton 2008). Contrary to global health workers' assumptions, for many men, definitively knowing their HIV status was not always perceived of or experienced as a form of empowerment and agency. Instead, the men's power derived from strategic and calculated efforts to maintain ignorance about their HIV status during HCT as a way of preserving dignity and normal behaviors. Circulating narratives framed the HCT program as being easy for "confident" women to participate in, while it complicated the lives of men. Local discourses served to justify both the ongoing social sanctioning of women who tested positive and the refusal of men to be tested in their homes.

GLOBAL HEALTH INFRASTRUCTURES, HIV, AND SEX WORK IN MAHALI, A STIGMATIZED PLACE

Mahali was imaged to be a stigmatized place not only because of PEV. People also located its badness in its high rates of HIV and the high number of sex workers and truck drivers there, both of which contributed to viral frictions as national politics of gender, class, and ethnicity intersected with global and government-driven HIV infrastructures, treatment, and care. For example, participants in a group conversation in a rural community near Mahali agreed with Eunice when she stated: "Other Kenyans think of us [in Mahali] as people who are useless, very sick; HIV is plenty. There is already an AIDS hospital [here]!" Others described Mahali as a "dumping ground" for HIV because the HIV clinic seemed to attract outsiders to the area, as one woman stated: "It is this facility— the HIV clinic. Information is going around that there is a facility in Mahali that takes good care of people who are infected with HIV. So when people—from far-off places—hear of this facility, they want to come and at least live near this facility, so they can access these drugs without having to travel . . . each month."

The HIV clinic, constructed to alleviate the problem of the high burden of HIV and AIDS-related deaths in Mahali, was described as creating new kinds of challenges. What made locals feel that Mahali was stigmatized was not always the clinic itself, which was also viewed as an important asset, but rather that it attracted undesirable "Others" who were painted as immoral. These "Others" included poor single women, sex workers, and people who were unwanted in and/or had been chased away from other communities and thereby were imagined as further staining the reputation of Mahali and its inhabitants. Some people were resentful as they described the extra burdens of having to deal with such "immoral" migrants. As we sat in an empty classroom after the students had been dismissed for the day, Achieng, a teacher, strategically made use of a pejorative term to describe the students' parents and assess their impact on the morality of the children to express her negative perception of Mahali: "The parents at our school are the prostitutes. Their children are not morally upright. You see, . . . the moral uprightness of the people in Mahali is not right. This town is a dumping ground for HIV. When people test positive, they come here to die [and] leave behind their children. Because the children are HIV+ and their mothers were prostitutes, the [extended] family will not take that child back. So we in Mahali are left with the burdens of so many orphans."

There were many orphan-headed households in Mahali. In 2019, I was brainstorming with my research team about future directions for our work, and one idea that came up was to collect narratives from people living in the community who had grown up in orphan-headed households. My research assistants identified this topic as long and grossly neglected by the global health community in Mahali. While the area once hosted a significant program to feed orphans and other vulnerable people, funding for the program had ended in 2011, leaving a large and still unfilled gap in HIV-related care and prevention. One assistant explained that a local strategy used to help close that gap was to encourage and train orphans to participate in the brewing, distributing, and selling of illegal forms of alcohol. While my research assistants considered this approach far from ideal, they perceived that it had diminished the levels of begging and petty theft in the community. In 2012, two of my research assistants, Emmah and Henry, took me on a tour of a large public cemetery in Mahali filled with numerous unmarked graves. Emmah and Henry remembered many of the deceased as single women who had died from different causes (including complications from AIDS, unsafe abortions, violence, and various accidents and diseases) and for whom no family members had come forward to claim their bodies to provide more proper burials. Historically, burials were done on ancestral land in rural, rather than urban, areas. For many of my interlocutors, AIDS and those suffering with it brought a seemingly unending cycle of disorder and moral chaos into the community. Moses described the "problem" related to the living conditions of the children he taught, which included those who were orphaned and those being raised by widows who earned their livings through commercial sex work, this way:

> Kids are being left alone by their parents [as orphans]. Most of them are being left in the house—alone! And the worst part [for the kids who are not orphaned] is really the parents. Because our parents have around three kids who are between eight and twelve years old, and this parent is bringing [men] into their house—to a single room. . . . It means that these [children] are growing up with a problem. Because they do notice that it is not their father. Because their father [already] died of AIDS, and so the mother is bringing—not even just one—many men [into the house for sex].

HIV was still perceived and sometimes experienced by people—even in a place where HIV care and ART had been accessible for years—as being associated with AIDS-related deaths and thus to have "unraveled the arrangement of social, material, and moral forces on which the orderly perpetuation of life itself depends" (Mbembe 2006, 336).

A concerned employee at the HIV clinic encouraged me to walk around Mahali at night so I would better understand what she meant by her comments that the community was perceived by outsiders to be a bad place. She linked the negative national and international attention and perceptions of Mahali specifically to the high rate of HIV, the high volume of truck drivers, and especially the large number of local single women because they were "looking for money" and had just stopped "caring about HIV":

> HIV in [urban] Mahali is somehow—so high. Listen, if you have time in the late evenings, move through the center, and all you will see is that most of the women in Mahali are single [and] divorced ladies who are just waiting. And most of them are jobless! And there are a lot of truck drivers here, like [in one] night you can get over 200 truck drivers. And most of [them] are [HIV] positive—because they have so many girlfriends ... all along this highway. I think that is what has really contributed to our high rates [of HIV in Mahali]. ... Most of our clients [at the HIV clinic] are ... commercial sex workers. If our clients are [HIV] positive and know [it], they stop caring about HIV. They just don't care anymore. ... Even if they are [HIV] negative—they don't care! They don't believe so much in even condoms. I mean—although they tell us they use [condoms]—I don't think [they do]. ... These [sex workers] are looking for money, and they do negotiate [prices and services]. The use of a condom and not using a condom are different prices. So somebody will give like 1,000 [shillings] for not using a condom, and using a condom is only 250 [shillings]. Maybe she has some problems that she has to sort out, so she'll just go for the 1,000—for the money. You know, at that point [when problems are many] the money becomes more important [than the safety of a condom]. And with most of these men, they [think], "How can I use a condom? [Sex] is not sweet with a condom," ... but they will not say so [directly]. Instead, they will just say, "I am allergic to rubber."

Perhaps the most challenging part of living in and around a "dumping ground for HIV," I was told, was that the people moving into Mahali were dangerous and suspected of malicious intentions. This was because they were "Others" (not locals): no one knew anything about their histories and/or family backgrounds. The influx of "Others" also meant that it was difficult for people to know if they were living with HIV or not.[5] Locals frequently assumed that "Others" were infected with HIV and therefore were untrustworthy, intentionally spreading the disease. One woman maintained that "foreigners just come to Mahali with that mentality to stay here only to spread their HIV." Another interlocutor stated that it was women—specifically, former wives who had been abandoned by their husbands—who came to intentionally spread the epidemic: "A number of our newcomers are sick [with HIV]. Because the women who come to this town, they only come when they are HIV+. If a man finds his wife is HIV+, he can't stay married to her. That would be a shame [to the man because it would be a sign that the wife had been unfaithful to him]. So the wife just comes to Mahali. And these women just come to spread [HIV]. They come once they are sick because they hear there is medicine in that HIV clinic."

Although the HIV clinic was not visible from the main highway, people living in the community could easily deduce that anyone going into or coming out of the building was infected and receiving HIV-related services. Consequently, I learned that those with the financial means to do so often traveled to clinics in other areas for treatment and care. Several clients of the HIV clinic in Mahali traveled significant distances from their homes and social lives in other cities and towns as a way of keeping their seropositive statuses private. But most residents had limited resources and thus had to rely on the HIV care provided nearby. The socioeconomic positioning of a person thus impacted who attended (and who was seen attending) which HIV clinic.

People from surrounding rural communities also commuted into Mahali to visit the HIV clinic. Faith, a social worker at the clinic who genuinely cared for and empathized with those in her case load, graciously allowed me to accompany her one day as she traveled into several rural communities to check on and deliver basic supplies to some of the most vulnerable PLWHIV. It was not an easy task to locate people to get the supplies to them, which Faith explained was a common, yet frustrating, component of her work. We knocked on doors that no one answered and then went from homestead to homestead, looking for people and asking where they might be—using names or descriptions of people no one seemed to recognize. Faith said that sometimes people registered at the clinic using different names to maintain privacy. We spent the whole day searching for several people and found only one and left a message for a second. It was March and it had rained only a handful of times late at night, so the days were still mostly dry and hot across the region. This made it possible for us to make our way along dirt roads (which are often washed out and inaccessible during the rainy seasons) and into rural communities, each of us riding on the back of a *boda boda*. But the termites had come, indicating to everyone that the drought was nearly over, so people were making plans and preparing to plant. The Kalenjin-owned tractors were back on the roads again, moving swiftly about the landscape. Vegetables were still hard to come by and, in Mahali, people were making jokes about being tired of eating the same foods at every meal. It also seemed that everywhere we went people were struggling with a *homa*, which I linked to the changing seasons.

Among those living in the urban center of Mahali, the significant increase in the numbers of outside police and security officers was also described as worrying and helped explain high rates of HIV, even among children. These outsiders were strangers and suspected by locals to have come to spread HIV, as Kimaiyo explained: "You will find also that security forces are often introduced here. Most of those security forces—the police—form relationships with our small girls, and these girls are given some small presents, maybe sweets, . . . to create room for later [sexual] relationships. And you find that these people who came here for the security purpose, we [locals] don't know their [HIV] status. So [they] contribute to the spread of HIV to our young children." For other people, the "Others" were truck drivers or people from abroad who were immoral because they were "known" to have come to Mahali with no other purpose than to engage in what locals referred to as "spreading sprees." Two people, first a health worker and later Simiyu (who identified himself as Luhya and worked at a local *hoteli*), told me about a man from Uganda who had been convicted of this crime in recent years, which pointed to the potential criminalization of people with HIV: "There was a [man] who came here from Uganda. I thought he was a [truck] driver. I was seeing [him] come to eat here and he always came with beautiful girls. And finally, I heard that he came from Uganda to spread the disease! He was later arrested in [a large city]. It was investigated and . . . they discovered it. He was arrested, taken to [a] cell, and diagnosed with HIV."

Many long-term residents of Mahali imagined that HIV came into the area from individuals living outside the community, which was a practice that people connected, in part, to the HIV clinic, or as an aspect of global health infrastructure. This belief was further rooted in xenophobic attitudes, or a general shared culture of fear and distrust of "Others" in a community where people paid very careful attention to social and sexual networks (and who went into and out of the freestanding HIV clinic) to determine and gossip about who was potentially infected. These beliefs mirrored and further aggravated existing tensions between insiders and outsiders that had been circulating in and around the place for decades and were at the heart of ethnic conflict and political violence. This unevenly compounded the experiences of stigma among migrants (see Steenberg 2020), especially single women who moved into the area. At the same time, this attitude toward migrants aggravated intrapersonal forms of stigma among wealthier, married, and long-term residents such as those described as being on the List. Mahali residents often (re)negotiated ideas about who belonged and who did not across the intersecting lines of ethnicity, gender, and class—a practice that Peter Geschiere (2009) referred to as the perils and politics of belonging. In a community with tremendous tensions over land and chronic eruptions of political, ethnic, and gender-based violence, HIV-related stigmatizing public discourses of blame played on these very local anxieties about immoral "Others" lured to Mahali because of the HIV clinic, who were also presumed to be intentionally spreading the disease. What was ultimately threatened among both those who were stigmatized and those doing the stigmatizing was the desire to feel and experience a sense of security and belonging somewhere, in an otherwise uncertain and dangerous world.

WIVES VERSUS SEX WORKERS: HIV AND GLOBAL HEALTH INCONGRUENCIES

Consistently across my years of research, interlocutors linked HIV to sex work or to careless or reckless sexual behaviors and practices. No matter which words were selected, they all communicated negative sentiments that it was the individual's fault for having become infected by engaging in some sort of immoral sexual activity (see also Rödlach 2006). As Jane once summarized things, "Okay, in Mahali today, we call it [long pause], in Mahali, we call HIV a sex worker disease. People know that [HIV] can get anyone, but . . ." In this section, I further examine the durability of the moralizing understanding of HIV as a sex worker disease to explain the persistence of HIV-related stigma and discrimination.

While people working at the HIV clinic in Mahali tried hard to normalize an exceptional disease—for example, circulating discourses like "HIV is a disease like any other"—other HIV-related programming (in)advertently communicated different ideas, suggesting that "HIV is a sex worker disease." While I am unable to pinpoint the source of this latter message,[6] there were two possibilities. The first was PEPFAR, which required any organization desiring money to sign a pledge opposing commercial sex. Since 2005, PEPFAR has especially rewarded programs willing to promote abstinence and marital fidelity (Parmet 2008; Parsitau 2009). Scholars previously working in Kenya have noted that in recent years, PEPFAR has encouraged churches to promote their own moral teachings through HIV prevention messaging (Parsitau 2009). Church leaders condemned sex work and promoted abstinence and fidelity in marriage, while also promoting HIV prevention strategies such as making HIV testing mandatory for people who intended to marry.

These discourses and contingencies had a real impact on the lives of people living in or passing through Mahali. For example, Makena, a single woman living with HIV, recalled—as we sat in a private room at the HIV clinic after her monthly appointment—having felt and experienced stigma at church because of her HIV status, which cut her off from a much-needed and desired community of faith. She described her feelings about learning that she was living with the virus and how others around her had responded. She spoke of a deep sense of shame because of her perceived failure to uphold the standards of her Christian faith. Unable to find employment, she had come to rely on a relationship with a man to help provide for her basic needs. She construed this not only as a personal failure but also as a contradiction in her life and in the context of our discussion about HIV and her church. She blamed herself for her infection (which led her to contemplate suicide) as others in her faith-based circles came to learn about her HIV status and pronounced her "a sinner." Ultimately, Makena was threatened by and cast out of her support networks at the church: "I had to leave my church because the church members knew [I was living with HIV] and told me that I had sinned. . . . I felt bad because I was saved [a converted Christian], and I was unable to stay alone [without a man for financial stability]. I thought, 'I will drown [myself] in water and die.' I felt I should jump inside a bore hole. I am just discouraged because recently I was almost taken to court for rudeness [because of my response] when one person asked me who my [sex] partner was."

The second possible source of the message that "HIV is a sex worker disease" was the NGO that offered HIV outreach services in the container clinic, where I spent a significant amount of time and got to know people working there. Through my work with them, I came to suspect that global health community programming may have intersected with local and national sexual identity politics to produce viral frictions. I spent much of my time during my preliminary research (May–August 2010) at one community-based organization, which at that time offered two types of HIV-related services: an orphan feeding program and a peer education program that promoted the empowerment of women to negotiate condom use with men, get regular HIV screenings, and regularly use reproductive health services and treatment (e.g., birth control and screenings for cervical cancer). The latter program initially targeted only sex workers in Mahali.[7] Recognizing that sex workers were not the only individuals susceptible to HIV infection and to reduce the stigma facing the women who attended the clinic, in 2009 this local organization extended its outreach services to include all vulnerable women. Given the effects of PEV, people working there correctly assumed that this included every woman in Mahali.

By the time I returned to Mahali to conduct a year of fieldwork in 2011–2012, this community-based organization had changed many of its programs to focus on health-related issues beyond HIV. Yet throughout my research (through 2020), HIV-related outreach to sex workers reemerged as a priority through efforts that operated out of the container clinic. With the support of several international entities that collaborated with the Kenyan government, the clinic took over the peer education program component and was almost exclusively targeting and offering services to truck drivers and sex workers. While this NGO did not directly state that HIV was "a sex worker disease," indirect messages along those lines were certainly delivered to locals. For example, activities in the clinic did not even begin until late afternoon or evening, when most married and respectable women were already at home, preparing supper for their families. But at this time, many people—including local men, truck drivers, and sex workers—were drinking, eating, and socializing in bars.

Common outreach events organized by the NGO in the area were so-called moonlight clinics, which were conducted very late at night and which I witnessed and participated in during 2012 and 2014. Tents were set up to serve as makeshift VCT stations, with employees poised to administer rapid HIV tests and supply almost instantaneous results. The work mostly, but not exclusively, drew on the labor of local sex workers trained as peer educators,[8] who brought men (mostly their clients) in for testing, offered public condom demonstrations, and distributed free condoms. With these local services dominating much of the regular HIV scene in Mahali (beyond the HIV clinic, school curricula, media articles, and formal presentations given at public events), I believe that it would be hard for locals to take away any message other than "HIV is a sex worker disease." This NGO in Mahali that targeted HIV during this period may have been working at cross purposes with those efforts and sending mixed messages that while "HIV is a disease like any other," it was simultaneously still a "sex worker disease."

HIV—including local experiences with and global and national health responses to it—was used as a device that blended into gender politics to produce viral frictions, which (re)produced gender inequalities and moralizing discourses about the disease. As conflicts erupted between people, especially between women, so did the use of categorical labels, including *HIV+*, *wives*, and *sex workers*. For example, among the many burial ceremonies I attended, one was for a single woman whose friends were invited to take a photograph next to the coffin. After her picture was taken, Muthoni, a divorced Kikuyu woman, overheard a group of women whom she described as "wives gossiping": "You see all of these ones [the friends of the deceased]? They are all HIV+ [because] they are all CSWs!" Muthoni retorted, "You [say] that you know we are HIV+, but your men do come to us, so if we are positive then you are positive!" The assumption that sex workers were diseased was not contested by Muthoni. Instead, she drew on the strength of this negative status to issue a counterattack, destabilize the gendered status quo and the notion that HIV was a sex worker disease, and disrupt processes of HIV-related stigma.

However, such fear-mongering tactics also worked in other ways. For example, Leah once showed me a text message she had received from the suspicious wife of one of her colleagues: "I feel sorry for you. I did not breast-feed [the name of the child].[9] And I know you and [my husband] don't use condoms." Gendered conflicts were not exclusively about HIV, but importantly, verbal threats of being infected with HIV—as well as accusations of being responsible for the spread of the virus, along with blame for spreading it—were sometimes deployed during contentious struggles between women, thereby blurring and complicating the lines between categories such as victim and perpetrator, wife and sex worker, good and evil, and HIV− and HIV+. HIV was described as a device in ethnic politics, as I explained in chapter 2, and appeared to have become normalized in everyday interactions. But it sharpened existing gender inequalities and differences while also perpetuating moralizing discourses about the virus and those living with it.

As people worked to gain access to limited resources, the distorting and bending of gendered categories became obvious when the notion that "HIV is a sex worker disease" produced an unintended and unexpected local outcome and opportunity. Muthoni, whom I came to know well, had successfully penetrated the HIV-related NGO in several nearby communities by strategically and consistently presenting herself as a sex worker.[10] She had been selected, trained, and employed as a peer educator, and she regularly worked during moonlight clinics. Muthoni had been taught and was intermittently paid to help in local efforts to distribute condoms in bars in the evenings and provide regular local condom demonstrations. She was like a handful of other women in the area, and over the months that I spent time with her, I never really thought much about her wide range of employment opportunities. One day, however, Muthoni confided that she did not identify herself as a sex worker. She explained that she had one long-term boyfriend who generously helped raise her children, but she had successfully capitalized on her status as a single woman who lived in Mahali. That is, she had presented herself to international and national organizations as a sex worker with the goal of landing employment in the NGO sector in the community. This had enabled her to gain capital—financial, social, and cultural.

On a handful of occasions, I observed that Muthoni used this presentation of herself to benefit those in her social network, which gave her additional prestige as a single mother. For example, one day she joined me in a social gathering with a group of relatively wealthy women that consisted primarily of her close friends who were single and sometimes referred to as local "high-class" sex workers. Muthoni began laughing and recounted an incident that had occurred the previous day. She said that she had been approached by a community leader who had been asked to help coordinate a "stakeholders' meeting," designed to assess the impact on various segments of the Mahali population of the temporary diversion of the highway being planned by a Chinese company and to be implemented by Chinese workers. She explained that she had been contacted by the leader and asked to serve as the representative of her group. Another woman inquired, "What group?" Muthoni responded, "As the leader of the CSWs!" I remarked, "Wow, you are famous!" Muthoni responded, "That is not a good title. But I told them that the road would really affect [CSWs] because we could all become infected with HIV by their [Chinese] employees, and so we needed to be assured that we would be kept safe and protected. I told them they needed to help pay to train us more about how to prevent the spread of HIV in the area." From Muthoni's point of view, the risk that her reputation would be tainted by association with the loosely and locally defined label of "the leader of the CSWs" was worth it, and she used the label to attach herself to the AIDS industry to financially benefit herself and her friends. This pointed to the viral frictions produced between local knowledge, the politics of living in a community and country with limited resources, and global health ideas about ways to draw dichotomized boundaries between individuals (e.g., wives and sex workers).

During a later research trip, Muthoni and I sat together and marveled at the numerous certificates she had accumulated over the years—evidence of her participation in the wide range of global and national programs, research projects, and outreach initiatives (see Prince 2012; McKay 2018) related to HIV and women's empowerment that had passed through Mahali and nearby towns and centers. Several of the certificates further showed off her HIV-related "technical know-how" as someone "exposed" to HIV-related knowledge, as well as her "technical know-who," or the personal connections she possessed that provided her access to the AIDS industry (see Prince 2014, 77; see also Whyte 2002). Muthoni commented that she had so many certificates that when she applies for (highly competitive) volunteer or temporary positions now, she has to be selective about which documents would demonstrate her qualifications because she simply had too many to take them all. Yet anthropologists working in Kenya have noted that the HIV-related knowledge gained during workshops and training sessions to acquire such certificates is largely rendered obsolete once they are awarded, because "knowledge is unstable and uncertain," and global health HIV information and interventions are constantly being updated and changed (Prince 2014, 77). Trainings that yielded certificates created significant gaps between those with professional knowledge and those with certificate-level knowledge. Still, in Mahali, some people had an uneven share of global health certificates: most had none at all. This highlights the awkward complexities of globalization—and the violent structural inequalities it (re)produces—that perpetuate the types of conditions in which witch hunts and accusations of witchcraft are experienced by people like Maggie and the responsibility and blame for the spread of HIV are placed on people like Wambūi.

5 • (RE)IMAGINING STIGMA AT THE INTERSECTION OF HIV AND MENTAL HEALTH STATUSES

In preceding chapters I emphasized how broad structural conditions and inequalities—explained as a result of the intertwined impacts of HIV, PEV, and economic marginalization—rapidly changed normal, everyday life and (re)shaped HIV-related public stigma and a wide range of subtle (and not so subtle) messages about HIV and those living with it at community and institutional levels. I also highlighted uncertain moments when stigmatizing discourses erupted unexpectedly into action to become felt and enacted forms of stigma and discrimination (see Jacoby 1994) that predominantly disadvantaged women but that also reinforced moralizing discourses that divided people into various ethnic, socioeconomic, gendered, and health categories. Consequently, we have seen how HIV was sometimes used as a device to blame and scapegoat particular groups during fierce local and national competitions for power. Amid these contentious circumstances, people worked to (re)negotiate their lives and relationships during a period of major uncertainty, political violence, socioeconomic vulnerability, change, and efforts to normalize an exceptional disease.

Anthropologists working in eastern Africa have suggested that in the contexts of economic struggles and conditions of uncertainty, it is useful to conceptualize PLWHIV as occupying a liminal "social space" where they are permanently suspended between the roles of potentially sick patients and normal, healthy people (McGrath et al. 2014, 314). Other scholars have demonstrated how patients are socialized for this social space through the chronic illness model that focuses on individualized forms and narratives of responsible self-care (Swendeman, Ingram, and Rotheram-Borus 2009; de Klerk and Moyer 2017). In this chapter, I focus on the creation and maintenance of this social space by exploring the changing nature of stigma alongside the implementation of anti-stigma interventions, ART, and efforts to normalize HIV using narratives of chronic disease and living positively with an HIV+ status. I consider how and why, during the age of treatment, circulating discourses centered heavily on concerns about the "unpredictable" mind of those living with HIV to (re)imagine and make sense of processes of stigma at intrapersonal and interpersonal levels. In this chapter and in chapter 6, I narrow the focus on stigma to concentrate on the perceptions, experiences, and responses of PLWHIV as they occupy this liminal social space while also negotiating wider social changes and inequalities. We begin by listening to and learning from Wanja.[1]

"BECAUSE I FOUND THAT I WAS NOTHING . . . SOMETHING DIFFERENT"

Wanja traced the various trajectories of her life as we worked to make chapatis (thin flatbreads served with a variety of dishes) in the freestanding kitchen where she was occasionally paid to help cook and do other casual work for the family of an employee at the HIV clinic. We were each wearing a *leso* (a decorated cloth worn as a covering and used by women for many purposes)[2] so we wouldn't get the skirts we were wearing underneath dirty. Wanja identified herself as Kikuyu and shared with me her memories of a time when she had been a married housewife and farmer. Her husband had a well-paying job, and together they had four children. When her spouse died suddenly, Wanja's life became more turbulent. She began moving across the country from one job to another and from place to place. The mobility required by her work initially placed considerable pressure on her, as a widow with several children, but that eventually eased when her children went to live with her mother at the family's rural homestead in the central region of Kenya. However, things became complicated when she learned that her youngest child and only son[3] had died. When she spoke of his death, her eyes filled with tears, which she dabbed at with the handkerchief she kept clenched in her fist. Wanja suspected that her mother had poisoned him because she was always complaining that he was "a burden" on her already limited and scarce resources. After a turbulent time of grief and a struggle to forgive her mother—a topic to which she sometimes circled back when we spoke—Wanja was grateful to finally land steady employment and housing provided by a family, working on their *shamba* (farm) in a rural area just outside Mahali. She believed that her life was moving in a more positive direction until she contracted HIV and came to feel "like nothing . . . something different." She told me about learning she was infected:

> [A man had been pursuing me for some time] . . . and people were saying that I was somehow abnormal [for not being in a sexual relationship with a man]. . . . That is when I came [to think], "Why should I live desperate when there are

men?" [So I felt] I should start socializing. So we made love! . . . So this man had a wife . . . but he never wanted me to know. So he was telling me, "I'll marry you." I couldn't believe or even think he had a wife. . . . Then when he told me, "If you are not going to give birth—to give me a kid—I think there is no interest. There is no need for me to stay with you." . . . I prayed [to] God and thought, "May you give me another boy [to replace the one who had been poisoned]." So I had decided! It is now that I decided, and I got pregnant.

When I [was] about to give birth [to a son], . . . I was told by another woman, "You know what? I never wanted to discourage you, but . . . do you know that you will be a second wife?" I never believed [that]. I thought that that lady was jealous! But then she kept on telling me such things [until eventually I came to meet the first wife, who was also pregnant]. After I gave birth, I told the husband, "Don't think I was interested to be married [to you]. Me, I was married to a person who gave dowry to my people, and I cannot go to another home. So let us say that we have wasted time with each other." And I told him [that] and I became very strict. I went on with my work. I stayed. I worked very hard. I worked! . . .

Until the time when the boy was around five years [and he] started becoming sick. He would even wake up at night and it was always something like pneumonia. . . . But as he grew, it disappeared! And we went on with life. But then [later] . . . it was me. . . . I started becoming sick. Feeling weak. I started feeling pain. . . . I came to the hospital. I was given medicine—all sorts of good medicine. . . . But nothing changed. Then I came across [a doctor who told me to have my blood checked]. I did and I was [HIV] positive. So I started worrying, where did I get it? . . . So that is when I brought even my child [to the doctor, and] he was found [to be HIV] positive. I told God, "Oh God, although the life will be short, give us happiness. That is all."

So I stayed there [in the rural community]. I came to the [HIV] clinic [and saw] the gentleman who [had] wanted to marry me—the father of my child. Yeah, I [saw] him at the [HIV] hospital. Sitting in line! . . . He also [started] calling me [on the phone and saying things such as], "You know, I am sorry! I have started a new life. I had no mind then." . . . But I told him, "So you knew it was this way [you were living with HIV]? And you were that way [HIV+]? And that is what you wanted? You wanted to waste me, [infect me on purpose]?" So I told him, "I'm sorry. [My son and I] are not going to die. Here is the boy and he is still growing!" So I left him [the man] in the queue [at the HIV clinic].

At the next [HIV clinic] visit . . . I met [his first] wife! I knew [for sure] where I had got the virus. It [was] from this man. And . . . that is the time I started becoming weak. And from there I started becoming a drunkard. I started drinking . . . because I found that I was nothing, something different.

During her pursuit of a fuller, more respected, or normal personhood—as a hard-working widow, desiring a spouse and son—Wanja contracted HIV. When we first met in 2011, she was a casual laborer, helping people with cooking, clean-ing, and farming and still drinking alcohol, an activity that she continued to indulge in at our last meeting in 2019. Although we did not discuss it, I could smell the distinct odor of local brews coming from her body whenever we engaged in the polite greetings that are typical in Kenya, which include hand-shakes and hugs. After her HIV diagnosis, it was her drinking that she (and one of her employers) viewed as the cause of a series of spiraling hardships, including losing several jobs, becoming homeless, and being raped while intoxicated. For Wanja, her heavy drinking was not triggered by her HIV diagnosis. Rather, it was a strategy through which she coped after a long series of stressful and traumatic life events, including realizing that she had been infected by a man who she believed had wanted to marry her. Wanja was distraught: she felt "different," like "nothing." She blamed herself for having been foolish. She saw herself as a responsible woman who never engaged in careless or reckless sex but who had been duped by a man who had only pretended to care about and want to provide for her and their child in the contexts of resource and employment scarcity, uncertainty, and extreme gender inequalities.

Wanja did not feel or experience stigmatization or discrimination because of her HIV+ status, but she felt criticized for what she described as being a "drunk-ard" and blamed for her "psychological problems" and "bad behaviors" that put others in the community at risk for HIV transmission. The ongoing self-stigma and blame combined with the gender-based violence that she endured to amplify her own susceptibility for HIV reinfection, as well as for contracting other sexu-ally transmitted infections and opportunistic infections known to have deleteri-ous consequences that accelerate the progression of HIV. Although researchers have largely treated mental health stigma and HIV stigma as separate phenom-ena (Hatzenbuehler, Phelan, and Link 2013), in the lived realities of people like Wanja, they sometimes converge to negatively influence health and the sense of well-being. Wanja's story therefore provides a solid backdrop for identifying viral frictions, as well as the crisis mentality that aptly characterizes what it is like for many people who are diagnosed, live, and experience long-term survival with a stigmatized chronic condition in sub-Saharan Africa (see Russell and Seeley 2010; McGrath et al. 2014; de Klerk and Moyer 2017).

UNDERSTANDING GLOBAL HEALTH ANTI-STIGMA CAMPAIGNS AND "PROPER KNOWLEDGE"

Over the past decade, the development and implementation of fleeting pilot or short-term interventions designed to address HIV-related stigma have been popular among global health entities working across sub-Saharan Africa (Kemp et al. 2019; Rao et al. 2019). Since such interventions have been conceptualized by people living in the Global North, social scientists have long promulgated the idea that these types of programs reflect the views of stigma among those who developed the programs and tools rather than the social and structural realities, logics, and moral particularities of the places where they are inserted and enacted (Liu 2009). To appreciate the impact of globalization in the lives of people in Mahali, I focused on how stigma has been imagined, measured, and addressed by the global health community.

According to Arthur Kleinman (1988, 159), stigma in "the West" has come to be associated more with individual disgrace than with physical characteristics. This shift, he argues, reflects the "psychologization of experience in the West, through which metaphors of distress and other human problems that were once bodily have become mental." Consequently, many contemporary stigma interventions have drawn heavily on psychological approaches to assess stigma at the individual level only, subsequently addressing the problem with education-based approaches (Stangl et al. 2019). Such initiatives have persisted in the Global South even though psychologists have long demonstrated that the exclusive use of education-based programs tends to do little more than teach people that stigmatizing beliefs and discriminatory practices are socially undesirable (Corrigan and Penn 1999; Penn and Corrigan 2002). This leads people to conceal rather than reject stereotypical beliefs about others living with stigmatized conditions, such as mental illness. Stigma reductions resulting from such interventions have thus tended to be short-lived and superficial (Corrigan et al. 2000).

HIV anti-stigma campaigns have been universalized into packaged and portable tools, described as "briefcase concepts" (Eves and Butt 2008, 5; see also Liu 2009). Popular global briefcase concepts for HIV-related stigma have generically advocated for individuals to "increase tolerance," "increase empathy and altruism," and "reduce anxiety and fear" toward PLWHIV. The concepts have also provided PLWHIV with basic counseling services to help them—as individuals—develop better "coping skills" to manage the effects of stigma in their personal lives (Parker and Aggleton 2003, 16). The underlying premise behind these panaceas is that individuals' scientific knowledge through education will translate to a reduction of stigma and will improve HIV screening rates and the uptake of biomedical care and treatments. Yet anthropologists have long demonstrated that briefcase concepts, though well intentioned, put the onus on individuals and their personal choices (Castro and Farmer 2005; see also Booth 2004; Fassin 2007; Marsland and Prince 2012), as I noted in the introduction. Sociologists and anthropologists criticize such approaches for being too narrowly focused and failing to consider the myriad broader structural forces and social contexts at play, in which those being stigmatized and those stigmatizing are both embedded (e.g., V. Das 2001; Link and Phelan 2001; Parker and Aggleton 2003; Castro and Farmer 2005; Yang et al. 2007). Anthropologists have paid less attention to the impact of individualistic anti-stigma and global health initiatives on the everyday social lives of PLWHIV and those living in a community inundated with national HIV programming and messaging. As illustrated in the case of Wanja, who is blamed (and who blames herself) for her intersecting mental health and HIV statuses, stigma was transformed in Mahali to become "more psychological nowadays," as several interlocutors put things for me, due to viral frictions. These discourses also indexed observations of the stressors associated with living with a chronic illness and an "unpredictable body" in a resource-constrained setting (de Klerk and Moyer 2017, 307). Given how HIV-related stigma might be ameliorated, a one-size-fits-all chronic disease model to address these phenomena might not have the intended and desired outcomes in every situation. Rather, it may produce unexpected ones.

I saw and heard artifacts of anti-stigma campaigns with their briefcase concept messages throughout the community, including in the HIV clinic. I saw stickers and posters about the dangers of stigma that proclaimed the need for "proper knowledge," which national campaigns claimed was the "only way to win this war" (see figure 5.1). I read in a manual at the clinic that stigma would be reduced through sustained efforts to educate the larger community with "proper knowledge" on how HIV is transmitted, prevented, and treated. The manual had been written by Population Services International–Kenya to train community-based health workers. In 2014, I also saw a video that regularly played in the waiting area at the container clinic. Its primary message linked stigma to fear rooted in ignorance. Stigma, the video proclaimed, was due to the lack of individual "proper knowledge" and could be removed if people, including both those who were living with HIV and those who were not, were better educated. I was struck by the constant refrain of "proper knowledge." While I knew the term referred to universal knowledge about HIV science and technologies, its use signaled how little attention was being paid to the important social knowledge possessed by people in Mahali about PEV, economic realities, beliefs about what constituted proper talk, and the politics of uncertainty. This use was thus dismissive of other things at community and structural levels that needed to be addressed for stigma to be ameliorated. Yet I also heard traces of anti-stigma campaigns echoed by people I interviewed. I asked them what could be done to further ameliorate stigma in the area. The only solution ever provided, other than the suggestion that I come up with a real cure, was a plea for more education.

The local cries for increased "proper knowledge" differed slightly from global health discourses in their emphasis, revealing viral frictions. People consistently requested increased educational training focused on modes of transmission other than sexual practices and behaviors (e.g., blood transfusions, accidents, and vertical transmission, or the passing of infection from mother to child during gestation, delivery, or breast-feeding). The disease was incessantly linked to what people described as the "immoral" behaviors of individuals engaging in "immoral" sex. For example, Josiah, who worked at a cybercafe, explained his rationale for the need to expand HIV education about the modes of transmission: "You know,

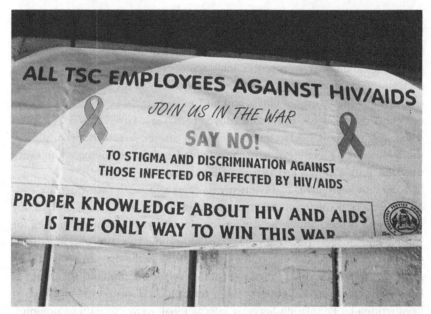

FIGURE 5.1. A sticker advocating an anti-stigma campaign on a door at a primary school in Mahali.

when people get to know that you are HIV+, it is like you become a social misfit in society. You become a total outcast, . . . they tend to look at you as being immoral. They don't actually look at the other avenues [through which] people can get HIV. They only assume that the only way people get HIV is just by sex." Cherop echoed this logic when discussing the need to conceal an HIV diagnosis: "If you are HIV+, you equal immoral. So I think because we have never changed and realized that you can get HIV through other means or ways other than through immoral sexual acts, . . . we still have to have those private parts of our lives. Because that will give you the confidence to continue on with your activities so that you are able to fit in society."

Comments and sentiments about the need to refocus education on alternative modes of transmission were astute. Anyone who just spent time in Mahali and glanced around would quickly gather that HIV was always transmitted through unprotected—or what locals had come to understand as "immoral" or "careless"—sex and behaviors. Residents and visitors read signs and posters highlighting the disease, encouraging individuals to make "good choices" as "responsible parents," abstain from unprotected sexual acts, be faithful to one sex partner, and practice condom use. People also heard moralizing speeches during all kinds of celebrations and ceremonies. In early January, I traveled with research assistants to a nearby rural community to attend the engagement negotiations and a party for Violet and her future spouse, Benson. Seated in the back corner in the hot and crowded living area of the small Kalenjin homestead of Violet's parents, I had graciously been invited to attend, listen, and observe as the relatives and closest companions from both sides of the new family not only formally presented gifts to one another but negotiated and had witnesses sign handwritten, detailed records in a notebook of the bridewealth to be paid (e.g., a large water tank, cattle, and furniture) by Benson and his family in exchange for Violet. The events helped cement relationships between the two sides of the family and outlined their responsibilities, roles, and obligations to each other. We exited the house and joined an even larger gathering of more distantly related family members, colleagues, friends, and neighbors outside, where there was a soft, welcoming breeze, the air smelled fresh, and the sky was almost perfectly blue. We shared a meal prepared by women in the extended family and coordinated by a hired caterer, who also prepared the meat. With the assistance of a former favorite teacher, Violet cut an elaborate cake and guests offered their wrapped gifts and good wishes to the new couple before settling into spots in the grass where they chatted and waited for the presentations to begin. Several speeches warned of the dangers of HIV and reminded listeners how to prevent its spread. For example, Omar (representing the HIV clinic) gave a speech about HIV. In all these kinds of educational messages, the onus was placed on individuals like Wanja and the women alleged to be on the List, rather than on the myriad (often cascading) social, structural, and ultimately stressful conditions that might have constrained their choices. The messages thereby inadvertently cast blame on anyone who became infected, especially those who chose to drink heavily as a coping strategy. Requests for education about HIV transmission were not actually pointing to deficiencies in the knowledge levels about the information being presented. Rather, the requests indicated that people had received the "proper knowledge" and the intended (often moralizing) messages that were communicated through the combined global and national health efforts, which were driving, instead of ameliorating, processes of stigma.

HIV messaging and anti-stigma briefcase concepts that promote the use of individual knowledge, responsibility, and agency (or the ability of people to exert control over their lives) in the prevention and treatment of HIV and stigma are important. However, they would be more helpful and effective if they were presented within the contexts of knowledge of the social determinants of health: the economic, social, and structural conditions that influence the health status of individuals and groups. Likewise, the "proper knowledge" accessible to people in Mahali while I was doing my research exposed several faulty assumptions about HIV epidemiology that have been documented by other scholars working in sub-Saharan Africa (Ashforth and Watkins 2015). The first assumption is that HIV is highly contagious, and that one unprotected sexual encounter will result in infection. The second is that anyone who has participated in adulterous sex is automatically infected, contagious, and dangerous. But these beliefs run counter to contemporary scientific evidence and knowledge about HIV and suggest that it is time to update prevention messages so people know that HIV is a difficult virus to contract (Ashforth and Watkins 2015) and that ART can suppress the virus in ways that prohibit its transmission.[4]

VIRAL FRICTIONS FROM INTEGRATING "PROPER KNOWLEDGE" AND LIVING POSITIVELY

To better cope with HIV and better manage stigma, people at the HIV clinic (and anywhere else that HIV testing occurred) were counseled and provided with "proper knowledge" regarding HIV, including ways to live positively, which also sometimes blended with economic and moral realities to produce viral frictions. When I asked people at the HIV clinic what it meant to live positively, the concept evoked the idea that a person needed to change his or her outlook toward life and normal everyday behaviors. People described living positively not as putting others before themselves, but as needing to focus more on themselves, citing a range of behavior changes that included being especially vigilant in avoiding stress and engaging in self-care (de Klerk and Moyer 2017), following the rules of safe sex (Rasmussen 2013) and all other instructions from health professionals, eating often and having a balanced diet, getting regular exercise, taking medicines every day, and making enough money to maintain one's health and well-being. Some of these messages and reminders were written explicitly on people's clinic appointment cards, which read, "Keep all appointments. Bring all medicines with you. Never run out of drugs." Yet it was difficult, at best, to meet all the requirements for living positively for many people living in Mahali, whether they were living with HIV or not. This fact amplified the stressors of everyday life among many PLWHIV.

Occasionally, patients or employees at the clinics mentioned the discomfort, strain, and guilty feelings associated with being (or potentially being) burdens (financial and otherwise) on their friends and family members because of their HIV, the demands of living positively, and their need to focus so many of their physical efforts and economic resources on themselves. HIV thus presented them with a new moral dilemma, one that emerged from their being diagnosed with a disease that continued to evoke accusations of immoral behaviors from others and caused moralizing public narratives and gossip to circulate. Caring for and supporting themselves were difficult in Mahali, a community characterized by high rates of poverty, limited resources, and an inadequate health care system, as well as suffering among many community members and their supportive kin (see also Lock and Nguyen 2010). For example, in 2012, Dorcas, an employee at the HIV clinic, became emotional as she recalled two patients she had recently worked with who dreaded the idea of becoming burdens on their families. This dread motivated their behaviors. For both clients, the strongly felt need and the moral and ethical obligations to avoid being (or even complain about being) a burden to others overshadowed their own health and survival. Dorcas said: "A client told me that she didn't want anyone in the family to know she was HIV+ because the mother had diabetes and had become a burden. She [the client] did not want to be a burden, so she said, 'Let me just die alone [before I become a burden].' Another client told me that she always had to borrow money for transportation [to the HIV clinic], so she said she felt that she was becoming too much of a burden to the others and she felt it would be better to die, rather than burden [them]."

As Josien de Klerk and Eileen Moyer (2017, 307) note for older PLWHIV in Mombasa, self-care was mediated by gendered and generational responsibilities and "always cast in social terms and never just as individual responsibility." Sometimes people in Mahali ceased living positively as a form of self-stigma but also as a strategy of being a good family member who did not burden others. This was an aspect of the "morality of care" that exposed "the hidden collective, the people not present in the consulting room" (de Klerk and Moyer 2017, 315). It was rooted in an ethic and values that prioritized the group over the individual. In these instances, PLWHIV sometimes assessed those in their immediate social network using logics that reflected historic legacies of "socialization for scarcity," or "the assumption that resources for poverty reduction and international health initiatives will be in perpetually short supply" and therefore are distributed unevenly and limit the possibilities and effectiveness of interventions (Greene et al. 2013, 61). Socialization for scarcity continues to dominate global health initiatives in Kenya and produces tensions within and between local people, including PLWHIV in Mahali. In the calculus of their own limited resources and those of their loved ones, PLWHIV sometimes placed themselves at the bottom of the hierarchy of who was worthy and deserving of using them. This was hard for the employees working at the HIV clinic to witness and accept. Gladys, another health worker at the clinic, recalled a client whose health had rapidly declined after the World Food Programme cut off her food relief:

Even in this area there was recently a woman who was tested and told that she was positive. . . . [She was on] food relief, [which] you are given for six months if you are weak . . . [but when] the relief stopped, she started to say, "Oh, I went to the pastors to be prayed for and I am prayed for and they have told me that I am not HIV+ [anymore]." But when you look at her, you just see that she is going down, down, down. She has lost weight, and even if she goes to the hospital, she will be told that her CD4 [cell count] is down. Before, when she was going [to the HIV clinic and using ARTs and getting food relief], she was very healthy, and you couldn't even notice she was sick. But [now], she has diarrhea, and if you tell her to go to the hospital [for this], she will just tell you that she is okay. She was even recently visited by a white person [a foreign doctor]. . . . But you will find that these people [who refuse ARTs] are so stubborn that even when they are given medicine, they don't [take] it. And my opinion is that these [HIV] counselors should be visiting these people [those refusing to use ARTs] often, so they will have morale to continue with life and always have someone to encourage them.

The woman described by Gladys (who was visibly upset when speaking about the woman's situation because she felt helpless to do anything about it) lacked the resources to live positively, or to maintain her hope and physical health after her food relief ended. Her health started to deteriorate, but she refused to complain about her predicament and instead used a story about how she had been healed while the virus ravaged her body. She was a victim of structural violence; her body within the larger social, economic, historical, and political contexts that enveloped it (Lock and Scheper-Hughes 1996)—was withering away slowly (Farmer 2004), not by her own choice, ignorance, mental incompetence, or even self-stigma. Her body was a product of historical legacies of socioeconomic inequalities that can easily transform the experiences of living with a chronic disease to those of living with a fatal condition, even when ART is available. This case demonstrates how bodies can be remedied by ART when sufficient social care and structural and material support are provided. Such care and support are essential components that need to be more evenly inserted into the current and heavily biomedicalized disease management system and model of HIV care being used to end AIDS in sub-Saharan Africa (McGrath et al. 2014; Russell et al. 2016).

However, these local ethical and moral dilemmas related to being, becoming, and not wanting to become burdens to others were rarely construed by health professionals as ethical or compassionate gestures toward family and friends. Rather, people who stopped using ART or failed to comply with the requirements associated with living positively were sometimes blamed by others in the community for making poor decisions. In the words of my interlocutors, they were accused of any number of "irrational" behaviors, such as having "stigmatized themselves," holding "faulty" cultural beliefs, and/or suffering "mental disturbances." Employees at the HIV clinic labeled people who missed appointments or stopped taking ART as "defaulters." They were seen as constant "problems" in efforts to end AIDS. These "defaulters" experienced various repercussions for failing to attend clinic appointments. At the end of each session of HIV support groups, a handful of people may be required to stay on, with each person questioned about why he or she had been late to the session or had missed a previous appointment. I overheard people saying that they could not find the transportation funds to make the trip, their employers would not let them take the time off, or that another life event (e.g., a child was graduating) had interfered with clinic attendance. But I also heard the riposte: these were not excuses. Frustrated employees asked, "Is your health not important to you?" After the verbal reprimand, patients were required to be the last seen by the health professionals for the day, a punishment for their negligence with the aim of teaching people not to repeat the error and further socializing them into the chronic disease model and how to live positively.

I do not doubt that employees at the HIV clinic had the best interest of their clients in mind. They did not want patients to run out of their ARTs or to develop resistance to the drugs. The employees were also limited by constraints on the resources at their disposal to address the many barriers that prohibited their clients from keeping appointments. However, by administering the reprimands, they cast blame on individuals for "defaulting" rather than on the social challenges and structural barriers that may have legitimately prevented patients from keeping appointments. As other scholars have pointed out, not everyone in the world is equally capable of living positively (Marsland and Prince 2012). Yet the expectation of doing so persists, sometimes on the part of health care providers, as does the felt and enacted stigma and blame that falls upon those who fail to meet such expectations.

ART AND THE TRANSFORMATION OF STIGMA

People consistently told me that stigma had changed over time. The changes were always linked to the increased presence of global health programs targeting HIV and the opening of the HIV clinic in Mahali. Nearly everyone I spoke with directly expressed a belief that stigma had been reduced, making remarks like "stigma is now going down—it is no longer like [it was] before" and "[stigma] is still there, but it isn't like before." Stigma was not imagined as having been reduced everywhere or equally across Kenya, especially in rural areas. For example, Mercy stated that "stigma is still in the other areas—it seems like people in other areas don't know the modes of transmission other than sex. In the villages, I know the stigma is still there. There are still those problems [because] people don't have the proper information." The challenge for many residents of urban areas was that people were rarely confined to one place. Many were highly mobile—moving about the country, and back and forth between rural and urban spaces—and boundaries were quite porous. This mobility complicated stigma and its experienced uncertainties and dangers. As I described in chapter 3, stigma was not a static characteristic in the minds of individuals, but was uncertain and contingent upon a person's social context, personal network, and situational circumstances (physical, geopolitical, and economic).

When I asked how and why stigma had changed, people mentioned only two things: increased global health education and the rollout of the national ART program. Cherop explained:

Because those last times [referring to early years of the epidemic and the first few years following PEV when ART distribution had been disrupted] . . . people [living with HIV] were totally rejected. But now anyone can live with that person because you cannot even know that the person is sick anymore. So long as the person knows early enough to get [ARTs], no one can ever know! . . . Before, people did not know what the problem was because those medicines were not there. You could always know that person [was HIV+] because . . . the rashes would be there. It could be very bad. But now people can live very well. You cannot even tell they are sick!

Social rejection and stigma were perceived to have been reduced by the introduction of free ARTs, which allows HIV to remain relatively undetectable in a body. This made it nearly impossible to know who to discriminate against or stigmatize. ARTs were viewed not only as having reduced the rates of death and dying in the community, but also as being useful in their ability to conceal what would otherwise eventually become a visibly stigmatizing condition.

What people told me needed to be hidden and concealed was no longer the obvious HIV-infected body, but rather the ARTs that enabled the body to remain healthy and symptom-free. Albert, a long-distance truck driver, who was watching television in Nduta's home when we first met, explained ARTs as follows: "ARTs—no one talks of them. People do not talk about them because then they would be suspected of using [them]. How would you know about them if you did not use them? People do not speak of [ARTs] because they don't want it to be known that they are HIV+."

Mwangi made an especially intriguing statement about how stigma "used to be," before ARTs. He compared the past with the present when he remarked that in the early years of the epidemic, diseased bodies were wrapped in polythene (plastic) both to hide them and to protect others from physical contagion. He continued: "We no longer put bodies in polythene. Now people are hiding the drugs—taking them out of the bottles and putting *them* in the polythene."

My research assistants told me that it was known to be a common practice among patients at the HIV clinic to put their ARTs in a plastic container or envelope and discard the bottle labeled with the name of the drug. The bottles were imbued with and seen as revealing of secrets like a seropositive status (Manderson et al. 2015). Discarding the bottles allowed people to take their ARTs publicly, while claiming that they were suffering from other, less stigmatizing, ailments. Between a bus stop on the highway and the clinic was a path bordered by bushes and littered with people's unwanted ART bottles (see figure 5.2).

The ability to conceal an HIV+ status with ARTs brought both relief and anxiety to people. Locals felt that ARTs had helped the community, because it had drastically reduced the number of deaths. Josphat explained: "Those ARTs are

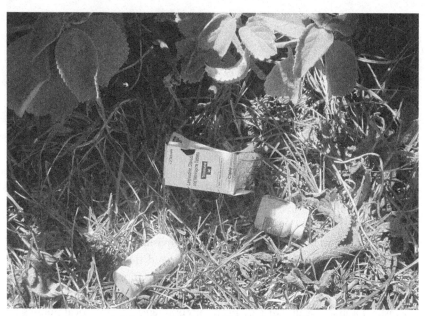

FIGURE 5.2. Antiretroviral drug bottles discarded in the bushes along a path near the HIV clinic in Mahali.

very important because if we [had] no drugs, we could have lost many. People are very grateful to [the HIV clinic] because [since it] came here, we have no deaths anymore.... Earlier, we were burying people every day, but now those [death] rates have gone down. Now it is only like one or two per month! It is very low.... Death now is only from the failure of the drugs." Relief from the number of burials, the restoration of hope for the future, and a boost to local morale were cited as having come along with ARTs. Njeri shared her observations of how the locals felt about ARTs: "People talk good about ARTs and that [HIV clinic]. You know, before, this disease was completely killing. If you were sick, you just died. The truth is that for many...they were revived at [the clinic].... If not for [the clinic] they could have been dead, and [it] may be that their kids would have lost hope in life, but now they are still surviving!"

However, this relief was not without new anxieties for some people. New types of stigmatizing discourses concerned the dangers associated with those living with HIV. The ability of a person to hide being HIV+ because of ARTs made others feel threatened. For example, Omariba, a young truck driver who regularly stayed in Mahali, shared his fear that women in particular using ARTs were more "admirable," and therefore could easily seduce men. From his position, this new form of power given to those living with HIV (or able to hide an HIV+ status) was a leading contributor to the higher rates of infection among men in Mahali and their eventual inability to find a marital partner, since people paid careful attention to others' social and sexual networks. In the container clinic, Omariba told me:

> There are many [people living with HIV] in Mahali. You can just go and look on the person and [she might] be finished [very sick inside] ... [but] ... because she is using medication, when you actually look at her ... face, the legs ... she is admirable. And normally, with men, we do look at the figure.... This lady will then just start to seduce the man, and he takes her home. And when this man comes to the point [later] that he needs marriage, he cannot find one lady in this area [to marry] because everybody [knows] that he slept with an HIV+ woman!

On a handful of occasions, people suggested that ARTs were becoming a problem for locals, because they allowed people to conceal the disease from others and secretly spread it. For many, the potential invisibility of infection provided PLWHIV with power over those not infected, and thus PLWHIV were construed as being particularly dangerous. The viral frictions produced between knowing (increased global and national health testing efforts and the push for disclosure) and concealment (the need for confidentiality and local politics of uncertainty and not telling) produced new sources of anxieties and tensions. This, in turn, intensified local gossip as well as the need to identify who was or might be infected with HIV. Kimaiyo suggested that I think about and really study the issue of ART: "I am positing this challenge, as you do the research on HIV and AIDS. I want you to go back and really study, and really do something about this issue of ARTs. With the ARTs being distributed, [it is] becoming a real setback to the fight against AIDS. So I don't know what you can do about it. But it also brings that other angle where people now feel like, 'ARTs—now we have found our solution!'"

One afternoon in December 2011, I was especially struck by the intensity and persistence of the gossip about and the perceived problem of ART. While I was sitting in a *matatu* and waiting for it to fill up so we could head to Eldoret, I noticed Kibe, a local man, passing by the vehicle with a woman I did not know. Another passenger, Lucy, suddenly made a remark loud enough for others to hear: "I feel sorry for Kibe's new wife. Everyone knows about Wangari [his previous wife]." Other people in the vehicle glanced over and took notice of the new pair. At one point, Wangari had been married to Kibe and they had had two daughters but they later divorced. Locals took it for granted that both Wangari and Kibe were living with HIV. While Lucy probably did not officially know the HIV status of Kibe's new wife, her comment demonstrated local expertise in speaking carefully about matters of sexuality and HIV, as well as the prevention strategy of paying attention to social networks in the context of a stigmatizing epidemic. According to Lucy's logic, her observation of the stranger walking with Kibe evoked the suspicion that the woman had entered the complex sexual history of Wangari and possibly was infected with HIV, which could taint her reputation in pitiable ways. While people often articulated what was emphasized during HIV prevention programs across Kenya—that HIV testing is essential and the only way to know if someone is infected—Lucy's assumption was a common one. After the vehicle was filled and we headed toward Eldoret, I looked out the window and noticed in the distance young Kalenjin men hunting, their bodies smeared with whitish clay showing that they had recently been circumcised and were in a state of liminality, "betwixt and between" (Turner 1967, 93) the social categories of childhood and manhood. I began to think about what they might be learning during this rite of passage. But my thoughts kept returning to the persistence of gossip related to HIV infections and what it would be like to constantly be at the center of such gossip.

THE DANGER OF MENTAL PROBLEMS AND THE "UNPREDICTABLE" MIND

Like Wanja's story, dozens of other interlocutors' narratives showed that stigma had changed since the introduction of ART. Local understanding about stigma had shifted from an original fear of physical contamination and pollution by a body to the fear that a person living with HIV had (or might have) a mental disorder (e.g., depression or a substance abuse disorder) and constant stress (de Klerk and Moyer 2017). In these narratives, the potential unpredictability of the minds of PLWHIV was accentuated. People in Mahali were witnessing and describing the new kinds of social and emotional challenges that accompanied HIV as a chronic condition and the required lifelong management of ART in a resource-poor place. The local experiences with HIV and perceptions of PLWHIV, alongside the advent of global health efforts, were described as dangerous in new ways.

The language of stigma (as well as the psychology of stigma) emanating from HIV and anti-stigma messaging and campaigns focused on the individual level had clearly been adopted by people in Mahali and was used to describe many of those who had been infected. However, the concept did not assume the same mind–body dualisms that tend to dominate Euro-American society and thought. Rather, locals blurred such boundaries in their refusal to imagine the physical body as distinct from both the mind and interpersonal relationships. For example, Joy, a farmer and casual laborer, reported that she rarely felt stigmatized because of HIV. On most days, she claimed, she could keep HIV out of her sense of self, her daily life (except when she needed to take her ART), and her interpersonal relationships. This was not true, Joy claimed, when she became noticeably ill and could not escape her internal feelings of stigma and fears of social abandonment. Whenever she became sick, her usual interpersonal dynamics with others suddenly changed. This, she reasoned out loud, was because people knew she was living with HIV, which meant that her body was "unpredictable" (de Klerk and Moyer 2017, 307), and others also knew that any illness could result in her demise. For Joy, the shift in how others responded to her verbally always made her feel considerably worse, rendering her mind "unpredictable" in ways she described as reducing her health. She recalled the last time she had experienced a shift in her relationships with others: "When I look weak, people say, 'You are about to die.' The last time this happened, it made me cry so much that I became even sicker and I even ended up [in] the hospital!" The state of her social relations with others (and their words) had a very real impact on her mental and physical health experiences associated with this malady.

When asked during an interview to clarify her statement that stigma had changed in recent years, Jane explained the transformation: "The stigma we had early for those infected with HIV—before the *wazungu* [plural of *mzungu*] and the ARTs came—was a big one. People were locked away so they would not infect anyone else. And if people learned that someone had HIV and was having sex with others, the community would kill that person to stop [him or her] from spreading the disease. Also, people [in Mahali] have always hated those with chronic diseases and mental problems. In the past, no one would allow a person with a mental problem to marry into their families—it was taboo." As Jane makes clear, stigma was manifested more intensely early in the epidemic. It took the form of physical isolation—even killing—as a local strategy adopted to stop the spread of the disease before the introduction of ART. Jane's statements about early attitudes toward incurable diseases and mental problems suggested a new manifestation of stigma since "the *wazungu* and the ARTs came" and implemented the chronic disease model. In other words, since the arrival of the global health initiatives (and as talk about the epidemic shifted from describing it as a deadly condition to presenting it as a chronic condition treated with ART), stigma and PLWHIV came to be equated with potential "mental problems." Stigma became manifested in new ways, influenced by global health programming, as local knowledge was used to think about those living with the virus. Bodies were no longer overtly physically isolated but rather were socially differentiated in more subtle ways, such as not being able to find a marital partner (see also chapter 6).

Many people echoed this shift in thinking. For example, one interlocutor recalled: "These days people are trying to accept [HIV]. I can remember stigma [before ART]. Anyone who died of AIDS was put in some polythene papers to send the message [to everyone else] that nobody should come near that body [and by extension, other bodies associated with it—lovers, caregivers, spouses, and so on]. The body was dangerous." In contrast, when people spoke about the predominant type of stigma in Mahali, they did so using the language of the psychology of stigma (importing words, discourses, and logics from briefcase concepts and other global and national health messages). Stigma was described as affecting (or potentially affecting) the minds of particular individuals. At least semantically, this relocated the danger from the physical body to the mind of PLWHIV.

To provide further evidence for this shift, locals mentioned various changes in stigma. Silas, a *boda boda* driver, told me that "nowadays it seems if [people find] that they are HIV+, it is like they get psychologically affected." Dickson, whom I had met at the HIV clinic, appeared surprised when I, as a researcher, asked him to clarify what he meant when he used the term *stigma*, but he defined the process in a similar way: "Stigma. Can I say that stigma is nowadays very psychological? It makes people feel that they are the odd one[s] out in the society, and you feel like you are not liked by other people because of how you are now." Cherop explained that locals were experiencing new forms of "problems nowadays" because of stigma. She offered this justification: "People with HIV have a lot of problems nowadays. They feel despised by the community . . . and because of that . . . , you find that [they now have] troubling thoughts. They have stress and they [suffer] even more sickness!" Some people felt that the psychological problems brought on by an HIV diagnosis made sufferers dangerous, not necessarily because of physical contagion, but because the disease made people likely to behave in morally and socially deviant ways: "If people have HIV, sometimes they are just going around—living in that other way—without even caring. . . . I have heard many stories of people leaving letters when they die of all the people they have infected—intentionally! It is just that they have psychological problems. They get psychological problems, and that does happen here so much." For others, the psychological problems associated with HIV were to blame for the extremely high rates of alcohol consumption that had, in recent years, come to characterize the community, as well as individuals like Wanja who internalized the blame and responsibility for contracting HIV and turned to alcohol to try to cope. In turn, this manifestation of the local "mental disturbances" helped people explain the increasing number of new HIV infections in Mahali. During an impromptu conversation with a group of people, Ibrahim told me rather frankly that he estimated that one-third of the population of Mahali was infected with HIV (people he claimed who had only themselves to blame), and thus he provocatively concluded that they were "insane":

People with HIV start drinking, so they can forget [that they are living with HIV] . . . so they may not be stressed and feel like [they] are in a normal situation [again]. Because . . . you are sick and you know that you are the cause of that sickness and that you have even infected your own wife. What would you do? You start drinking. The moment your wife [discovers] that she is also sick, what will she do? She will come only to have a mental disorder. And that is what makes someone become addicted to alcohol. And that is why you can see that at least one-third of the population in [Mahali]—they are insane!

Likewise, David spoke of his experiences working at the HIV clinic. He construed "testing positive" as a local "emergency." He went on to explain at length that it was an "emergency" because the news that a person was infected with HIV caused him or her to deviate from local norms and the general rules of social interaction because of an ongoing association of the disease as deadly and without a cure—an association that he made, too:

> The emergency of testing positive! I think that is the word—emergency of testing positive. It is an emergency! [It must be] addressed immediately. . . .
>
> There is no stigma. There is the reaction. Everybody will tell you that he was shocked [upon learning he was HIV+]! Okay, okay after the shock, what do you do? Okay, . . . I was shocked. I was shocked to know that I was HIV+. So I started remembering. Who were my girlfriends? Who could have infected me? [But] . . . you don't continue staying in the shock for a year! . . . The shock is you knowing that, knowing that you have a deadly disease. That is only the reason for shock. This is a deadly disease and it has no drugs [that cure it]. That is the only shock. . . .
>
> But after realizing the shock, what do you do after? . . . Many men . . . if they are sincere will tell you, "After I realized I was HIV+, I started suffering." After shock, [you can ask people] "What did you do?" So after the shock, [the] response of the shock. It depends on the individual. Some would think to go and murder themselves. Suicide. Hmm? Drinking spree. Hmm? Causing chaos? Hmm? Start selling everything! Squandering everything. Divorcing! Hmm? Because after the shock, some feel, "I cannot stand telling my wife that I am HIV [positive]. So the best thing is to divorce." Huh? Yes. [You] start chaos with your kids. You isolate yourself. There is [that] isolation. Huh? But all of these are coming because of [the] diagnosis.

For David, stigma was no longer the problem. Rather, the problem was the intrapersonal, psychological reaction of a person learning that he or she was living with HIV—a condition described not as normal but as exceptional and requiring special emotional attention, social support, and care.

In Mahali, stigma, like an HIV diagnosis, evoked notions of uncertainty and potentially dangerous psychological reactions in the context of a country where some scholars have argued that mental health stigma is even greater than the stigma associated with HIV (Jenkins et al. 2013). This cast the HIV-infected body as dangerous in new ways. An infected person allegedly might commit suicide, which was considered a shameful form of death when ART existed; become a "drunkard"; or go about spreading the disease intentionally. ART had the potential to conceal a seropositive status, and this made PLWHIV even more dangerous in the minds of some people living in Mahali. ART brought about new local manifestations of stigma and anxieties.

Although people living in Mahali had access to free, comprehensive HIV treatment and care, they did not all have reliable access to social support, food, or even basic mental health services (beyond counseling on how to cope with HIV and live positively). PLWHIV were told to eat a balanced diet (see Kalofonos 2010; Prince 2012), but many were not able and did not receive the support to do that, despite the fact that links between HIV and mental health disorders had been well documented (Boarts et al. 2006; Ng'ang'a 2011) and support systems were recommended. As Wanja's experience illustrates, this neglects the reality of how diseases, and sometimes their associated stigmas, interact with myriad other diseases and violent social conditions to become syndemic and produce negative health outcomes, especially for the most marginalized individuals in a society (Singer and Clair 2003; Mendenhall 2017; Pfeiffer et al. 2017). Unfortunately, neglect is too often typical of local realities in resource-constrained settings where vertical global health programs prioritize only one or a few diseases over others like mental health disorders (Kleinman 2009), and in the absence of more robust primary health care and health insurance systems. As I demonstrate in the next section, this prioritization, alongside the biomedicalization of HIV, also produced viral frictions.

STIGMA AND THE INJUSTICES OF VERTICAL GLOBAL HEALTH PROGRAMS

Due in part to vertical global health programs, or the very heavily prioritized attention given to HIV by the global health community, PLWHIV were sometimes seen as benefiting unfairly from their health status in ways that uninfected people did not. Consequently, PLWHIV in Mahali were sometimes accused of having infected themselves on purpose, as an immoral strategy designed to illegitimately gain access to the perceived privileges and wealth being inequitably distributed at the HIV clinic. Vertical global health programming and information thus moved out horizontally (Benton 2015) to mix with local knowledge and national politics to produce new and unexpected tensions and interactions between PLWHIV and those who did not have the virus.

While community members and employees at the HIV clinic at times inadvertently blamed individuals for their "mental problems" and/or "defaulting" or failing to live positively, I also noted a general discourse within the community that those living with HIV were believed to be the most well-off residents. Although ironic, these discourses mirrored findings from quantitative studies in the region that reported a higher quality of living and less depression among PLWHIV on ART compared with their uninfected peers, likely due to having access to better health care (Martin et al. 2013; Negin et al. 2013; Russell et al. 2016). In Mahali, the rationale behind this belief was based on the local perception and sometimes experience that global health initiatives offered their clients a multitude of benefits and advantages, to which people who were not infected did not have access, a phenomenon that also has been documented among people living in refugee camps in northern Uganda (Wilhelm-Solomon 2013). Some community members felt that HIV+ patients were unfairly prioritized over those who were HIV- simply because there was treatment for HIV (see also Kaler and Watkins 2010; Moyer and Hardon 2014). For example, Mercy spoke of the benefits and attention that PLWHIV received in the community, noting that this produced distinctions and inequalities between those who were infected and those who were not: "Those who have HIV and AIDS are much better than us because they are treated so well. A lot of care is given to them! They get a lot of attention. Even when someone is sick, he doesn't need to pay any money to be treated! For example, if he has typhoid, he just goes to the hospital. He is diagnosed and given drugs [snaps her fingers]. Free!" Another woman told me that PLWHIV had greater access to employment opportunities, her resentment palpable as she thrice referred to people working at the HIV clinic as "sick" and refused to imagine their health as restored on ART: "The staff working at [the HIV clinic] are really the sick people [those living with HIV]. So they cannot be greeted by somebody like me [who is not infected with HIV and looking for a job]. Like I have children [and am single], but I cannot go to [the HIV clinic] and get a job. They are favoring those who are sick. [They] only hire those who are sick so they can help themselves. I cannot be given that type of employment."

In a community marked by extreme poverty, inequitably distributed wealth and other resources, and an inadequate and compromised general public health care system (with the exception of HIV care programs), PLWHIV were perceived to have access to monies being channeled into the country by international donors. Consequently, they were believed to benefit in ways construed as unjust. Sharon explained what happened when someone was seen talking to a person known to be living with HIV. She pointed to what were most threatened in Mahali—health, opportunities for an improved life, and money—for both the stigmatized and those doing the stigmatizing that helped to justify and sustain the logic behind the practice of excluding and avoiding PLWHIV among those who were not infected:

If someone is HIV and AIDS and you are seen talking to him or her, after that person disperses and you have finished your discussion ... someone [will tell] you to "Take care!" They will whisper to you, "You know that man [has] HIV and AIDS? He is not normal. So [avoid] him!" Then, if it is a woman—a friend of yours—and someone finds you drinking a cup of tea in her house, she will call you and tell you, "Don't you know that person is HIV and AIDS?" It is not fair for you to be drinking in that house because you don't know what is the content of her sickness. Maybe she [has] TB [tuberculosis], and you can get it. Because she is also HIV+, she will get her free treatment—but you, living without HIV, you will be eaten [financially destroyed] getting rid of your TB!

Another related stigmatizing discourse that intersected with class inequalities and politics was the fact that PLWHIV were sometimes suspected of having been infected on purpose, so they could receive benefits and attention through global health research projects and clinical trials. One of my interlocutors suggested that people strategically became infected so they could benefit from the global health projects at the HIV clinic: "People talk very much about people [living with HIV and AIDS]. They say that somebody has HIV because he is too sexed or because he is ignorant. Others say that people contracted the virus intentionally so they could be used by and benefit from the researchers. People do gossip about researchers because they say when a person talks to a researcher, they are infected because that is why the researcher wants to talk to them. People living with HIV are treated positively—they are given much more attention by the medical community."

The tensions between infected and uninfected residents, especially regarding the perceived inequitable distribution and acquisition of resources, sometimes made its way into the experiences of PLWHIV. In particular, the beliefs circulating about global and national health programs' providing free care and other humanitarian benefits sometimes produced viral frictions in the lives of those who lived with the virus but did not receive any of those provisions, beyond the distribution of free ART. As Charity, a casual laborer, and I sat in a consultation room at the HIV clinic, she spoke of the contradictions produced in her own life as local beliefs butted against global and national realities and the limitations of foreign aid and relief. She presented herself as existing in a state of liminality and of having fallen in the cracks of uncertainty produced by local, national, and global efforts. Charity described her fear of being pushed out of her "social space" within the chronic disease paradigm (McGrath et al. 2014, 314). Caught in a state of "continuous uncertainty" (Moyer and Hardon 2014, 267), she felt depressed, stuck at the margins of care, and unable to "ascribe clear meaning to the life that had been saved" by ART (Moyer 2015, 269). Her moral world was confused and her life and future were uncertain, as she described:

I am depressed. . . . I am okay with the medicines, but the appetite is so much. But I am given no food. I am not supported because my husband says that I must go to my brothers for support. But the brothers say, "No—you must go to the husband." My father says that the HIV clinic gives free food, money, and medicine, so I should be going there. But I do not get money there. My family does not give me support for transportation to get my ART, and so they don't want to be associated with me anymore. . . . They say they don't care if I eat or not, because I am on my way [dying]. Everyone thinks I am on my way [dying].

This kind of talk about food and people being cut off from it exposes inequalities (Prince 2012), even when the body is "okay with the medicines." As Steven Russell and Janet Seeley (2010) have argued, returning to normal life for many people on ART is plagued by economic insecurity in Uganda. In the age of treatment, sometimes people are "expelled" from all essential social networks because of "economics and geopolitics" (Moyer 2015, 261). The notion that PLWHIV were pampered and fed at the HIV clinic and by international organizations was thus a convenient way for their families, friends, and other community members to withdraw their support and resources. Their reactions also were about jealousy—related to the uneven distribution of resources—and served as a local form of self-preservation in a resource-poor place. This toxic combination of factors contributed to the persistence of HIV stigma.

6 · "WHAT HAS HAPPENED TO YOU?"

HIV and the (Re)Making of Moral Personhood

In *Stigma: Notes on the Management of Spoiled Identity*, Erving Goffman (1963, 3) highlights the relationship between stigma and personhood when he defines a stigmatized person as someone "possessing an attribute that makes him different from others in the category of persons available for him to be, and of a less desirable kind. . . . He is thus reduced in our minds from a whole and usual person to a tainted discounted one." But what does it mean to be a "whole and usual person" or a "tainted discounted one"? This chapter centers on these questions and opens with a story of two siblings, Martin and Ruth, to provide an important backdrop for expanding the analysis of HIV-related stigma using the analytical lens of personhood in sub-Saharan Africa. During my research, I observed and participated alongside Ruth as she extended the robust social support and care necessary to help mend her brother's physical and mental health and well-being, as well as his social and moral personhood that had been temporarily damaged by an untreated HIV infection. In this chapter, I emphasize the challenges that processes of HIV stigma brought to people who were "neither ill nor back to normal life" (de Klerk and Moyer 2017, 315) but who were socialized—through global and national HIV programming aimed at ending AIDS—to occupy new liminal social spaces (McGrath et al. 2014). These socialization efforts, as they interacted with shifting local ideas about—and generational conflicts related to understandings of—how the world works, I argue, created social tensions that influenced the lines being (re)drawn around who was a normal person (or not). As the case of Martin will begin to illuminate, some people found new ways to develop, construct, and imagine themselves and their identities that demonstrate how HIV and stigma were slowly transforming local subjectivities and socialities and creating new forms of therapeutic citizenship that are revealing of viral frictions.

One day, as I was walking toward her house, Ruth appeared at the wooden gate of her compound and said, "I have been telling you that AIDS stigma has gone down, but here it is again in my own house!" Her elder brother, Martin, had come to Mahali from the opposite side of the country: he had become very ill and needed a family member to care for him. Ruth had agreed to take on this task and, using money from her own pocket, had hired someone to replace her temporarily at work so she could stay home to care for Martin and not lose her job. She had cleaned out a tiny, dark food storage area and added a single bed that almost filled the entire room in preparation for Martin's arrival. Ruth told me that Martin was normally quite robust but had lost almost 50 percent of his weight.

As the story went, Martin's house helper in Kitui had called his wife, Patience, who lived in Nairobi, to report that he had not left the house compound for many days. Instead, he had been seen "drinking heavily," "refusing to eat," and even "locking himself in his own room." Patience had called Ruth and asked her to help investigate the situation. Ruth then contacted another relative to bring Martin to Mahali, where she would get to the bottom of what had been described as unusual, suicidal-type behaviors and care for Martin. In this case, Martin's health and well-being were a family affair.

Ruth spent the first day with Martin at a large public hospital, where a rapid test confirmed what had been silently suspected: he was living with HIV. They were referred to an HIV clinic for more extensive services. Ruth was convinced that her brother already had full-blown AIDS, evidenced by his severe wasting, but she could not say such a thing out loud because it would be inappropriate for her to do so as his younger sibling and because he was "already so down" (very sick). According to Ruth's logic, this rendered Martin more vulnerable to stress and other "mental disturbances" that she, like others, believed were caused and/or aggravated by negative news. Although Ruth suspected that Martin already knew he was infected, she believed he could not say directly to her or his wife, "I am HIV+," because of a conviction that delivering such direct news was rude and could potentially devastate another person. Ruth figured that Martin had used the more subtle strategy of letting the HIV test communicate to her what was going on. She wanted him to attend the HIV clinic in Mahali—where she believed there was less stigma than any other place—since "everybody in the community is already either infected or affected." But just as important, the services provided at the local clinic were described as superior to those provided elsewhere in Kenya.

Patience had not been told that Martin was living with HIV, and Ruth kept silent and denied possessing such information, engaging in an elaborate process of what Whyte (2014, 35) has described as "knowledge management." Ruth rationalized that it would be an inappropriate time to disclose such information, given all the tension, the geographic distance between husband and wife, and especially the uncertainty of the situation (that is, the unknown outcome for Martin). She also did not know what Patience might do with the information. Her reaction could be dangerous, even deadly, if the news "disturbed her mind." What seemed to have complicated matters even more for Ruth was the fact that the last time she had seen Patience, she recalled that Patience had also lost a significant amount of weight, which meant that Patience might also already be infected with the virus. From Ruth's perspective, any direct suggestion that a person had engaged in sexual relations with someone infected with the disease could suddenly shock a person to the point of death. Thus, the bearer of the news would be responsible for the other person's ill health and possible demise. As Corinne Squire (2015) argues, sometimes people conceal rather than share private information, not with the intension to harm, but instead to prevent potentially devastating consequences that can accompany the direct revelation of secrets.

Soon after Martin arrived at Ruth's house, she asked me to get him a few costly food items from a larger city that would be good for him but could not be purchased in Mahali—imported oranges and Ribena, a drink made from black currants, that would boost his immune function and morale. When I brought the items to her, she presented them to Martin, introduced me to him, and left us to talk. I found his cramped room, with the single window closed, hot and stuffy. Still, a large hole in the window let in a dusty beam of sunlight that illuminated Martin's shivering body under several wool blankets. Although he appeared uncomfortable, he graciously thanked me for the items. I was glad that he was in Ruth's home and not sharing a hospital bed with another person, which was sometimes necessary at the public hospital when wards became overcrowded with patients. After I had spent a short time visiting with Martin, Ruth came and ushered me out of the room. Apparently, a handful of friends and neighbors had also come to give their regards to Martin. The guests had been seated in Ruth's living area while I chatted with Martin and, according to Ruth, "had started whispering about why [I] was taking so long." She told me that this could inadvertently (and nonverbally) expose the fact that Martin had HIV, because *wazungu* were always especially interested in that particular disease and those infected with it. This latter statement underscored the oversaturation of global health experts who had disproportionately focused on HIV and had been passing through Mahali for some time. Ruth was very carefully and strategically navigating the public perceptions of her brother.

Over the next several months, Ruth spent significant amounts of time and money and leveraged a noteworthy amount of social and cultural capital by attracting physicians and other health care professionals to come and offer home services to Martin. I was simultaneously impressed and overwhelmed by the resources and energy expended by Ruth, who fortunately had the means and social networks to care for her brother in that way. But I was also disheartened to see firsthand the realities of what was needed to manage and maintain quality care for someone who was so ill, especially given that most people lacked access to such resources.

Ruth helped administer Martin's prescribed ART, which she carefully wrapped in a plastic bag and stored behind dishes and various other items at the back of a large cupboard on one wall in the main living area. (The cupboard is an artifact in Kenyan homes that often symbolizes that a woman has married: it is a common engagement gift prepared and given to a newlywed woman, usually by her mother, to start a new household.) After taking ART, Martin very slowly grew stronger and gained weight until finally he was able to go back to his home and return to his job with the Kenyan postal service. He would make the lengthy commute and return to Mahali each month for an appointment at the HIV clinic, which would help ensure his privacy. Martin was pleased by the fact that no one in Mahali ever looked sick, including those waiting in line at the clinic. And it was true: it was rare to see an extremely ill patient at the clinic. ARTs had restored many of the physical bodies that passed through—something that brought great relief to those living in Mahali and significantly reduced overt expressions of social stigma. Martin also felt that the clinic seemed to really respect the privacy of patients and that people (including other patients) were encouraging and supportive. Such experiences, Martin reasoned, could not be duplicated in clinics closer to his home, where he had heard horror stories about the maltreatment of HIV patients. I had also read such reports in the media—stories highlighting the tragic effects of stigma across the country, like the forced sterilization of HIV+ women in one community and the firing of a man in another town because of his seropositive status. These examples were consistent reminders that stigma was a possibility in Kenya and that people should be wary of its uncertainties and potential dangers.

Martin's caregiving story, while exceptional in many regards, is important in that it points to the centrality of the linked management of HIV, caregiving, social relationships, and other nonmedical aspects of well-being (Russell et al. 2016) that are essential to sustaining human existence and processes of person-hood everywhere. I met Martin after he had purportedly attempted suicide by drinking heavily and not eating, which reflects the perceived corporeal and social death (the felt, experienced, and/or anticipated loss of a sense of normal-ity and thus a diminished sense of personhood) that accompanied the infection. But the strategic, careful, costly, and long-term commitment to support him made by Ruth and others within Martin's social and kin network also protected his personhood and preserved his life and psyche. While ART was certainly responsible for improving Martin's physical health, it alone could not have accomplished the equally important work of repairing his social and moral per-sonhood. In sub-Saharan Africa, PLWHIV with consistent access and deter-mined adherence to ART can have the same life expectancy as those who are not infected with HIV (Mills et al. 2011). Yet as we have seen, due to conditions of political and gender-based violence, uncertainty, and poverty, HIV remains a challenging condition to manage (McGrath et al. 2014; Moyer and Hardon 2014). Because all human lives are composed of mutually constituting processes— biological, social, moral, historical, psychological, political, economic, and linguistic (through storytelling and people's words)—medical anthropologists often use a holistic, or biosocial, approach to make sense of and understand human health, the body, and healing in societies around the globe. This is the theoretical imperative behind conceptualizing novel, holistic ways to eradicate stigma, one that can get lost in the intense biomedicalization of HIV, discourses about ending AIDS and HIV as a chronic disease, and efforts to normalize an exceptional condition in a resource-limited place.

PERSONHOOD, HIV, CURSES, AND SOCIAL CHANGE IN SUB-SAHARAN AFRICA

What constitutes a "whole and usual person" (Goffman 1963, 3) can be understood only in relation to the larger social and structural contexts into which a physical body is born and embedded (Rosaldo 1980; M. Jackson and Karp 1990; Carrithers, Collins, and Lukes 1996; C. Piot 1999). Simply having a human body and being human are not the essence of personhood. Rather, personhood is about having a human body and being human in relation to others in particular and meaningful ways (Landsman 2009). Consequently, anthropologists have come to conceive of personhood, like stigma, as a process. Meyer Fortes (1973, 287) argued that becoming a person is never a passive act but instead requires the individual to "appropriate the qualities and capacities, and the norms governing [personhood's] expression to himself." It is hard work to become a person, a task that is socially learned and accomplished through the broader culture available to and the messages that surround us. We depend on other people to teach us how to be (or how not to be) in the world. Some individuals can be viewed as more or less human than others (Goffman 1963; Whyte and Ingstad 1995; Landsman 2009), as persons are placed in hierarchies that are contingent and can lead to contentious power struggles that are played out both within and between individuals. Such processes are further complicated as people seek to make their ways and develop themselves into legitimate persons in communities that are embedded in countries (like Kenya) with complex histories and that are experiencing rapidly shifting social, economic, and political conditions brought on by globalization. For the remainder of this chapter, I emphasize the ways that ideas about and experiences with HIV, the body, caregiving, and processes of stigma and personhood converged and were transformed at the nexus of local, national, and global circulating discourses and practices.

In their classic article on the topic in sub-Saharan Africa, John Comaroff and Jean Comaroff (2001, 271) argue that personhood was conceived of and enacted as a complex and lifelong process of "being-through-becoming." Using the case of Tswana adults in South Africa, they argue that persons worked to "build themselves up" by "acquiring wealth in [relationships with] people" and by protecting themselves from enemies and rivals (270). The Comaroffs write: "Construction of 'the person' was a constant work-in-progress . . . no self could be static. Stasis meant social death." These anthropologists contend that people built themselves up relationally through the "great works" that they accomplished (271). "Great works," the authors suggest, depend on social ties and are accomplished through hard labor, such as employment, farming, participation in rituals, and marriage. In Mahali, I found that PLWHIV and those who were HIV− engaged in this praxis of self-construction in their everyday activities and social interactions. I noted that people still attempted to "build themselves up" as individuals by pursuing "great works"—mediated by their ethnic, economic, generational, and gendered positions—by marrying, reproducing, raising offspring, farming, caring for and being generous to others, practicing their faith, and engaging in business, to name a few of life's important endeavors in this setting. However, the ways people went about accomplishing these shared and important life goals were varied and sometimes produced social tensions and conflicts between people and groups.

To the Comaroffs (2001, 272), processes of "becoming" persons were complex and exceedingly dangerous, as the construction of the self was constantly under threat from countervailing forces that could terminate self-production. Since the body was not imagined to be limited to the corporeal body—but rather was defined through the sum of all relationships (seen and unseen) encountered by the body—personhood was felt to be constantly at risk and vulnerable. Accordingly, the only time a person stopped "becoming" was when he or she fell "victim" to witchcraft or was "eaten" by someone or something more powerful, at which point the person became absorbed by a new personality. Stacey Langwick (2011, 90) might refer to these unfortunate processes in East Africa as explainable through the notion of a "malady of person."

As in many cultures, in Kenya and elsewhere in sub-Saharan Africa, eating is often a reference to sex. The term *eating* can also be used as a metaphor for one person (or something more powerful) inflicting harm (sometimes financial) on another person (John Comaroff and Jean Comaroff 2001; Rödlach 2006). In addition to referring to the provision of nourishment to a body, discussions centering on food and/or feeding can demarcate social relationships while also implying the duties, responsibilities, and obligations between those who eat together or feed one another (C. Piot 1999). Put another way, talk about one person offering food to or feeding another can be a statement about social ties, caregiving, and thus the composition of one's own personhood. Conversely, any mention of not being fed or of being made to eat food alone in some contexts is about inequality (Prince 2012) and can be an articulation of not belonging and/

or of a disintegration of social (often kin) ties, and therefore of a potentially diminished personhood. People in Mahali sometimes spoke of being "eaten" by external forces or not being fed or having to "eat alone" if they had HIV. Once, while caring for Martin, Ruth made a fleeting comment about being "eaten" by HIV. She was not making a literal statement about a virus in her body. Instead, she was making a statement about the financial and emotional drain that caregiving was taking on her own, finite resources.

Among numerous ethnic groups across eastern Africa, there are documented common threads related to conceptualizations of the body as intimately tied to ideas about personhood, health, and disease causation (Cogburn, Strong, and Wood 2019). For example, as described by the Comaroffs (2001), people are sometimes imagined as having an individual, physical body that is linked to a broader social body. Explanations about the etiology of an illness can thus be construed as the result of either a physiological problem or a disturbance of the social body. Consequently, various health problems, including those related to infertility or complicated pregnancies, might be explained as the consequence of violated social or moral norms, such as committing adultery, failing to share resources for the good of the group, or making incomplete bridewealth payments (Allen 2002; Cogburn, Strong, and Wood 2019). In my own research, while sharing the story of the birth of her third child, Leah explained the source of her difficult and prolonged labor as connected to her mother-in-law's being unhappy about the pregnancy, which caused the unborn baby to feel unwelcomed:

> The labor was very complicated, and I was very much worried I would be taken to the theater [taken to the operating room for a C-section], which I could not afford. It was like there was something that was going on. You know sometimes in Kikuyu . . . because I am a Kikuyu, we have beliefs that if one of the parents is not happy with the pregnancy, there will be something wrong with the baby coming out. Unless the parent releases you. So I thought that maybe something [like this was] happening. There is somebody who is rejecting the baby now. So the baby feels that he or she is not welcomed. And so when my mother[-in-law] came and saw me [in the hospital], I thought she had something to do with this.

As described in chapter 3, there has been a decline in the conceptualization of HIV as caused by others and outside malicious forces, which aggravated stigma and placed blame on individuals who contracted HIV. According to Langwick (2011, 156), this sort of decline represents "a world in which life is increasingly conceived of through modern notions of persons and bodies that are self-contained rather than relational." I suggest that these new conceptualizations of HIV reflect a shift to viewing it as a malady of God brought on by an individual's actions.

Still, a growing body of anthropological work on HIV in the era of treatment in eastern Africa centers on PLWHIV as "embodied subjects" and emphasizes that patients still experience the (in)abilities of their bodies in relation to the state of their social relations (Whyte 2014, 11; see also de Klerk and Moyer 2017). Sometimes people from various ethnic groups claimed that HIV was perceived as the result of a "curse from God." While curses were documented in early ethnographic accounts in Kenya (Kenyatta 1962; Langley 1979), this kind of talk led me to inquire about its more contemporary meanings. I began by asking a research assistant to help me better understand the concept, to which her initial response was, "When people say that, that is a serious one—it means the person has done something that was very wrong." We added a question about curses to our follow-up semistructured interviews and learned that intergenerational tensions were an important aspect of understanding how curses were imagined to play out in the context of a community experiencing rapid social and structural changes. This sentiment was echoed by several interlocutors. An herbalist remarked: "You know, the older generation thinks that this disease [HIV] is a curse. It is a total curse. It has come to clear the next generation. So the old people are very much worried about this curse . . . that God has sent to clear the world. And what they are really saying is that people have become such sinners and that God is angry [with] them. So HIV is the wrath to them." Others suggested that curses from God were the result of individuals who engaged in behaviors that defied the moral teachings of their elders: "Curses come from parents—you cannot be cursed by a stranger—it is the parent who can either curse or bless you." Talk of people being "cursed" was one way of articulating the tensions and conflict between generations as a consequence of globalization and development in Kenya.

The decision to curse could be based on the "child" (regardless of actual age) being perceived by a parent or another relative or ancestor to have blatantly disobeyed or disrespected a kin member—for example, a person who had engaged in an activity or behavior that went against the wishes of the parents or other members of the family, such as marrying a person a parent did not approve of or, more recently, cohabiting with a partner instead of being officially married. Cohabitation had become quite common in Kenya, especially when economic constraints made it difficult for people to afford marriage. I also observed and overheard parents arguing with their daughters about the clothes they were wearing. Some people complained about schoolgirls wearing "trousers" or slacks and skirts that exposed their knees and thighs, which they described as unacceptable and evidence of a moral decline among Kenyan youth. These kinds of anxieties were exacerbated through the media, including a set of news stories that circulated in 2012 after a reported protest about uniforms at a secondary school in the central region of the country. The protestors were later suspended for allegedly demanding their right to wear "miniskirts" to school. This news sparked controversy, outrage, and debate among educators, politicians, faith leaders, and citizens in general. A sense of moral panic was further fueled when Education Minister Mutula Kilonzo publicly supported the protestors with a statement that went viral across a variety of media outlets: "I am in total agreement with them [students]. Why do you dress a schoolgirl like a nun? These girls do not want to be nuns; they want to be modern!" (quoted in Macha 2012).

Another reason for a curse was violation of social and cultural norms and expectations. These violations might come in the form of sexual deviance like rape, adultery, or sex work or as breaking other taboos such as those against murder or inflicting other harm intentionally on another person. Gladys, whose family lived in a rural community just outside the urban center of Mahali, had invited me to join her to visit her niece, who had just had a baby. As we journeyed to the home where the niece was recovering after giving birth, carrying the typical gifts of sugar, soap, rice, cooking oil, and new baby clothes, Gladys offered an example of how she imagined curses that echoed the "discredited" status of women who engaged in sex work and were treated as "not quite human" (Goffman 1963, 5), even in death: "Sex workers are believed to be cursed [for violating social norms]. When a person is found in the family to be a sex worker, she can become excommunicated because that is taboo work. We just had a sex worker [in the community] who died recently, and no one in her family even came to the burial, which is [the result of] a curse."

Curses were not only associated with blatant disobedience toward a parent and/or a violation of social norms. In addition, they could be sent if people were perceived to be failing to perform their respective duties, which were shaded by issues of ethnicity, age, and gender, among other factors. One Kalenjin man gave the following example of why a parent might send a curse to offspring: "If you are a man and have a farm, it is good to cultivate. The man is to be the provider. . . . He must work hard to see that his family has clothes, that they have eaten, and that they have been educated. Because he is the head, he must provide it all. That is the law . . . and if you don't play your part . . . that is a curse."

As HIV testing was increasingly promoted in the area, people described being asked to reflect not only on their own past and behaviors but also on those of others in ways that felt individualizing and sometimes mentally taxing. One woman spoke about the tendency of locals to engage in such reflections: "People are saying that [HIV] is a curse. So they have to ask themselves, 'Where did this disease come from? What is the origin?' Some will say that HIV came to them because of something that happened in the past. So people do spend their time trying to figure out what happened." Because of the economy, especially since PEV, many women and men were often unable to perform some of their normal duties. Curses served to explain why some people were unable to uphold their respective social obligations and provided a way of making sense of how previous individual actions—in relation to their social roles, expectations, and relationships—were linked to present circumstances. These evaluations extended to those who contracted HIV in ways that sometimes heaped blame on and scapegoated infected people. Still, some people felt that there was little they could do to remedy the effects of curses. Mwangi once spoke of this inability as a violent social conundrum thrust upon people in Mahali that kept residents just out of reach of being considered fully enlightened, and morally good Kenyan citizens: "It is like we are stuck in the middle—we no longer know our traditions, but we also aren't fully modern yet."

HIV AND TRANSFORMING LOCAL SUBJECTIVITIES

Chepchirchir, who was living with HIV when we first met in 2012, was in my view a very successful woman. In her fifties, she had been educated and had a high-paying job. Her family had land, and she had raised and educated her children. Chepchirchir was a widow and still in good standing with her in-laws. She was able to provide for her family members and therefore also able to fulfill her moral obligations to others. At various points in our time together, I asked her about her experiences of being diagnosed with and seeking care and treatment for HIV. While the experiences had not been easy, she maintained that living with HIV had never caused any noteworthy or troubling experiences with another person (among her kin or in her church, professional, or other social networks), with her medications, or in her work. I connected this positive outlook and attitude to the fact that Chepchirchir worked in the AIDS industry. She disclosed her seropositive status freely and did not live with the constant fear that someone might see her taking ART or using services at the clinic. On a handful of occasions, she repeated that she had never been bothered by, felt, or experienced any episodes of stigma or discrimination. I was surprised, therefore, when she added the following comment at the end of our time together: "For now, I continue on with my [antiretroviral] treatment [for HIV]. But I long for a brighter future where I will be the same with other people again." With this comment, Chepchirchir gave voice to the social space opened up by ART for people who were neither sick nor normal (McGrath et al. 2014; de Klerk and Moyer 2017). Living in this liminal space fueled and sustained intrapersonal feelings of not being "the same with other people," as well as more intense forms of self-stigma for some (but not all) PLWHIV.

Not feeling "the same" or normal was a common sentiment articulated in many of the stories I collected among PLWHIV. For example, Wanja described turning to alcohol after a long string of stressful life events, including an HIV diagnosis, and she concluded that "I was nothing . . . something different." One man explained that when "[you have] that disease . . . you . . . are hated because you have done something that was not normal." Many of these types of comments echoed the content of circulating gossip about PLWHIV that I describe in preceding chapters. Kipkemboi—a young man who had traveled from Nairobi to attend the HIV clinic in Mahali, where no one knew him—recalled his recent diagnosis as not only a personal crisis, but also as a dangerous rite of passage or a realization that he had become a completely different person:

> It is a really hard experience. It is very serious. And it is very, very dangerous. You fear very much that anyone might come to know ... because they will start announcing to everyone [whispering]: "Someone is sick!" And then the discrimination will start. Slowly people will start to fear you. Slowly people will be avoiding you. And you know for me, it is really dangerous because I am young. I am not married yet. I do not have kids. And I do not yet have a job. If people find out that I am HIV+, they will have to ask, "What has happened to you?"

For Kipkemboi and others, the potential threat of being avoided and cut off from various forms of social and interpersonal relationships (for example, marriage or cohabitation, having children, and finding employment) because of an HIV+ diagnosis evoked a sense of danger and of being abnormal, and therefore it was a potential marker of the beginning signs of the breakdown of the person (see also Lock and Nguyen 2010). While notions of personhood in Kenya were slowly changing because of global processes, social relationships were still believed to be at the heart of and ultimately responsible for transforming a human body, over time, into a legitimate, respected, and normal adult. Having HIV, therefore, often made people feel not normal. As Kipkemboi stated, it potentially set people apart from others, cutting them off from some of the most significant forms of social relations considered essential to cultivation of the person. What HIV most threatened for Kipkemboi (especially because he was a young man) were his social relationships. That threat was related to his own shifting sense of identity as a normal person, and he anticipated those around him beginning to openly question him about this transition: "What has happened to you?"

Understanding this logic helps make sense of statements by PLWHIV that they would "take the pledge" or "die alone." "The pledge" was a formal promise that they would not engage in certain activities of normal social life as a way of protecting other people in the community. These were common statements made by people to indicate that they had accepted the fact that they were destined for lives that would be (in various ways) segregated from particular domains of social life and marital and kin relations. Like the lifestyle change requirements associated with living positively, taking such a pledge (formally or informally) would make any person feel different. Conversely, some people—such as those who were imagined to have gone on rampant "spreading sprees"—were frequently characterized as "refusing" such a pledge and not wanting or refusing to "die alone." This latter description was used to negatively reference and identify a particularly dangerous person in the community because of his or her refusal to become the (somewhat sexually and sometimes financially) isolated individual that locals believed he or she needed to be for the safety and betterment of the community.

Sometimes people spoke about the negative, unintended consequences of the HCT program, when HIV counselors circulated throughout the community offering in-home testing and counseling. Citing examples of social disruptions as evidence, several people claimed that the HCT campaign was a "disaster." For example, Chepkorir, a secondary school teacher, spoke of the importance of local social and moral rules and concerns about preferred ways of talking about sensitive information. In particular, she discussed how HIV results should be disclosed, advice should be given, and trust should be established and maintained within the hierarchies of a household. She complained that the HCT counselors violated these basic social norms and rules by ignoring people's ethnic, linguistic, and generational backgrounds and marital status. To further illustrate her point, Chepkorir explained the negative, unintended consequences during HCT when an HIV test revealed a sexual mishap involving an older woman in her rural community:

> During the HCT testing, this [grandmother] came to realize that she was HIV+.... Now this lady is so embarrassed.... Now everyone knows that grandma is HIV!... [S]he talks very badly now ... [and] tells her children ..., "Bring me food!" because ... she was told that when you have [HIV], you need to eat properly. "I need to eat! I need to eat! Bring me food!" And sometimes she refuses to pick up her *jembe* [tool used for subsistence farming].... "[Grandma], what is wrong with you?" [Her reply:] "The HIV has [kept me from working on] the [farm]!"... It is like she has become mentally disturbed [and] traumatized. I think this HIV and AIDS thing needs to be handled with a bit more confidentiality.

Chepkorir seemed to believe that the HCT campaign facilitated the grandmother's engagement in a particular "sick role" performance (Parsons 1951, 440)—of living positively, evidenced by her refusal to participate in labor and demand for extra food and attention. Therefore, HCT opened a space through which she could be exempted from conforming to social and cultural norms and performing roles and household duties. At the same time, HCT was characterized as "traumatizing" and offering the grandmother a new set of responsibilities beyond the clinic and in her home—as a good patient who engaged in self-care—to live healthily with an exceptional, chronic condition. Chepkorir's call for "more confidentiality" seems to be rooted less in a concern about individual human rights and more in anxiety about and reaction against the counselors and the local contradictions they produce. She believed that HIV disclosure and the recommended lifestyle changes among those infected could socially disrupt an entire household in an economically and politically vulnerable community.

PERSONHOOD IN WORK, MARRIAGE, AND REPRODUCTION

As Kipkemboi pointed out, three of the biggest threats to the development of a person living with HIV were failing to find work and sexual partners and to secure and/or maintain a spouse. While ART helped many individual bodies physically feel more normal, people still faced social challenges that interfered with both interpersonal relationships and their intrapersonal sense of being normal when compared to others. For example, when I sat in the HIV clinic with Achola as she described her recovery process after starting medication, she said that she felt more like a real person then, albeit with one exception: she knew she could no longer engage in intimate relations with others in the same way as normal people did. Abstaining from sexual relationships to ensure that she did not infect others was an ethical concern and priority for Achola as she endeavored to be a moral person. During our time together, she also morally comforted herself and negotiated with God, using the fact that she had not behaved badly as a wife or engaged in sex work when she contracted the virus that, in combination with ART, helped restore her sense of being a "real person":

> ARTs have made me feel more like a real person. I have started to gain weight and am feeling the body is healthy. I was feeling that my body [did not] want to work anymore. I was feeling tired. But now I am more like a real person . . . [because] if I am feeling bad and not like a person, it is of no help. The one thing I tell God, "I know I didn't prostitute [myself] to have this sickness—I was in the house [a married and faithful woman] when it got me. I will not infect someone [else]." I will stay alone that way [abstaining from sex] until God does what he wants with me.

Work and Making Money

The challenges of earning a living in Kenya were greater for PLWHIV than for others and made them worry about the normalcy of their personhood. Despite the claims I heard throughout my research that PLWHIV were more readily hired in the AIDS industry (see chapter 5), I noted a simultaneous public perception that PLWHIV could not remain employed once their status became known by others. As one man said rather matter-of-factly, "If your employer knows that you are HIV+, you will get sacked. And who wants to be sacked in today's economy?" In a similar way, Dorcas, an employee at the HIV clinic, spoke about the experiences of her clients with regard to work. She emphasized the trouble that women had in finding and maintaining employment as house helpers. She told me that "no one wants an HIV+ to look after their kids! If anyone finds out [you are HIV+], they will chase you away. But if no one knows, then you are just okay." I believe that this belief came from common knowledge that female house helpers sometimes had sexual relations with their male employers or teenage boys living in the household. Knowing that a house girl was living with HIV would be like "inviting the disease into the family," as some people put it. Yet, this tacit framing ignored the behaviors of the men and boys living in the households that employed house helpers, thereby absolving them of responsibility and shifting the blame to young women as the source of new infections. Felix, a police officer, reiterated this belief, adding:

> A big challenge for people [living with HIV]—for those who have some form of employment, if they are formally employed—whenever the boss discovers that this person is HIV+, they are normally sacked. They are put off. . . . Especially in some sectors—the hotels [restaurants], employment at home [house help]— whereby people feel that [the employee is] becoming a threat to their children and their social setting [restaurant or house]. They are just dismissed. Because [the employee with HIV is] a threat, once [the employer has] big boys at home or if it is a male employer . . . [the employee] becomes a threat to the [men] in the house [Felix is assuming here that one job of the house help is to have sexual relations with the men in the house]. And then everyone will get HIV [in that house]!

Cherop felt that it was difficult for PLWHIV to work. However, for her the reasons were based on deeply rooted stereotypes that the employee would no longer be able to sustain the necessary energy levels, because everyone infected with HIV was seen as chronically sick. Consequently, the employee's ability to physically work hard would cease once his or her infection worsened. Again, the possibility of PLWHIV being restored to full health on ART was frequently denied, thus transforming them into something new. The result for a person who was physically unable to work, Cherop continued, was that he or she would be construed as a different type of person. What made these people different was their inevitable inability to fulfill their respective duties and social obligations (providing for and contributing to the well-being of the larger family), which would ultimately lead to social isolation and rejection. When I asked her to tell me how HIV was affecting family life, she said:

> When [you become] sick [with HIV], you'll not be the same person again. Maybe you are using your health [to work and earn] money [by doing physical labor, such as] kibarua, digging in the shamba, [or] taking the stones and building houses. . . . The really hard [physical] works. When you are sick, at that time you'll never do those hard works again. . . . [T]he body starts going down—your energy, the strength of your body. So at that time, if you [were] used to helping your family, the family will lack your help because you will be too sick. . . . When you can't work, there is rejection in the family. And then in the community.

PLWHIV corroborated these general community beliefs and public perceptions, which were sometimes supported by their employment experiences. Some people spoke of the strategies they used to continue eking out a living despite the virus. The efforts of one truck driver to conceal a seropositive status revealed that what was most at stake for him was his method of maintaining his chances for future work and employment, and thereby his personhood and reputation in both his family and community. But PLWHIV also used other tactics to earn a living. Wangechi, who worked as a casual laborer, told me that because local people knew she was living with the virus, she could not find employment in the immediate urban area. To deal with this dilemma, she looked for odd jobs in rural areas farther from her urban apartment, where no one knew her or her seropositive status. This was especially inconvenient to Wangechi because she had small children: "Those in this area can't call me for work [when it is available]. Not for work cultivating the *shamba*. They just tell me, 'You can't work— you are HIV+. How are you going to [work]?' To find my work, I travel to the rural areas. So at times, . . . there are very many hardships."

On the other hand, some PLWHIV emphasized that the only time the malady crept into their interpersonal relationships was during the work associated with ethnic rituals and ceremonies. Nancy, who sold secondhand clothing, offered the following information about being excluded when she visited the rural community where she was born: "Even today I am discriminated [against]. When we have a celebration in my village, I am not given work to do—I can't even serve the visitors, and cooking is prohibited for me. One time, I went to a wedding ceremony. I was given a part in the preparations, but a person who knew that I was HIV positive called out to me and told me to go away because I could cut myself and the blood could flow into the food."

Others spoke of the challenges of living with HIV and participating in local "merry-go-round" groups, which are creative, quite elaborate, and highly organized ways in which locals lend significant sums of money to one another (Oware 2020). These rotating credit groups are common all over the world and go by a variety of names, such as *stokvel* in South Africa. Every month, each member contributes an agreed-upon amount of money, and one person receives all of the money to pay for things such as school fees, engagements, fertilizer, burials, or medical expenses. This process is repeated every month until everyone in the group has been the person to receive the pool of money. Jacob, a farmer, told about a recent incident in which he described himself as being discriminated against, thereby making it clear that what was most at stake in this case, for both the stigmatized person and the person doing the stigmatizing, was money in the context of extreme economic inequality. Jacob was quite aware that he was being discriminated against because of his HIV+ status. However, his need to borrow money made him willing to be mistreated. On the other side of the coin, those doing the stigmatizing were equally concerned about money and needed to borrow from other people. Therefore, the discriminatory behaviors they exhibited toward Jacob were construed as practical, logical, and fair from their view of things. Jacob also highlighted how unexpected verbal assaults toward those living or associated with HIV were quickly and easily made, albeit in ways that felt random and uncertain to him and that drew on the insulting notion that ART—rather than the discriminatory behaviors of others—influenced the temperament of people. Jacob recalled:

> When I first started a merry-go-round group, I was the last one to get the money because the others feared that I would die before I repaid their money. But I needed the extra money, so I needed to keep associating with them. I took their offer [to go last] even though I know they were discriminating against me. We went for many rounds without me dying! But they still maintain, up to today, that I be the very last one every time. Most of the members feel that I deserve to go last [because of HIV], and one time when I got into an argument with another group member over a book I had borrowed, he threw words and said that the only reason I was arguing was because my ARTs were interfering with me and making me hot tempered!

Marriage and Reproduction

Perhaps the biggest threat to the development of personhood was the difficulty people had in finding marital partners if others knew they were living with HIV. When I asked about the possibility of someone living with HIV getting married in the community, I was consistently told that a positive status posed a major challenge. Juma, a store clerk, said that the idea of a person living with HIV getting married was almost unfathomable: "Nowadays, it is not accepted to be married to an HIV+ person because even if you wanted to get married, you must first be tested, and if you are found positive, marriage is automatically disqualified. Even in the church you must produce a VCT card for marriage to take place. Unless you run away and stay together [elope]—but that is illegal—you will never be given a marriage certificate."

When I went on to ask about the possibility of marriage between discordant people—one person living with HIV and the other not infected—people were visibly appalled. Mercy's immediate response was that being married to a man who is living with HIV "would be like sticking my head in a pot of boiling water!" A man responded equally quickly and with initial shock to the same line of questioning: "Hey—if anyone knows [the man has HIV and is marrying a woman]—it is bad! That is a bad one! Because they know that [the woman being married] will die—automatic! That is a serious one." These types of comments suggest that HIV continued to be seen as a fatal condition among general community members, even in the age of treatment. Other people were more polite in tempering the surprise they may have felt at my question. For example, James responded, "According to me, it is not good for an HIV+ to marry into my family unless everyone else in my family is also HIV+ already."

Simply asking about discordant marriages violated a basic local logic that marriage was about reproduction and thus not a context for condoms, abstinence, and/or many of the safe-sex practices promoted by global and national responses to HIV. It also violated ethical and moral concerns about potentially spreading HIV to others. After Cherop poured hot water over my hands for washing and the used soapy water dripped into a small collection basin, she unwrapped fresh *mandazi* that she had purchased earlier that morning, placed them on two small plates, and filled two cups with steaming chai from a thermos that had been resting on a wooden coffee table between us. As we ate and drank together, she explained the importance of having children: "It is a blessing to have kids. Because without kids there is no marriage. In the Kalenjin community, if you don't bear kids, you are left, and the husband marries another wife, and mostly you are chased away. So for the good and continuity of the marriage, there have to be kids and the sharing of responsibilities [between a husband and a wife]." Kimaiyo offered strikingly similar remarks: "You know, Kalenjins believe that procreation is first in marriage. To Kalenjins, marriage is not actually for companionship. The factor number one is that marriage is for procreation. And in our culture, what happens is that if the man is impotent, and he has age mates—those people who . . . belong to the same age set [and with whom he was circumcised]—the man will just allow the friend—the age mate—to help him sire kids." As these quotes make clear, reproduction was at the heart of the marital union, and therefore living with HIV posed a major threat to and complicated the processes of personhood in the lives of many people.[1] This was because the only safe way to have sexual intercourse, according to prevention messages across the community, was with a condom or if (through attending the HIV clinic and taking ARTs) a person's viral loads were suppressed or he or she was offered PrEP. But these strategies were described as challenging ideas about normal marriage.

A common theme across many stories that I collected was the friction and social tensions that HIV sometimes produced between husbands and wives. I noted that HIV, HIV testing, and ART sometimes (but not always) produced rifts in marriage. For example, in 2012, Dorothy, who was HIV+, pointed to what was most at stake for many women and men living in Mahali as they worked to develop themselves as legitimate persons. She wanted to have more children with her husband to show the collective productivity of the couple. By conceiving another child, she hoped to both bolster and amplify their reputations and status, as well as their collaborative and mutual participation in the work expected from conjugal relations. Dorothy was her husband's second wife. He never told her that his first wife had died of complications associated with AIDS and maintained that the disease's presence in the family was Dorothy's fault. Although she learned about the first wife's death through conversations with kin, she seemed to have come to terms with the fact that she must accept the blame, as evidenced by her strong desire and motivation to use her ART to "feel better" so she could "go back to him." She explained:

DOROTHY: When I first came [to the Mahali HIV clinic] in 2011, I [had been] sick [since] December 2010. My brother saw that I had sores, and he told me that he would not treat me [pay for care] unless I was tested for HIV. He had been telling me to be tested from 2007 [an indirect way of telling someone he or she probably has HIV]. . . .

INTERVIEWER: Where do you live?

DOROTHY: It is fifty shillings [to travel by *matatu*] to get here. I moved from my matrimonial home and came to Mahali first for the herbal medicine because I was needing a baby [she had been unable to conceive after giving birth to her first child]. That is when this disease came out and [herbalists] started saying it was a big cancer. That is when I went for testing and was found to be HIV+. . . . I called the husband to tell him, but he said that the disease had no effect on him and that he did not need to be tested. He told me, "This is your fault. You know where you brought the disease from." So I [have] stayed away from him. But I want to be feeling better and to eat well so that I can go back to him. So I am staying away from him [for now]. But we only have one kid, and he has had three with the first wife—the one who died of AIDS. But the husband had kept that one private [that the first spouse had HIV]. He never wanted me to know that the first wife had HIV—he never wanted me to know that she died of HIV. . . .

INTERVIEWER: How are things going now?

DOROTHY: These rashes have come out [referring to the rashes that were visible on her body] since I started using the ARTs. The disease is everywhere in the body. And I am having trouble with food. We who have HIV must eat a lot—at every moment. But I have not been given food [a way of saying that she is not yet being well provided for by her family and/or husband]. And when I am given food, it is to be eaten alone. . . . When I talk to people who have HIV, I encourage them to persevere— because I was almost made mad before—I wanted to hang myself or to cause an accident. That was until I realized I must accept this situation and go on with my life.

Dorothy had been cut off from most of her social and kin support because of her HIV+ status, evidenced through her experiences of being denied food or being required to "eat alone." Still, at the moment of our meeting she was feeling hopeful. Willing to "accept this situation" and the blame from her husband for bringing the disease into the family, Dorothy desired to restore matters as a way to potentially regain her status as a productive woman and wife.

Later in my research, I learned of a discordant couple in which the wife was living with HIV and the husband was not. The wife had stopped taking her ART, and the husband explained his numerous strategies of trying to convince her to resume her treatment. He ultimately threatened to divorce her and return her to her parents and natal home. He rationalized that he did not want to be accused of preventing her from taking her medications and being labeled an unsupportive or negligent husband. This marital story is still unfolding, as HIV and its associated global and national HIV programming and messages continue to transform social relationships and the way people negotiate shifting rationales about how, why, and where to place blame for the spread of this virus.

(RE)IMAGINING PERSONHOOD AND THERAPEUTIC CITIZENSHIP

People with HIV in Mahali were not completely paralyzed by their concerns about becoming a different kind of person. Over the course of my fieldwork, I noted how locals creatively and strategically used national health programming to at least partially restore their social relations—and thus continue to become persons—that were initially imagined as having been lost or out of reach when they became infected with the virus. For example, Njoki, who was living with HIV and had been widowed when her husband died of AIDS in 2002, said the stigma she had been subjected to by her in-laws had been reduced once she conceived a child, even after the death of her husband.[2] In 2012, Njoki explained that she and her late husband had been unable to conceive a child, even after trying various remedies. In the end, they had opted to adopt a child, just prior to the man's untimely death. However, it remained unclear to Njoki whether the problem with conception was a result of her own body or that of her husband. She went on to share details about using her involvement in an HIV support group in an attempt to determine whether or not she could actually conceive. She continually repeated that she (and her late husband) had truly loved the adopted child, but she added that as a woman, she did not feel completely productive or normal since she had not actually given birth:

> I had the need of getting another child and didn't want to infect anybody with the virus. I approached one of the members of my HIV support group and we became friends . . . and after some time I requested him to try to help me have a child . . . to see if I could get a child of my own because I was not feeling proud [as a woman] of the adopted child. . . . But after some time I missed my period [and] consulted the doctors, who did a pregnancy test and told me that I was two months pregnant. I became very happy. I eventually gave birth to a baby girl. When I told my in-laws that I was expecting, they were very happy, and they encouraged me so much and they [even] visited me when I was at the hospital.

They love the child so much. I needed another child, regardless of whether I was HIV+ or not. I know it was dangerous and that I could have gotten another strain of HIV or an STD . . . [but] I wanted to prove to the whole world that I was productive. . . . I was not respected as a woman because I hadn't birthed a child. Now I am HIV+, but I am at least respected because I am the mother of a one-year-old daughter. I say amen.

Njoki's perceived need to birth a child so as to feel productive as a woman exceeded her own health concerns and the information she had received in the clinic. Still, she worried about infecting those who were not already living with HIV. Her social relations with those in her support group at the clinic helped her (re)imagine herself as a respected woman among her kin network in locally and socially meaningful ways.

People therefore strategically used support groups and the HIV clinic as social spaces for identifying sexual, reproductive, marital, and emotionally supportive partners. Likewise, they sometimes formed their own merry-go-round groups to help one another financially. These practices allowed them to continue building themselves up through their relations with others in new and unexpected forms of therapeutic citizenship (Nguyen 2010). Employees at the clinic said they encouraged these practices so their patients would "feel less isolated from normal life." Physicians and health workers thus "improvised" (Livingston 2012) their HIV services by extending what Annemarie Mol (2008) has termed a "logic of care," whereby they not only offered physical care and biomedical treatments but also empathized with patients and tried to address their social needs, concerns, and well-beings. At the same time, the HIV clinic staff (re)socialized people to manage HIV, relationships, and stigma in an otherwise precarious social space (McGrath et al. 2014; de Klerk and Moyer 2017) that was coproduced by global and national HIV programs and their resource-poor community setting. A physician mentioned that when counseling teens and youth who were living with HIV, he advised them to find sexual partners who were also infected because they would "better understand each other" since they were "in that same environment." Omar, another health worker, had explained this approach several years earlier:

[Reproduction and marriage] . . . are some of the many challenges that we have. [Clients think], "Because I am positive, I can't be married. There is nobody who will get married to me." But when they reach [the HIV clinic], we normally advise them just to take their drugs, and at a certain CD4 count they can [safely] be pregnant. But normally we advise them to look for [spouses] who [are] also positive because they will share a common agenda. We do not encourage them to look for [partners who are] negative because they will not rhyme in any way with an HIV–individual. Personally, I normally encourage them. If you need a partner, look for somebody [who is also HIV+], who really understands your status. We even have some here, and they do weddings. They meet at support group and they wed. They wed! It is really amazing. You have to learn to mobilize these people here . . . at every step so they feel less isolated from normal life, . . . from their normal life-styles. Let them feel that the only difference is that they are taking drugs.

As Martin described it, in many ways, the HIV clinic in Mahali was a place of temporary respite, where people could feel accepted and valued before having to return to their regular lives, where stigma, hostility, gossip, and secrets abounded. Still, while Omar wanted patients to feel normal, a process he promoted by encouraging relationships exclusively between PLWHIV and reminding them that "they will not rhyme in any way with an HIV– individual," this latter type of comment reinforced the notion that people attending the HIV clinic were different. Another clinic employee described working hard to provide a climate in which people felt included, united, and supported because they had the same HIV status. Likewise, a social worker, when talking about the goal behind insisting that patients state their HIV status during support groups, described disclosure as a theoretically redundant yet performative act that benefited both the teller and the listener (Davis and Flowers 2014; Davis and Manderson 2014) at the HIV clinic. Such performances created and maintained a shared sense of intimacy and identity among PLWHIV as a social group (Manderson et al. 2015). Disclosure, in this setting, was sometimes about distinguishing between categories of people—those who were living with HIV and those who were not—and flipped the script of what it means to join an exclusive members' club. Samuel said:

[During a support group] you have entered into a room of thirty people and you are told to stand up and declare [your HIV status]! And if you don't—I just send you out! [I tell them], "This is a members' club [for people living with HIV]—if you are not a member [HIV–]—you go out!" So . . . when I am doing the recap [at the end of the support group] I ask, "Before you came from home or before you reached [the HIV clinic], how many people knew that you were HIV+?" [They usually reply], "Only two!" [And then I ask], "And right now, how many people know that you are HIV?" [They reply], "Only two!" Then I ask them, "And who are these people [referring to the other members of the support group]? You just stood and told them that you are HIV, too!" So after that, it is like [breathes a sigh of relief], "I have told all these people I am HIV." And that is why you are always seeing us [employees during support groups] repeating the concept that when you come to support group, you tell a lot of people. It's like you cannot tell your . . . relatives and friends that you are HIV. But when you come to [the HIV clinic in Mahali], you feel that you are in the right environment. This environment is a conducive environment, and you can say anything. You can laugh. You can hear people laughing! Chatting. Discussing. "What, how was your entry point?" ["How did you learn you had HIV?"] Unlike outside [the clinic where you can't discuss such matters openly]. Yeah, when you come to [the HIV clinic] you feel like you are a part of the family. But what makes you feel that you are a part of the family? It is the welcome that you have been accorded. [And] that is when you feel, "Oh—this is the right place!"

Samuel, like other support group workers, tried to make clear to PLWHIV that they had a common bond and identity because they are all infected with the same virus and thus are "part of the family" of people on ART (see also Davis and Flowers 2014). Furthermore, he noted how differently people living with the virus were treated within the walls of the clinic, as opposed to "outside" or in the larger community, where they were unable to safely talk about HIV and their experiences. The HIV clinic offered a momentary sense and space of belonging and relief from the stigma that persisted beyond its walls, at least among those who did not default and could keep living positively.

Global health knowledge and technologies, national programs, and local health provider efforts to help people continue the processes of regaining personhood worked together to reconfigure the ways that marital, kin, employment, and other social networks were imagined as possible in the community. People were being differentiated because they harbored a virus, thereby contradicting claims made that HIV was a disease like any other. Such disclosure performances were not restricted to the bodies and people living in Mahali but rather were being taken up by people across Kenya, in a variant of what Mark Davis and Paul Flowers (2014, 79–80) call a "technosexual imaginary," or ideas about what is socially possible for PLWHIV on ART. The term is used to describe how online, social media disclosures of an HIV status and identity "reveal productive and creative biopolitical action on the part of those affected by HIV." Perhaps mimicking what appeared in global, online sources, these practices were observable through the print media in Kenya. When I read *The Daily Nation* on any given Saturday (or *The Star* on any day) during my trips in 2011, 2012, 2014, and 2019, I regularly saw classified ads for people seeking relationships with others. For example, I pulled this ad at random from the *Daily Nation* from Saturday, December 3, 2011: "I am [person's name], a businessman aged 40 and a widower with two kids. Looking for a lady aged between 37 and 40 from any Kenyan tribe. She should be HIV negative." In the very next entry, I was likely to find another post that differed in one crucial way: "HIV positive. Never married. Healthy and very strong. Senior driver but currently not working. . . . Seeking a 27–40 year-old HIV+ lady who is very financially stable and ready to support. Should be Luo or Luhya and ready to settle this coming holiday."

Clinics and national media venues, where programming and socialization were concentrated, served as key sites for both building people up through their relationships and differentiating citizens (by their HIV status), a phenomenon referred to as "biological citizenship" (Petryna 2002; Nguyen 2010). Though contrary to the notion that people conceptualized their biological statuses and developed their identities in relation to an imagined global world that existed beyond the nation-state, personhood and identities were being constructed in relation to a set of criteria that included an HIV status and several other characteristics—age range; ethnicity; gender; economic, marital and employment status; and location—that can be read as distinctly Kenyan.

"AIDS IS REAL, BUT NOT A CURSE FROM GOD"

Wangechi was a single mother and casual laborer who had spent her whole life in Mahali. She and her children were known to be living with HIV, which from her perspective always seemed to complicate her life. Over the past ten years, I observed that she was often treated poorly by others in the community, and understandably she was regularly upset about that. Despite this, Wangechi had learned that she was living with HIV after giving birth before ART was available and might be described as a survivor who got a "second chance" (Whyte 2014) once treatment programs were rolled out in Kenya. She was confident that she had been infected by her husband, from whom she had quickly separated because of the disrespect he showed her, but only after pleading with her relatives for permission to move out of the conjugal home and return to her natal family. She recalled her marriage and the way it ended:

> You know, I got married when I was very young. When I was just sixteen years. . . . Then the man started frustrating me. He went for another woman. Then I just said [to him], "Am I not right for you?" So I just beat the marriage. I stayed single [lived without him]. It's a bitter pill to swallow, but you have to swallow it. You have to persevere. Now I am looking after my kids all alone. And you have to accept that. This is life. You know [that husband] is the man who brought HIV into my house. So I do not like that man! Even now, if we meet, I'll never talk to him . . . [because] he blamed *me* [for bringing HIV into the marriage]! And he said, "You [are] just a prostitute!" When he realized that I was HIV+, I just got embarrassed. I told him, "You know, your life is yours, mine is mine. Just go to your people. Then I'll go [back] to mine. Whoever will die early, will be buried by his people." And I never went back [to him]. Even now, I don't like him. I forgave him, but I don't like him.

After her HIV diagnosis and separation from her husband, Wangechi had had tumultuous relationships with various relatives. One day, she tracked me down at the HIV clinic because she wanted to give me a handwritten copy of a poem she had written in English. I had recently conducted a series of life-history interviews with her, and she felt that the poem would help to further contextualize her life for me. It also allowed her to share her experiences as a PLWHIV in Mahali. Wangechi recalled that she had started to read the poem out loud during a World

AIDS Day community gathering, but that she had been cut short and criticized for being rude and inappropriate for "shouting" about her experiences in a public setting. Her poem points to many of the things at stake and presents the challenges for PLWHIV as they work to develop themselves as legitimate persons in the contexts of uncertainties, insecurity, social changes, and inequalities. These local challenges intersected with global and national health efforts to (re)produce the viral frictions described in her poem:

AIDS IS REAL, BUT NOT A CURSE FROM GOD
I was young when I became an orphan;
Feeding, clothing, and shelter there—all alone.
Many things turned in my young mind, unknown.
AIDS is real, but not a curse from God.

This big monster tread alone in my mind
And erased my young soul without any kind.
Where on earth do I belong—an infected kid?
AIDS is real, but not a curse from God.

I was taken to witch doctors [traditional healers] for cure.
My grandparents, scared of shame, neglected care.
[The Mahali HIV clinic] my rescue center—you gave me hope.
AIDS is real, but not a curse from God.

ARTs my daily booster—I have and cherish you ever.
If you are not infected, you are affected—I will preach forever.
Remember take your drugs—going backward—never!
AIDS is real, but not a curse from God.

AIDS—you are transmitted in many forms:
Sex, blood transfusion, unsterilized objects and needles—also open wounds.
Go for a test today—though many will die of the stigma, it remains.
AIDS is real, but not a curse from God.

I will always "keep the promise":
Die alone—and never break this pledge.
Respect life and dignity of others, without prejudice.
AIDS is real, but not a curse from God.

CONCLUSION

Beatrice, Jane, and I went "footing" (walking) along a dirt road that led us uphill toward a rural village. We were going to attend the burial of an elder community member and friend of my two companions. Each of us carried a *leso* so we would have something to sit on during the long ceremony. People were planting maize, so as we traversed the rolling landscape it felt open, and we could see houses that had been hidden from view a few months earlier by the tall crop. The road connected us to a smaller footpath that wound down into a valley where cattle were grazing on greening grass and then back up again, past sloping *shambas*. We had to step over the occasional rope that tied a goat to a tree or fence post so that it would not wander off and eat a neighbor's crops. The disappearance of part or all of a crop could cause conflict and lead to trouble for the owner of the animal. The air and sun were warm, but the breeze was cool and steady. Our conversations were intermittently interrupted by giggling children as they chased after us and yelled "*mzungu!*" At one point, we overheard a group of younger children arguing about whether I was *mzungu* or *mchina* (a person from China or of Chinese descent). I looked different, but those following behind us were not clear about how to classify me. As we approached the homestead where the burial ceremony was already under way, we spotted a large white tent and several parked cars, and we found a significant gathering of people who were eating a meal of rice, chicken, vegetables, and chapatis that had been prepared for visitors. We later sat in the grass, where we listened to eulogies and prayers and watched various groups of visitors, including some whom Beatrice and Jane joined to pose for photos next to the casket. Eventually, as we joined a crowd of burial attendees and walked shoulder to shoulder with them to witness the lowering of the casket into the grave, the air became filled with emotional cries and the sounds of women wailing. The person being buried had been respected and was beloved by those in attendance. On our way home, just before the dirt road we were following spilled us back out onto the noisy tarmac highway that would take us back to the busy urban center of Mahali, we passed through a forest. There, Jane pointed to a few remaining indigenous trees, including a variety she referred to as *Emitik*. The *Emitik* tree, she explained, was a hardwood—strong, independent, and resilient—that lived for a long time and could endure harsh conditions. The imported trees that people had begun to plant, she continued, were inferior to the *Emitik*: their wood was softer, and although they grew quickly, they were weak. Because they could not tolerate wide variations in environmental conditions, they were fleeting. Africans, with proper training, could become like *Emitik* trees, while *wazungu*, because of their lifestyle and upbringing, were usually like imported trees.

Over my years in Mahali, I heard people decry the continued erosion of traditions, rituals, and social networks that had historically ensured the proper training and discipline of people. This erosion was linked to processes of globalization and was offered as evidence of a rapidly declining morality in Kenya. One day in early 2012, when Moses and I had planned to meet at the school where he worked so that I could begin conducting a series of life-history interviews with him, I witnessed two instances of instilling proper behavior in young people, instances that I found unsettling.

Upon my arrival at the school, an administrator escorted me past several classrooms, each packed with a lively group of students who sat in pairs at small wooden desks. We passed one room where several older students were reciting poetry in preparation for an upcoming regional competition. After serving as an international audience for the impressive performers' practice, I was directed to a meeting room. This room was small, dark, and cramped, with a locked file cabinet in one corner and a table surrounded by a handful of chairs at the center. A wooden door led to an even tinier room at the back where books were stored. The cinder block room doubled as Moses's office, and I was instructed to wait there for him. Moses suddenly entered the cold, makeshift office briefly and uttered a single frantic command, "Watch her!" To my surprise, Moses was holding the arm of a small girl dressed in a school uniform, her hair neatly shaved like all schoolchildren. Moses offered no additional words or explanations but instead silently pulled up the girl's skirt to show that one of her thighs had recently been burned by the edge of some sort of flat object, leaving behind uniform wounds that were raw and gruesome.

Moses had received an urgent text message from the child's mother, Wanjiku, a former student and AIDS orphan who was now an adult. Wanjiku had texted Moses saying that she needed immediate assistance "mediating a situation." Moses suggested that I wait with the girl while he looked into the matter. Inside Moses's office, the little girl and I were left staring awkwardly at each other as her eyes filled with tears. She looked frightened until I offered her a piece of grape yogurt candy I found in my pocket. Outside the room, we could hear shouting and furniture being shoved around.

As the little girl and I waited in Moses's office, I looked out a small barred window into the school courtyard, where I saw about five older girls being instructed by a teacher to lie on their stomachs. I was shocked to see the teacher strike each girl in turn—hard—several times with a solid stick. Each girl maintained a stoic face as she received the blows. While I knew that corporal punishment was still practiced in Kenyan schools, seeing it firsthand, and so closely, unsettled me. The Kenyan government had banned the use of physical punishment in schools in 2001, but such practices had persisted (Mweru 2010). I was told that this was because of a belief that growing up properly—or being molded into respectable, moral adults—required firm discipline to teach proper respect and to ensure training in the esteemed values of being a hard worker, obedient, and resilient, as well as having the ability to endure suffering without complaint. Routine beatings at school, by parents, and even of wives by husbands, was a way of teaching respect and proper behavior, relations, and talk between individuals in various life stages.

After the noises and voices in the next room had subsided, Moses re-entered the room and explained the situation. Wanjiku was the youngest child in her family. When her mother, a single parent, died from complications associated with AIDS, Wanjiku was raised by her older brothers instead of by another family member or adult. The current dispute was between Wanjiku and her in-laws. The in-laws claimed that Wanjiku had not been raised properly as an AIDS orphan and wanted justice. They were angry at Wanjiku—and had physically attacked her—for burning the thigh of their granddaughter (the little girl), who, from their point of view, had the potential to provide them with future security.

Wanjiku's brief explanation of why she had burned the little girl's thigh with a hot *panga* (machete, or long bush knife) was because the girl had lost three library books in a short period of time and Wanjiku had been fined for each book. She could barely afford to pay one fine, let alone three. Believing that the child lacked discipline and was in need of severe punishment, and hoping to end the expensive practice of losing her library books, Wanjiku had punished her daughter in the same way that she had been punished by her brothers as a child.

With a frustrating and corrupt legal system, the in-laws turned to violence as a tactic for obtaining guardianship over the little girl and to ensure that she was raised properly. They knew that there would be few, if any, ramifications for harming their daughter-in-law. Practices of people working together in groups for justice were common, and there was little the legal community could do. As one police officer told me, after harsh beatings of wrongdoers, "We are simply left to take the bodies to the mortuary. The problem we find is that there is never any evidence."

As the mediator, Moses had demanded that the in-laws cool off and take matters to the police. He needed to escort Wanjiku to the police, to see if they would lock her in a jail cell for protection until the hostilities ceased. It was still early in the afternoon, but I decided to head home, worn out by the events of the day. On my way, as I tried to make sense of what had happened, I recalled the conversation I had had with Jane about *Emitik* trees and Kenyans' desire for and methods of proper upbringing. When I returned to the privacy of my own room, I closed the door and wept. I felt very small and weak, engulfed by the violence, uncertainty, and suffering in our globalized world. I think my tears also reflected my self-doubt in that moment, my fear that I did not have what it took to do fieldwork in Mahali. I felt like an imported tree.

VIRAL FRICTIONS AND THE PERSISTENCE OF HIV STIGMA

These examples of intense efforts to ensure proper support of and behavior in children highlight three important insights about living in our shared, contemporary, and interconnected world, and they help summarize the answers to the central questions driving this book: How and why is it that HIV-related stigma persists in Kenya during the age of treatment? First, everyday life in Mahali's urban trading center (located along a busy highway), as in many parts of the world, is unevenly and chronically uncertain and filled with social tensions, contradictions, and inequities that have been brought about by much broader globalizing and historical forces. This point is salient for understanding and contextualizing viral frictions and the persistence of stigma in the very small town of Mahali, where everyday material, social, and moral existences seemed to be threatened and were marked by uncertainty. Community violence and national and regional conflicts—ethnic, age-related, gender-based, political, and/or socioeconomic—erupt without warning. Some people are obviously very sick with HIV, while others have HIV but do not appear to suffer any overt symptoms. A small number of people have privileged access to officially sanctioned HIV knowledge or gain paid or volunteer employment in the AIDS industry, and thus have the potential for upward mobility and status as modern and enlightened citizens. Most people in Mahali do not have access to such work or these sources of capital. Many of the people living with HIV are in a state of "permanent transition" and are unable to fully return to their normal physical and social lives on ART (Mattes 2014, 272). Still others, especially those facing food insecurity and extreme poverty, are unable to thrive on ART (Moyer 2015). In this latter group, a few get cut off from local, national, and global relationships and are stripped of their rights as citizens and persons, also losing their already limited sources of care and support. While carefully selected and spoken words are believed to be powerful enough to heal, they can also terrorize and even devastate a body physically, mentally, morally, and socially. Such violent and uncertain conditions have long been documented in sub-Saharan Africa. For example, Jean Comaroff and John Comaroff (2006, vii) wrote: "Yes, postcolonies are especially, excessively, distinctively violent and disorderly. Yes, they are sinking ever further into a mire of conflict, coercion, and chaos. Yes, this does seem to be a chronic, not a temporary, state of being."

People living in these kinds of precarious conditions, like everyone every-where whether living with HIV or not, want to have a secure sense of belonging in the world. During my research in 2011 and 2012, I overheard people talking about changing the name of Mahali (meaning "place") to Mahali ya Amani (meaning "peaceful place"). The hope was that doing so might somehow alter the fate of the place and the life trajectory of its residents. While I was staying in Mahali in 2019, I was lulled to sleep by distant sounds of the peaceful and melodic voices of an interethnic group of committed women who gathered regularly to sing and pray for the community throughout the night. Women and men alike are acutely aware of the ills afflicting them, which include but extend well beyond HIV infections. They are seeking to take charge and attempting to move the community in new directions using the limited resources available to them.

Second, daily life in Mahali matters deeply, as evidenced by the ways people are in motion and engaged in constant practices of "being through becoming" (John Comaroff and Jean Comaroff 2001, 271), with shared dreams of becoming like *Emitik* trees—strong and resilient. But as globalization rapidly transforms social life, many things are at stake every day alongside such changes, including the needs and dreams to earn money; to attain a secure sense of belonging and safety; to experience promising opportunities to maintain their health and improve their lives; to establish and maintain reputations, statuses, and relation-ships; and to put ethical and moral principles into practice (Kleinman 2006; Yang et al. 2007). The struggle to define the meaning of those shared dreams is difficult at times. Occasionally, people use HIV as a device to win a conflict with a rival or to gain an advantage over a competitor. And sometimes the only things people can imagine doing—perhaps out of a sense of justice or community, in an attempt to resolve social contradictions, or to reduce the experienced and perceived threats to what matters most—is to seek revenge, accuse another per-son of being a witch, kill themselves, scald the legs of their own child, drink heavily, or leave behind lists of names of the people they imagined had been infected with HIV. What matters most to people can be seen clearly in the arenas of health, healing, and illnesses (Langwick 2011) and through circulating stories about HIV and stigma.

Third, HIV—both the disease and those living with and/or associated with it, such as sex workers—had come to be perceived by people as intimately linked to, sometimes responsible for, and at other times both the cause and the inevi-table result of social tensions and changes in the community that were actually brought on and shaped by much larger structural inequalities. The perceived and experienced chaos brought on by the AIDS epidemic flooded into relationships and identities in very real and sometimes deadly ways through the constant swirl of (often moralizing) stories and messages about HIV. People had clearly adopted the global health discourse that HIV is a disease like any other (Moyer and Hardon 2014). But the longer I was in Mahali, as Hansjörg Dilger (2008) learned over a decade ago in Tanzania, I found that residents, including health workers, still distinguished this malady from other diseases. They conceived of and sometimes experienced its spread and the suffering it caused (or could cause) in social, moral (Geissler and Prince 2010), economic, political, and historical terms. This was because everyday life was unevenly plagued by chronic inequities that produced frictions within and between people, and the disease was therefore described and experienced as being simultaneously normal and exceptional (Mazanderani and Paparini 2015). This produced a contradiction that people in Mahali had to negotiate. These negotiations rendered processes of stigma uncertain and contributed to its persistence across every overlapping level and form—individual (intrapersonal, interpersonal, and courtesy), community (public), and structural (myriad institutional levels).

In the age of treatment, living a normal life with HIV is theoretically attainable because of biomedical interventions and technologies. It therefore becomes an important aspiration among many PLWHIV across the Global South and Global North (Moyer and Hardon 2014). Globally and nationally circulating rhetoric related to ending AIDS reminds us all, including Kenyans, of this possibility and of the potential of ART to reduce stigma. At the time of this writing, however, AIDS and the spread of HIV have not been eliminated, and HIV-related stigma has not ended (McGrath et al. 2014; Moyer and Hardon 2014; Mattes 2019; Walker 2020), even in a community like Mahali with free and readily available access to HIV treatment and care. Instead, by the end of 2019, the HIV epidemic was still generalized, meaning that it continued to impact people across populations, and there were 1.5 million people in Kenya who were living with the virus (Avert 2020). In the same year, among those living with HIV, approximately 75 percent of adults and 63 percent of children were on ART, but still 42,000 new infections and 21,000 AIDS-related deaths had occurred. Deaths had declined sharply since I first began conducting research in Kenya in 2010, when more than 60,000 people died. Yet, while Kenya is a prevention success story in many ways, these numbers remain unacceptably high, and the country still harbors one of the largest HIV epidemics in the world. Despite reports of declining discriminatory attitudes toward PLWHIV in eastern and southern Africa (UNAIDS 2021) and strikingly high levels of HIV and AIDS awareness in Kenya, stigma has persisted (Avert 2020).

As I have illustrated throughout this book, when global and national discourses and practices related to normalizing HIV through the chronic disease paradigm, such as the individualizing messages contained in notions of living positively and anti-stigma interventions, are inserted into uncertain and inequitable conditions, frictions are produced and universal or global knowledge is transformed. These frictions (re)shape local experiences and socialities, or everyday forms of interaction. They help maintain the exceptional status of HIV (Moyer and Hardon 2014) and result in added tensions and challenges for

PLWHIV who were already living in precarious circumstances before their diagnoses. This is because patients, as well as those who love and try to support them, are expected to embody, perform, and behave as though HIV is a normal, chronic disease, even while they are experiencing or caring for someone with an exceptional condition (Walker 2020). Those who are unable to achieve normalcy or adjust physically, socially, and/or psychologically to highly biomedicalized regimes of living positively are left to experience new forms of stigmatization. These tension-filled experiences open up "social spaces" in which PLWHIV occupy a liminal state and remain just out of reach of being and feeling normal (McGrath et al. 2014, 314). In these social spaces, PLWHIV must constantly work to diligently manage and balance their "unpredictable" bodies (de Klerk and Moyer 2017, 307), as well as their unpredictable minds and social relationships that are situated within the unpredictable conditions of their family, community, region, and nation-state. The infection and disease, local expertise, structural conditions, national programs and politics, and viral global health knowledge, science, technologies, and discourses all work together to produce viral frictions and sustain HIV-related stigma.

HIV, A HIGHWAY, GLOBAL HEALTH, AND STIGMA

One windy morning in March 2014, I walked with Henry from the house where I was staying, which was behind a row of shops, toward the HIV clinic. It was early enough that the sounds and sights of people engaged in their morning activities were audible and visible. People were sweeping, and we could see others leaned over buckets of water, washing dishes and clothes. The daytime activities of life in Mahali's urban center were only beginning to pick up. We used a shortcut that took us through an area that was constantly littered with trash and had overwhelming smells, which Henry referred to as "no man's land." He used this term because the area was where some people dumped their garbage, since the government did not evenly provide such services to all residents in Mahali. Our path through "no man's land" intersected with a makeshift grass "road" that had been created over time by the collaborative efforts of vehicles that regularly passed along the route. At the intersection we turned left, heading down a small hill to the HIV clinic. With the main highway now directly behind us, I could still hear the steady, low rumble of trucks as their drivers pulled out of the trading center, jostled over speed bumps, and headed toward their next destinations. When we arrived at the HIV clinic, the metal front doors were already propped wide open, but there were only two employees, who were working diligently, inside. Outside, a small number of people whom I did not know sat alone, scattered across the lawn. I imagined that they had arrived early for their monthly appointments in the hopes of being seen first by the clinic staff and avoiding the queues that sometimes kept people waiting.

The HIV epidemic and the presence of global and national health efforts to address HIV in Mahali were facilitated in part by the highway running through its urban center. This road, like stories about HIV, transformed the place and local lives, as well as the bodies and psyches of people living in and passing through it, in rather unexpected ways. The daily global momentum passing through Mahali via vehicles, as well as the words, ideas, beliefs, products, and technologies carried by the people inside them, were slowed by the immense speed bumps that met everyone coming into the area. Akhil Gupta and James Ferguson (1997) encourage anthropologists to think critically about and problematize notions of "the field" and "the local" due to the interconnectedness of the modern world. I have demonstrated throughout this book that as viral, global health knowledge about HIV first rattled across the speed bumps and collided with local knowledge and institutions, as well as national and regional policies, programs, and politics, it produced friction (inflected the motion) and was distinctly and very locally processed, expressed, negotiated, and transformed through the circulation of spoken (and sometimes silenced) words (Bauman and Briggs 1990; Urban 2001). This friction reconfigured how people thought about themselves and their community. Viral frictions determined the shifting borders around ideas about who belonged and who did not, as well as about those who were normal or who were not. Consequently, viral frictions molded both how people imagined the (im)possibilities of their relationships (including kin, gender, marital, health status, and other social relationships) and how people living or associated with HIV understood and experienced the virus and HIV-related stigma.

I completed this book isolated in my house amid the most recent global pandemic confronting humanity. A report from UNAIDS (2020b) warns of the potential for COVID-19 to "blow us even further off course" in terms of worldwide progress toward "ending AIDS as a public health threat by 2030." Acknowledging that pandemics expose and rest along the fault lines of inequality, this report importantly views COVID-19 as a "wake-up call to do things differently" and outlines UNAIDS's reinvigorated commitment to social justice and a refreshed "vision for the global HIV response to achieve three zeros: zero new HIV infections, zero AIDS-related deaths, and zero discrimination." A more recent item published by UNAIDS (2021) calls on individuals to "challenge the stigma: pursue your right to health." Yet, this individualistic approach assumes the manifestation of a generic form of stigma and lacks specificity in terms of what "the stigma" and challenging it may mean, look, and feel like to people living in diverse places. At the same time, this report echoes strikingly similar calls to the global community made by UNAIDS (2003) for tackling HIV-related stigma and discrimination. That was the year when UNAIDS and WHO began a "3 by 5" initiative to provide three million PLWHIV in low- and middle-income countries with ART by the end of 2005. The accompanying World AIDS Campaign (with its 2002–2003 anti-stigma slogan and theme for World AIDS Day

2003, "Live and let live"), launched nearly two decades ago, advocated for the creation and use of educational materials that promoted hope among those infected, emphasized the harmful impact and consequences of stigma and discrimination, and promoted efforts that challenge ignorance, fear, and denial related to the epidemic.

What insights might the concept of viral frictions offer these efforts and calls "to do things differently" in the future? The stories shared by people in Mahali point to the idea that local bodies—as well as social, historical, economic, and political relationships—need healing from HIV, not only as a biological infection or epidemic but also as a malady. As many people living in Mahali made clear to me, this requires significantly more than a mere physical restoration of the body and healing of the individual at the psychological level. In this way, like Jane's explanation of the sudden reconstruction of a building on an insecure foundation, ART has only "smeared over the cracks" (see chapter 3).

Since 2003, global health has served as an "anti-politics machine" (Ferguson 1994), simultaneously biomedicalizing HIV—using ART and the chronic disease paradigm—and imagining people as though they are living outside of the many important economic, political, and historical contexts that help explain how and why processes of HIV-related stigma and discrimination persist in the Global South. Those transnational, health-related efforts have been determined, encouraged, and supported in part by global mandates (including those of UNAIDS), working in tandem with the impressively hefty amounts of funding made available through global structures to address and biomedicalize HIV (such as PEPFAR, the Global Fund, and the Bill and Melinda Gates Foundation). These international entities use complex mathematical models and global metrics to create big epidemiological data sets to help uncover the latest at-risk groups and to monitor and track interventions, compliance with them, adherence to ART, and discriminatory laws and policies, overt episodes of discrimination, and levels of discriminatory attitudes in selected countries. While impressive and important, this approach has largely neglected or failed to take seriously the insights offered by those working in the social sciences (Moyer 2015), including their fine-grained ethnographies of communities where the latest HIV interventions are inserted, piloted, assessed, and completed as new ones are implemented. Yet the kinds of information yielded through close, careful, and long-term community-based ethnographic research reveal the limitations and unintended consequences of the models and global metrics approach. Ethnographic insights add value and nuance to the findings generated through the use of big data that otherwise are unable to account for the local specificities and particularities that help to explain how and why it is that stigma and discriminatory attitudes are declining in some regions and rebounding in others (UNAIDS 2021). This omission has impacted the way HIV and stigma have been conceptualized, talked about, and attended to in sub-Saharan Africa in the age of treatment. HIV is a treatable biological condition, and social stigma and discrimination have been considerably more challenging to overcome (Moyer 2015). A highly biomedical-ized paradigm and approach has not succeeded in addressing these issues uni-formly across countries and communities with distinct power dynamics.

Although global health researchers have long noted that stigma operates at multiple levels, at the time of this writing (in early 2021), most HIV-related stigma frameworks used in low- and middle-income countries like Kenya have drawn on psychological approaches and primarily targeted stigma at the levels of the individual (or intrapersonal or interpersonal forms of stigma) and/or com-munity (or public stigma) (Kemp et al. 2019; Rao et al. 2019; Stangl et al. 2019). Efforts to address stigma have relied on short-term or pilot interventions that use education-only approaches and media campaigns geared toward equipping those who experience or perpetuate stigma with more universal scientific knowledge and information about HIV. This narrow lens for thinking about and addressing stigma has contributed to viral frictions. The processes of stigmatiza-tion are exceedingly complex and demand focused attention in order to under-stand the broader social determinants and structural inequities that produce the conditions, tensions, and contradictions that people at individual and commu-nity levels are trying to resolve when they stigmatize or are stigmatized by others. Research and interventions that center on individuals and communities and focus on the virus as detached from social, historical, and political contexts oversimplify a complicated set of circumstances that keep the processes of stig-matization in motion. This neglect has limited researchers' ability to study, understand, and inform the multilevel models and interventions that will be required to meaningfully influence sustainable change (Stangl et al. 2019; Walker 2020). The viral frictions I have presented in this book demonstrate that globally circulating viral discourses about and vertical practices related to the biomedi-calization of HIV, ART, and stigma "creep[ed] and seep[ed]" horizontally (Ben-ton 2015, 7) into and out of deeply rooted national and regional politics, conflicts, identities, and inequalities. These politics erupted at the intersecting lines of eth-nicity, gender, sexuality, and class that were being fiercely debated intra- and interpersonally among locals, which kept all forms of discrimination in motion during a period of major change. It is thus not surprising that I have documented the same circular HIV and stigma narratives and conclusions for over a decade. HIV testing, treatment, retention in care, and rates of viral suppression were nega-tively impacted by stigma because, it was argued, Kenyans (especially poorer people) lacked proper knowledge and had local problems related to their beliefs about HIV, PLWHIV, science, treatment, risk, and prevention. However, despite the high levels of knowledge about HIV that people had access to and that I encountered in Mahali, PLWHIV still did not feel totally normal. Instead, people described the sometimes subtle and sometimes overt aspects of normal social life from which they feared (and occasionally experienced episodes of) being excluded. This is why stigma persisted and why UNAIDS needs to keep calling on the global community to tackle and address this problem.

The exclusive focus on the virus and the use of universal or global HIV-related scientific knowledge to reduce stigma ignores the limitations of and frictions produced by global health knowledge, technologies, and narratives as they move into local communities characterized by poverty, regional political violence, and national uncertainties. Yet global health relies on a diverse range of actors working across overlapping levels and sectors and with a great variety of priorities and needs to deliver responses to HIV, which complicates the successful implementation of services (Dionne 2017; Hershey 2019). Future global health professionals, researchers, and policy makers will need to expand their focus and develop measures to assess and address stigma collaboratively and across individual, community, organizational, and structural levels so more comprehensive models can be envisioned and implemented (Rao et al. 2019). If the UNAIDS goal of "zero discrimination" is to be taken seriously, global health efforts will need to move beyond medicalization and place people back into their social, moral, historical, and political environments, using the socially relevant and culturally appropriate tools necessary to fight stigmatization.

Recently, the global public health researchers Anne Stangl and colleagues (2019) proposed the Health Stigma and Discrimination Framework as a guide for use among global health experts and at scale for the future development of interventions, measurements, research, and policies designed to ameliorate various forms of health-related stigma. This multilevel framework incorporates theories of stigma from across disciplines to outline a plan that encourages researchers and professionals to move away from the exclusive focus on stigma as it operates at the individual level. The model accounts for the relationship between stigma associated with a variety of health conditions and the broader social determinants of health and structural inequalities related to race, gender, sexuality, class, and occupation. However, the viral frictions presented in this book suggest the need for caution in using the global mandate to scale up or universalize global health models—an approach that can impede local effectiveness (Adams, Burke, and Whitmarsh 2014) if it ignores the democratic principles of participation and representation (Dionne 2017) and prioritizes the concerns of funding agencies over locally identified needs, concerns, and priorities (Hershey 2019). While global health programs value the creation of models that can be rolled out at scale so they can be funded, measured, and compared across many diverse settings and national contexts, this approach neglects the impact of globalization on national and local endeavors. The Health Stigma and Discrimination Framework is a first step toward improving models of stigma, but the viral frictions that shape local experiences of HIV suggest the need to engage in "slow research" (Adams, Burke, and Whitmarsh 2014) that allows us to account for local particularities. Addressing these specificities will help create more effective and sustainable global health interventions: "Slow research assumes that the local can always speak back to larger fields of funding, resource management, policy, and agenda-setting in global health arenas in ways that are not only critical but also positive in the sense that they are aimed at improving outcomes" (Adams, Burke, and Whitmarsh 2014, 182). To more effectively study and address HIV-related stigma, "slow research" and slow data, like that generated by ethnographers working closely and collaboratively with local people, may in the end enable global and national programs to be more productive and get us more quickly to the UNAIDS goal of "zero discrimination."

Ethnographers typically assume that there is a local perspective that is passively consumed by and through the forces of globalization. In contrast, while global health practitioners make claims about collaborations with resource-poor partner countries, they often take for granted the universals of science and technology and neglect the social conditions and inequalities that make global health efforts necessary in the first place (Geissler 2013) and that sustain inequitable power relations. Viral frictions highlight the actual, practiced fluidity and active, partnered interdependency of these local, regional, national, and global domains and produce unexpected HIV outcomes and social changes. As scholars and practitioners united by and committed to understanding and ameliorating the HIV epidemic, we have a theoretical imperative to reconcile universality with localism and to dismantle a wide range of dualisms—local and global, rich and poor, wife and sex worker, HIV− and HIV+, social and biological, stigmatized and stigmatizer, belonging and not belonging, and the like—that continue to limit contemporary global health efforts and interventions. We can complicate these dualist ontologies by emphasizing instead a contextual focus on "a language of relationships" (Goffman 1963, 3) and with the acknowledgment of their interconnectedness and the fact that they may work together to help maintain persisting forms of stigma and discrimination. Attempts to dissolve the current, artificially imposed dichotomies used to think about and respond to HIV will demand that practitioners, scholars, and policy makers support and engage in "slow research." This will require taking seriously the need to develop hybrid lenses that make visible the range of democratic, intersecting forms of proper (local, regional, national, and global) knowledge, logics, experiences, and priorities as they interact and are found in different parts of the world (Dionne 2017). These new lenses can then be used to think about, develop, adapt, and enact future programs and policies centered on ameliorating the many intersecting forms of discrimination and rooted in a social justice framework that promotes equity within and across populations.

ACKNOWLEDGMENTS

This book would not have been possible without the knowledge and support of many generous people and institutions. My greatest debt is to the people of Mahali, Kenya, who graciously welcomed me into their community and lives and shared their important stories with me. They are the backbone of and inspiration for this entire project. I am very grateful to my key interlocutors, who answered my repetitive and sometimes culturally inappropriate questions with kindness and shared their expertise, memories, and companionship with me, as well as their time, families, homes, personal experiences, and humor. I am especially thankful to and inspired by Beatrice, Emmah, Henry, and Irene, my wise and energetic research assistants, for their dedication and constant determination to make our project stronger. They each provided me with invaluable lessons about life in Kenya, as well as assistance by connecting me to and allowing me into their local social and kin networks and ensuring that I never felt lonely while abroad.

I am grateful to people working for the institutions and agencies that generously supported my research and provided financial support over the years. This research was made possible by funding from the Kinsey Institute for Sex, Gender, and Reproduction, the National Institutes of Health/National Center for Research Resources—Indiana Clinical and Translational Sciences Institute—TL1 Program (TL1 RR025759; Anantha Shekhar, principal investigator), and fellowship support and grants from the College of Arts and Sciences, Department of Anthropology, and African Studies Program at Indiana University Bloomington. The project was also supported by Award Number T32AI007637 from the National Institute of Allergy and Infectious Diseases. Follow-up trips and the time spent writing this book were made possible through the support of Rhode Island College, the Rhode Island College Foundation, and the Rhode Island College Alumni Affairs Office. I am responsible for the content shared in this book and any mistakes therein; it does not represent the views of my supporting institutions.

My overall graduate studies at Indiana University Bloomington, language training, postdoctoral research fellowship at the Indiana University School of Medicine, and this book benefited tremendously from the generous intellectual support, wisdom, and unique expertise and contributions of several mentors: Sarah D. Phillips, Beverly Stoeltje, Jeanette Dickerson Putman, Brian Gilley, Maria Grosz-Ngaté, Bernice Pescosolido, Thomas Inui, Harrison M. K. Maithya, Violet Naanyu, John Sidle, Susan Shepherd, Mary Ott, Kara Wools-Kaloustian, Jonathan Choti, Alwiya Omar, and the late Naomi Shitemi. Several anonymous peer reviewers provided honest and productive feedback, and their critiques on previous drafts of this book significantly transformed the manuscript's content. As a junior scholar and first-time book author, I am extremely grateful to Lenore Manderson for her mentorship. Her feedback on early drafts of each chapter greatly shaped and improved this work. I would also like to express my sincere gratitude to Joanna Broderick for her mentorship, friendship, and emotional support, as well as her careful technical editing of countless drafts of this book.

I want to acknowledge the influence and encouragement that my friends and family members have given me over the years. Thanks to my friends in Indiana, Rhode Island, Kenya, and beyond who helped care for and love my children while I did the ethnographic research and writing for this book. To my parents, Robert Smith and Susan Parent, thank you very much for supporting and always being interested in this project. I am grateful to my brother, Court Smith, for the hours he spent listening to me process this work on the phone. I am indebted to my three children—Adi, Theo, and Joel—for the numerous study breaks that helped keep me grounded and their constant cheerleading as I worked to finish this book. Finally, to Mark, thank you for encouraging me to work in sub-Saharan Africa and for your unconditional love, support, and commitment to our family.

NOTES

INTRODUCTION

1. Mahali and all other names of local places (with the exception of major cities and towns, like Nairobi and Eldoret) are pseudonyms. I use the English first names of my research assistants, who I thank in the acknowledgments and describe in the preface, but I refrain from using last names at their request and thus to respect their privacy. All other names of people are pseudonyms. To further maintain anonymity and protect the confidentiality of my study participants, I have changed many, but not all, descriptions of people, events, seasons, and settings, all of which should be read more as composites that I wove together by combining details about the many individuals with whom I engaged and the places and activities in which I participated (see also the preface, where I briefly describe the methodologies used to collect and present the ethnographic data included in this book).

2. The terms *prostitute* and *prostitution* are outdated and considered derogatory. They have been replaced with the terms *sex worker* and *sex work* or *commercial sex work* and *commercial sex worker* (CSW) across the HIV and social science literatures and in documents published by institutions such as WHO and the Joint United Nations Programme on HIV/AIDS (UNAIDS). In Mahali, while most people working in the AIDS industry typically used "sex worker" or "CSW" to describe (predominantly) women who earned a living by selling sex, many members of the general public continued to use derogatory terms. In addition, funding from the U.S. President's Emergency Plan for AIDS Relief (PEPFAR) required recipient countries to sign an "Anti-Prostitution Pledge" (see chapter 1).

I have left "prostitute" and "prostitution" in the text when quoting respondents or written documents of funding institutions. It is not my intention to offend anyone. Instead, I do this to emphasize the importance and power of language in shaping and reinforcing processes of stigma. Furthermore, in this quote, keeping the term *prostitute* adds depth and meaning to the larger story. Ruth, who almost always used the term *CSW* in other settings, strategically used *prostitute* in the pejorative sense here as a way of emphasizing the status loss of the married woman who had been buried and to underscore the rationale and attitude behind the harsh treatment, discrimination, and neglect that she had received from the church during the burial.

3. Kitenge is an East African cotton fabric with a wide range of patterns, colors, and distinctive borders. Pieces of the fabric are sometimes used to convey messages to others, including support for politicians, political and religious ideologies, or health messages.

CHAPTER 1

1. For more thorough histories of the origins of AIDS and the history of the disease in Africa, see Cindy Patton (1990, 2002), Vinh-Kim Nguyen (2010), John Iliffe (2006), and Didier Fassin (2007).

CHAPTER 2

1. Portions of this chapter were previously published in *Global Public Health* (Pfeiffer and Maithya 2018).

2. It was also considered bad because of the immoral outside "Others" (e.g., sex workers, truck drivers, and imported police officers) who were described as moving into the area from far away (see chapter 4).

3. In addition to global health initiatives, other NGO activities centered on peace-building initiatives.

CHAPTER 3

1. I do not provide a citation for these quotes or a year to maintain confidentiality and protect the exact location of Mahali.

2. Portions of this chapter were previously published in "Dangerous Bodies, Unpredictable Minds" (Pfeiffer et al. 2017) and *Culture, Health & Sexuality* (Pfeiffer and Maithya 2021).

3. The person who collects money from the passengers.

4. This latter type of comment and question reflected for me the history of the struggle to make ART accessible to people of the Global South.

5. It should be noted, however, that people of all ethnicities, genders, and education and income levels did not reject witchcraft as an explanation for other maladies or ailments.

6. Formal training, teaching, and talking about HIV and printed matter promoting awareness were very common in Mahali.

7. People explained that this had happened during PEV and frequently worried about ART being cut off internationally because funds would stop or economic sanctions would be imposed.

8. Unfortunately, Ndegwa died in a road accident before PrEP was rolled out in the community. Therefore, it is not clear how PrEP might have transformed these relationships.

CHAPTER 4

1. Portions of this chapter were previously published in *Global Public Health* (Pfeiffer and Maithya 2018) and in *Culture, Health and Sexuality* (Pfeiffer and Maithya 2021).

2. These goals expired in 2015 and were replaced by the SDGs. As summarized on the UN website, "The eight Millennium Development Goals (MDGs)—which range from halving extreme poverty rates to halting the spread of HIV/AIDS and providing universal primary education, all by the target date of 2015—form a blueprint agreed to by all the world's countries and all the world's leading development institutions" (UN 2016). The SDGs build on the previous goals in the agenda for 2030 (UN 2015).

3. It is common practice in Kenya, especially among the Kikuyu, for children to be named for their grandparents. It is also common for the new mother to receive postpartum care at the home of the baby's father's parents or of her own mother.

4. Mothers are often called "Mama [name of the first-born child]"—in this case, Mama Beatrice.

5. I heard countless stories saying that it was common practice for a person in Kenya to move away from a community when it became obvious that he/she had HIV or if a spouse or lover was publicly known to have died of complications associated with HIV.

6. The statement echoed the history of the epidemic in Kenya (see the introduction and chapter 1), when early outreach focused almost exclusively on at-risk groups—especially sex workers.

7. This part of the program reflected initial public health development initiatives rooted in Western and extremely individualistic biomedical models of HIV prevention (Parker 2001). It

focused almost exclusively on targeting prevention messages being used in the United States toward the epidemiological category of at-risk groups (Kane 1998). In Kenya, the initial and dominant at-risk group was female CSWs (Kielmann 1997; Hunter 2002; Booth 2004).

8. While I was in the field in 2014, several interlocutors told me about a workshop designed for sex workers living and working across Kenya. I did not hear who sponsored the workshop, but it was held in Nairobi. Those who were selected to participate in the workshop were described as being paid generously to attend the week-long training. They were also given food and housing in an upscale hotel. Only a small number of individuals from Mahali met the selection criteria, one of which was the ability to speak English, which meant that they had to be quite educated. This disqualified and disappointed some women who identified themselves as sex workers.

9. This was an indirect way of saying that someone was infected with HIV.

10. She was able to do this because she was single, which regularly led to the suspicion that a woman was a sex worker.

CHAPTER 5

1. Portions of this chapter were previously published in *Global Public Health* (Pfeiffer and Maithya 2018) and in *Culture, Health & Sexuality* (Pfeiffer and Maithya 2021).

2. The *leso*, sometimes called a *kanga*, is associated with East African womanhood. It is a common gift to new mothers for covering their bodies after giving birth and is used as a baby carrier. Women often carry *lesos* for practical uses—as a towel, curtain, scarf, or shawl, and something to sit on during outdoor gatherings.

3. Having a male child is considered prestigious, important, and very desirable in Kenya, and it is a way in which a woman can elevate her social standing and reputation.

4. During a trip to Mahali in 2019, I was surprised to find that my research assistants were still unaware that ART could suppress viral loads and thus eliminate HIV transmission between discordant couples.

CHAPTER 6

1. Many youths in Kenya today form companionate or romantic marriages. However, having children is still an important way of demonstrating the productivity of the relationship to others and themselves.

2. Among the Kalenjin, children birthed by a married woman are considered to be heirs of the man and his kin group, even if the father did not provide the semen.

REFERENCES

AA (Alcoholics Anonymous). 2009. *Origin of the Serenity Prayer: A Historical Paper*. New York: General Service Office of AA. https://www.aa.org/assets/en_US/smf-129_en.pdf.

Adams, Vincanne. 2016. *Metrics: What Counts in Global Health*. Durham, NC: Duke University Press.

Adams, Vincanne, Nancy J. Burke, and Ian Whitmarsh. 2014. "Slow Research: Thoughts for a Movement in Global Health." *Medical Anthropology* 33(3): 179–197. doi:10.1080/01459740.2013.858335.

Adams, Vincanne, and Stacy Leigh Pigg, eds. 2005. *Sex in Development: Science, Sexuality, and Morality in Global Perspective*. Durham, NC: Duke University Press.

Adichie, Chimamanda Ngozi. 2009. "The Danger of a Single Story." TEDGlobal talk. July. https://www.ted.com/talks/chimamanda_ngozi_adichie_the_danger_of_a_single_story.

Allen, Denise Roth. 2002. *Managing Motherhood, Managing Risk: Fertility and Danger in West Central Tanzania*. Ann Arbor: University of Michigan Press.

Altman, Lawrence K. 1999. "In Africa, a Deadly Silence about AIDS Is Lifting." *New York Times*, July 13. https://archive.nytimes.com/www.nytimes.com/library/national/science/aids/071399hth-doctors.html.

Anderson, Benedict 2006. *Imagined Communities: Reflections on the Origin and Spread of Nationalism*. Rev. ed. London: Verso.

Angotti, Nicole. 2012. "Testing Differences: The Implementation of Western HIV Testing Norms in Sub-Saharan Africa." *Culture, Health & Sexuality* 14(4): 365–378. doi:10.1080/13691058.2011.644810.

Apter, Andrew. 1999. "Nigerian Democracy and the Politics of Illusion." In *Civil Society and the Political Imagination in Africa: Critical Perspectives*, edited by John L. Comaroff and Jean Comaroff, 267–307. Chicago: University of Chicago Press.

Ashforth, Adam. 2004. "AIDS and Witchcraft in Post-Apartheid South Africa." In *Anthropology in the Margins of the State*, edited by Veena Das and Deborah Poole, 141–164. Santa Fe, NM: SAR Press.

Ashforth, Adam. 2005. *Witchcraft, Violence, and Democracy in South Africa*. Chicago: University of Chicago Press.

Ashforth, Adam. 2009. "Ethnic Violence and the Prospects for Democracy in the Aftermath of the 2007 Kenyan Elections." *Public Culture* 21(1): 9–19. doi:10.1215/08992363-2008-018.

Ashforth, Adam. 2015. "Witchcraft, Justice, and Human Rights in Africa: Cases from Malawi." *African Studies Review* 58(1): 5–38. doi:10.1017/asr.2015.2.

Ashforth, Adam, and Susan Watkins. 2015. "Narratives of Death in Rural Malawi in the Time of AIDS." *Africa* 85(2): 245–268. doi:10.1017/S0001972015000017.

Avert. 2020. "HIV and AIDS in Kenya." August 25. http://www.avert.org/hiv-aids-kenya.htm.

Bakhtin, Mikhail M. 1982. *The Dialogic Imagination: Four Essays*. Edited by Michael Holquist. Translated by Caryl Emerson and Michael Holquist. Austin: University of Texas Press.

Bakhtin, Mikhail M. 1986. *Speech Genres and Other Late Essays*. Translated by Vern W. McGee. Austin: University of Texas Press.

Barkan, Joel D. 1993. "Kenya: Lessons from a Flawed Election." *Journal of Democracy* 4(3): 85–99. doi:10.1353/jod.1993.0045.

Barnett, Tony, and Alan Whiteside. 2006. *AIDS in the Twenty-First Century: Disease and Globalization*. 2nd ed. Basingstoke, UK: Palgrave Macmillan.

"Battered Men Silent for Fear of Being Rebuked." 2012. *Daily Nation*, February 14.

Bauman, Richard, and Charles L. Briggs. 1990. "Poetics and Performance as Critical Perspectives on Language and Social Life." *Annual Review of Anthropology* 19: 59–88. doi:10.1146/annurev.an.19.100190.000423.

Bayer, Ronald, and Amy L. Fairchild. 2006. "Changing the Paradigm for HIV Testing: The End of Exceptionalism." *New England Journal of Medicine* 355(7): 647–649. doi:10.1056/NEJMp068153.

BBC (British Broadcasting Company). 2019. "Garissa University College Attack in Kenya: What Happened?" June 19. https://www.bbc.com/news/world-africa-48621924.

Benton, Adia. 2015. *HIV Exceptionalism: Development through Disease in Sierra Leone*. Minneapolis: University of Minnesota Press.

Biehl, João. 2007. *Will to Live: AIDS Therapies and the Politics of Survival*. Princeton, NJ: Princeton University Press.

Biehl, João. 2008. "Drugs for All: The Future of Global AIDS Treatment." *Medical Anthropology* 27(2): 1–7. doi:10.1080/01459740802022777.

Biehl, João, and Adriana Petryna. 2013. *When People Come First: Critical Studies in Global Health*. Princeton, NJ: Princeton University Press.

Biruk, Crystal. 2018. *Cooking Data: Culture and Politics in an African Research World*. Durham, NC: Duke University Press.

Blunt, Robert. 2004. "'Satan Is an Imitator': Kenya's Recent Cosmology of Corruption." In *Producing African Futures: Ritual and Reproduction in a Neoliberal Age*, edited by Brad Weiss, 294–328. Leiden, the Netherlands: Brill.

Boarts, Jessica M., Eve M. Sledjeski, Laura M. Bogart, and Douglas L. Delahanty. 2006. "The Differential Impact of PTSD and Depression on HIV Disease Markers and Adherence to HAART in People Living with HIV." *AIDS and Behavior* 10(3): 253–261. doi:10.1007/s10461-006-9069-7.

Boellstorff, Tom. 2009. "Nuri's Testimony: HIV/AIDS in Indonesia and Bare Knowledge." *American Ethnologist* 36(2): 351–363. doi:10.1111/j.1548-1425.2009.01139.x.

Boone, Catherine, and Jake Batsell. 2001. "Politics and AIDS in Africa: Research Agendas in Political Science and International Relations." *Africa Today* 48(2): 3–33.

Booth, Karen. 2004. *Local Women, Global Science: Fighting AIDS in Kenya*. Bloomington: Indiana University Press.

Bor, Jacob. 2007. "The Political Economy of AIDS Leadership in Developing Countries: An Exploratory Analysis." *Social Science & Medicine* 64(8): 1585–1599. doi:10.1016/j.socscimed.2006.12.005.

Borneman, John, and Abdellah Hammoudi. 2009. *Being There: The Fieldwork Encounter and the Making of Truth*. Berkeley: University of California Press.

Bornstein, Erica. 2005. *The Spirit of Development: Protestant NGOs, Morality, and Economics in Zimbabwe*. Stanford, CA: Stanford University Press.

Bourdieu, Pierre, and Loïc J. D. Wacquant. 1992. *An Invitation to Reflexive Sociology*. Chicago: University of Chicago Press.

Brada, Betsey. 2011. "'Not Here': Making the Spaces and Subjects of 'Global Health' in Botswana." *Culture, Medicine, and Psychiatry* 35(2): 285–312. doi:10.1007/s11013-011-9209-z.

Brandt, Allan M. 2013. "How AIDS Invented Global Health." *New England Journal of Medicine* 368(23): 2149–2152. doi:10.1056/NEJMp1305297.

Brass, Jennifer N. 2016. *Allies or Adversaries: NGOs and the State in Africa*. New York: Cambridge University Press.

Bratton, Michael. 1989. "The Politics of Government-NGO Relations in Africa." *World Development* 17(4): 569–587. doi:10.1016/0305-750X(89)90263-5.

Brewis, Alexandra, and Amber Wutich. 2019. *Lazy, Crazy, and Disgusting: The Undoing of Global Health.* Baltimore, MD: Johns Hopkins University Press.

Briggs, Charles, and Clara Mantini-Briggs. 2003. *Stories in the Time of Cholera: Racial Profiling during a Medical Nightmare.* Berkeley: University of California Press.

Buggenhagen, Beth. 2004. "Domestic Object(ion)s: The Senegalese Murid Trade Diaspora and the Politics of Marriage Payments, Love, and State Privatization." In *Producing African Futures: Ritual and Reproduction in a Neoliberal Age,* edited by Brad Weiss, 21–53. Leiden, the Netherlands: Brill.

Burke, Timothy. 1996. *Lifebuoy Men, Lux Women: Commodification, Consumption, and Cleanliness in Modern Zimbabwe.* Durham, NC: Duke University Press.

Bwayo, Job, A. Mohamed Omari, Ann N. Mutere, Walter Jaoko, Christine Sekkade-Kigondu, Joan Kreiss, and Francis A. Plummer. 1991. "Long Distance Truck-Drivers: 1. Prevalence of Sexually Transmitted Diseases (STDs)." *East African Medical Journal* 68(6): 425–429.

Bwayo, Job, Francis Plummer, Mohamed Omari, Ann Mutere, Stephen Moses, Jeckoniah Ndinya-Achola, Priscilla Velentgas, et al. 1994. "Human Immunodeficiency Virus Infection in Long-Distance Truck Drivers in East Africa." *Archives of Internal Medicine* 154(12): 1391–1396. doi:10.1001/archinte.1994.00420120123013.

Carrithers, Michael, Steven Collins, and Steven Lukes, eds. 1996. *The Category of the Person: Anthropology, Philosophy, History.* Cambridge: Cambridge University Press.

Castro, Arachu, and Paul Farmer. 2005. "Understanding and Addressing AIDS-Related Stigma: From Anthropological Theory to Clinical Practice in Haiti." *American Journal of Public Health* 95(1): 53–59. doi:10.2105/AJPH.2003.028563.

CDC (Centers for Disease Control and Prevention). 1981. "*Pneumocystis* Pneumonia—Los Angeles." *Morbidity and Mortality Weekly Report* 30(21): 1–3. https://www.cdc.gov/mmwr/preview/mmwrhtml/june_5.htm.

CDC (Centers for Disease Control and Prevention). 2021. "Let's Stop HIV Together: HIV Stigma: Ways to Stop HIV Stigma and Discrimination." https://www.cdc.gov/stophivtogether/hiv-stigma/ways-to-stop.html.

Chege, Sam. 1999. "Donors Shift More Aid to NGOs." Global Policy Forum. https://archive.globalpolicy.org/component/content/article/176-general/31445.html.

Cherutich, Peter, Reinhard Kaiser, Jennifer Galbraith, John Williamson, Ray W. Shiraishi, Carol Ngare, Jonathan Mermin, et al. 2012. "Lack of Knowledge of HIV Status a Major Barrier to HIV Prevention, Care and Treatment Efforts in Kenya." *PLoS One* 7(5): e36797. doi:10.1371/journal.pone.0036797.

Cogburn, Megan, Adrienne Strong, and Summer Wood. 2019. "Choiceless Choice in Tanzania: Homebirth, Hospital Birth, and Birth Registration." In *Birth in Eight Cultures,* edited by Robbie Davis-Floyd and Melissa Cheyney, 49–87. Long Grove, IL: Waveland Press.

Cole, Jennifer, and Lynn M. Thomas, eds. 2009. *Love in Africa.* Chicago: University of Chicago Press.

Comaroff, Jean, and John Comaroff, eds. 1993. *Modernity and Its Malcontents: Ritual and Power in Postcolonial Africa.* Chicago: University of Chicago Press.

Comaroff, Jean, and John L. Comaroff. 2006. Preface to *Law and Disorder in the Postcolony,* edited by Jean Comaroff and John L. Comaroff, vii–x. Chicago: University of Chicago Press.

Comaroff, John L., and Jean Comaroff. 2001. "On Personhood: An Anthopological Perspective from Africa." *Social Identities* 7(2): 267–283. doi:10.1080/13504630120065310.

Cooper, Frederick. 1996. *Decolonization and African Society: The Labor Question in French and British Africa.* Cambridge: Cambridge University Press.

Corrigan, Patrick W., and David L. Penn. 1999. "Lessons from Social Psychology on Discrediting Psychiatric Stigma." *American Psychologist* 54(9): 765–776. doi:10.1037/0003-066X.54.9.765.

Corrigan, Patrick W., L. Philip River, Robert K. Lundin, Kyle Uphoff Wasowski, John Campion, James Mathisen, Hillel Goldstein, et al. 2000. "Stigmatizing Attributions about Mental Illness." *Journal of Community Psychology* 28(1): 91–102. doi:10.1002/(SICI)1520 -6629(200001)28:1<91::AID-JCOP9>3.0.CO;2-M.

Crane, Johanna Tayloe. 2013. *Scrambling for Africa: AIDS, Expertise, and the Rise of American Global Health Science.* Ithaca, NY: Cornell University Press.

Crenshaw, Kimberle. 1989. "Demarginalizing the Intersection of Race and Sex: A Black Feminist Critique of Antidiscrimination Doctrine, Feminist Theory and Antiracist Politics." *University of Chicago Legal Forum* 1989(1): article 8. https://chicagounbound.uchicago .edu/cgi/viewcontent.cgi?article=1052&context=uclf.

CSIS (Center for Strategic and International Studies). 2009. *AMPATH: An Integrated Model of Healthcare in Rift Valley Province, Kenya.* https://www.csis.org/blogs/smart-global -health/ampath-integrated-model-healthcare-rift-valley-province-kenya.

Dalal, Warren, Daniel R. Feikin, Manase Amolloh, Ray Ransom, Heather Burke, Fillet Lugalia, Alice Ouma, et al. 2013. "Home-Based HIV Testing and Counseling in Rural and Urban Kenyan Communities." *Journal of Acquired Immune Deficiency Syndromes* 62(2): e47–e54. doi:10.1097/QAI.0b013e318276beao.

Das, Moupali, Priscilla Lee Chu, Glenn-Milo Santos, Susan Scheer, Eric Vittinghoff, Willi McFarland, and Gant N. Colfax. 2010. "Decreases in Community Viral Load Are Accompanied by Reductions in New HIV Infections in San Fransisco." *PLOS Medicine* 5(6): e11068. http://www.plosone.org/article/info:doi/10.1371/journal.pone.0011068.

Das, Veena. 2001. "Stigma, Contagion, Defect: Issues in the Anthropology of Public Health." Presented at the conference on "Stigma and Global Health: Developing a Research Agenda," Bethesda, MD, September 5–7. https://web.archive.org/web/20130318041954 /http://www.stigmaconference.nih.gov/FinalDasPaper.htm.

Das, Veena, and Deborah Poole, eds. 2004. *Anthropology in the Margins of the State.* Santa Fe, NM: SAR Press.

Davis, Mark, and Paul Flowers. 2014. "HIV/STI Prevention Technologies and 'Strategic (In) Visibilities.'" In *Disclosure in Health and Illness*, edited by Mark Davis and Lenore Manderson, 72–88. New York: Routledge.

Davis, Mark, and Lenore Manderson. 2014. "Contours of Truth." In *Disclosure in Health and Illness*, edited by Mark Davis and Lenore Manderson, 153–165. New York: Routledge.

Davison, Jean. 1989. *Voices from Mutira: Lives of Rural Gikuyu Women.* Boulder, CO: Lynne Rienner.

Davison, Jean. 1996. *Voices from Mutira: Change in the Lives of Rural Gikuyu Women, 1910–1995.* 2nd ed. Boulder, CO: Lynne Rienner.

D'Costa, Lourdes J., Francis A. Plummer, Ian Bowmer, Lieve Fransen, Peter Piot, Allan R. Ronald, and Herbert Nsanze. 1985. "Prostitutes Are a Major Reservoir of Sexually Transmitted Diseases in Nairobi, Kenya." *Sexually Transmitted Diseases* 12(2): 64–67.

De Klerk, Josien, and Eileen Moyer. 2017. "'A Body Like a Baby': Social Self-Care among Older People with Chronic HIV in Mombasa." *Medical Anthropology* 36(4): 305–318. doi: 10.1080/01459740.2016.1235573.

De León, Jason. 2015. *The Land of Open Graves: Living and Dying on the Migrant Trail.* Oakland: University of California Press.

Dilger, Hansjörg. 2008. "'We Are All Going to Die': Kinship, Belongings, and the Morality of HIV/AIDS-Related Illnesses and Deaths in Rural Tanzania." *Anthropological Quarterly* 81(1): 207–232. doi:10.1353/anq.2008.0009.

Dingfelder, Sadie F. 2009. "Stigma: Alive and Well." *Monitor* 40(6): 56. https://www.apa.org/monitor/2009/06/stigma.

Dionne, Kim Yi. 2017. *Doomed Interventions: The Failure of Global Responses to AIDS in Africa.* Cambridge: Cambridge University Press.

Druyts, Eric, Mark Dybul, Steve Kanters, Jean Nachega, Josephine Birungi, Nathan Ford, Kristian Thorlund, et al. 2013. "Male Sex and the Risk of Mortality among Individuals Enrolled in Antiretroviral Therapy Programs in Africa: A Systematic Review and Meta-Analysis." *AIDS* 27(3): 417–425. doi:10.1097/QAD.0b013e328359b89b.

Eaton, David. 2008. "Ambivalent Inquiry: Dilemmas of AIDS in the Republic of Congo." In *Postcolonial Disorders*, edited by Mary-Jo Del Vecchio Good, Sandra Teresa Hyde, Sarah Pinto, and Byron J. Good, 238–258. Berkeley: University of California Press.

Edelman, Marc, and Angelique Haugerud. 2007. Introduction to *The Anthropology of Development and Globalization*, edited by Marc Edelman and Angelique Haugerud, 1–27. Malden, MA: Blackwell.

Elie, Paul. 2020. "(Against) Virus as Metaphor." *New Yorker*, March 19. https://www.newyorker.com/news/daily-comment/against-the-coronavirus-as-metaphor/amp.

Engel, Jonathan. 2006. *The Epidemic: A Global History of AIDS.* Washington, DC: Smithsonian Books.

Epstein, Helen. 2007. *The Invisible Cure: Why We Are Losing the Fight against AIDS in Africa.* New York: Picador.

Epstein, Helen. 2009. *Spotlight on Prevention: Uganda's Zero Grazing Campaign.* Washington, DC: United States Agency for International Development AIDSTAR-One Project. https://publications.jsi.com/JSIInternet/Inc/Common/_download_pub.cfm?id=18892&lid=3.

Evans-Pritchard, E. E. 1976. *Witchcraft Oracles and Magic among the Azande.* Oxford: Oxford University Press.

Eves, Richard, and Leslie Butt. 2008. Introduction to *Making Sense of AIDS: Culture, Sexuality, and Power in Melanesia*, edited by Leslie Butt and Richard Eves, 1–23. Honolulu: University of Hawai'i Press.

Farmer, Paul. 1992. *AIDS and Accusation: Haiti and the Geography of Blame.* Berkeley: University of California Press.

Farmer, Paul. 2001. *Infections and Inequalities: The Modern Plagues.* Updated ed. Berkeley: University of California Press.

Farmer, Paul. 2004. "An Anthropology of Structural Violence." *Current Anthropology* 45(3): 305–325. doi:10.1086/382250.

Farmer, Paul, Margaret Connors, and Janie Simmons. 1996. *Women, Poverty, and AIDS: Sex, Drugs, and Structural Violence.* Monroe, ME: Common Courage Press.

Farmer, Paul E., Bruce Nizeye, Sara Stulac, and Salmaan Keshavjee. 2006. "Structural Violence and Clinical Medicine." *PLoS Medicine* 3(10): 1686–1691. https://journals.plos.org/plosmedicine/article/file?id=10.1371/journal.pmed.0030449&type=printable.

Fassin, Didier. 2007. *When Bodies Remember: Experiences and Politics of AIDS in South Africa.* Translated by Amy Jacobs and Gabrielle Varro. Berkeley: University of California Press.

Fassin, Didier. 2012. *Humanitarian Reason: A Moral History of the Present.* Translated by Rachel Gomme. Berkeley: University of California Press.

Fassin, Didier. 2018. *Life: A Critical User's Manual.* Cambridge: Polity Press.

Feldman, Douglas A., ed. 1994. *Global AIDS Policy.* Westport, CT: Bergin and Garvey.

Ferguson, James. 1994. *The Anti-Politics Machine: Development, Depoliticization, and Bureaucratic Power in Lesotho.* Minneapolis: University of Minnesota Press.

Ferguson, James. 2006. *Global Shadows: Africa in the Neoliberal World Order.* Durham, NC: Duke University Press.

Fisher, William A., Taylor Kohut, and Jeffrey D. Fisher. 2009. "AIDS Exceptionalism: On the Social Psychology of HIV Prevention Research." *Social Issues and Policy Review* 3(1): 45–77. doi:10.1111/j.1751-2409.2009.01010.x.

Fortes, Meyer. 1973. "On the Concept of the Person among the Tallensi." In *La notion de personne en Afrique Noire*, edited by G. Dieterlen, 283–319. Paris: Centre National de la Recherche Scientifique.

Frank, Emily, and Alexander Rödlach. 2013. "To Disclose or Not to Disclose, That Is the Question! Antiretroviral Therapy, Access to Resources and Stigma in Southern Africa." *Journal of Southern African Studies* 39(1): 119–133. doi:10.1080/03057070.2013.767087.

Fylkesnes, Knut, Ingvild Fossgard Sandøy, Marte Jürgensen, Peter J. Chipimo, Sheila Mwangala, and Charles Michelo. 2013. "Strong Effects of Home-Based Voluntary HIV Counselling and Testing on Acceptance and Equity: A Cluster Randomised Trial in Zambia." *Social Science & Medicine* 86(June): 9–16. doi:10.1016/j.socscimed.2013.02.036.

Garrett, Laurie. 2007. "The Challenge of Global Health." *Foreign Affairs* 86(1): 14–38.

Geertz, Clifford. 1973. *The Interpretation of Cultures.* New York: Basic Books.

Geissler, Paul Wenzel. 2013. "Public Secrets in Public Health: Knowing Not to Know While Making Scientific Knowledge." *American Ethnologist* 40(1): 13–34. doi:10.1111/amet.12002.

Geissler, Paul Wenzel, and Ruth Jane Prince. 2010. *The Land Is Dying: Contingency, Creativity and Conflict in Western Kenya.* New York: Berghahn Books.

Geschiere, Peter. 1997. *The Modernity of Witchcraft: Politics and the Occult in Postcolonial Africa.* Charlottesville: University of Virginia Press.

Geschiere, Peter. 2009. *The Perils of Belonging: Autochthony, Citizenship, and Exclusion in Africa and Europe.* Chicago: University of Chicago Press.

Geschiere, Peter. 2013. *Witchcraft, Intimacy, and Trust: Africa in Comparison.* Chicago: University of Chicago Press.

Gilley, Brian J., and Elizabeth J. Pfeiffer. 2017. "'White Man's Disease': American Indian AIDS Conspiracy Theories and the Refusal of Synthesis." *Medicine Anthropology Theory* 4(3): 1–20. doi:10.17157/mat.4.3.456.

Gitahi, Nyawira, Sheila Juliet Eshiwani, Kenneth Mutai, Jared Ongechi Mecha, and James Njogu Kiarie. 2020. "Preconception Care Uptake and Immediate Outcomes among Discordant Couples Accessing Routine HIV Care in Kenya." *Ostetrics & Gynecology International* 2020: article 1675987. doi:10.1155/2020/1675987.

Global Fund (The Global Fund to Fight AIDS, Tuberculosis and Malaria). 2019. "Global Fund Donors Pledge US$14 Billion in Fight to End Epidemics." https://www.theglobal fund.org/en/news/2019-10-10-global-fund-donors-pledge-usd14-billion-in-fight-to-end -epidemics/.

Goffman, Erving. 1963. *Stigma: Notes on the Management of Spoiled Identity.* London: Penguin Books.

Goldstein, Diane E. 2004. *Once upon a Virus: AIDS Legends and Vernacular Risk Perception.* Logan: Utah State University Press.

Goldstein, Donna M. 2003. *Laughter out of Place: Race, Class, Violence, and Sexuality in a Rio Shantytown.* Berkeley: University of California Press.

Goodman, Allan. 2016. "Disease and Dying While Black: How Racism, not Race, Gets under the Skin." In *New Directions in Biocultural Anthropology*, edited by Molly K. Zuckerman and Debra L. Martin, 69–87. Hoboken, NJ: Wiley.

Gostin, Lawrence O. 2013. "PEPFAR's Antiprostitution Pledge: Spending Power and Free Speech in Tension." *Journal of the American Medical Association* 310(11): 1127–1128. doi: 10.1001/jama.2013.276527.

Green, Edward C. 2003. *Rethinking AIDS Prevention: Learning from Successes in Developing Countries.* Westport, CT: Praeger.

Green, Edward C., Daniel T. Halperin, Vinand Nantulya, and Janice A. Hogle. 2006. "Uganda's HIV Prevention Success: The Role of Sexual Behavior Change and the National Response." *AIDS and Behavior* 10(4): 335–346. doi: 10.1007/s10461-006-9073-y.

Greene, Jeremy, Marguerite Thorp Basilico, Heidi Kim, and Paul Farmer. 2013. "Colonial Medicine and Its Legacies." In *Reimagining Global Health: An Introduction*, edited by Paul Farmer, Jim Yong Kim, Arthur Kleinman, and Matthew Basilico, 33–73. Berkeley: University of California Press.

Grosz-Ngaté, Maria, and Omari H. Kokole, eds. 1997. *Gendered Encounters: Challenging Cultural Boundaries and Social Hierarchies in Africa.* London: Routledge.

Gupta, Akhil. 1998. *Postcolonial Developments: Agriculture in the Making of Modern India.* Durham, NC: Duke University Press.

Gupta, Akhil, and James Ferguson. 1997. *Anthropological Locations: Boundaries and Grounds of a Field Science.* Berkeley: University of California Press.

Hammonds, Rachael, Gorik Ooms, Moses Mulumba, and Allan Maleche. 2019. "UHC2030's Contributions to Global Health Governance That Advance the Right to Health Care: A Preliminary Assessment." *Health and Human Rights* 21(2): 235–249.

Hannig, Anita. 2017. *Beyond Surgery: Injury, Healing, and Religion at an Ethiopian Hospital.* Chicago: University of Chicago Press.

Hardon, Anita, and Hansjörg Dilger. 2011. "Global AIDS Medicines in East African Health Institutions." *Medical Anthropology* 30(2): 136–157. doi:10.1080/01459740.2011.552458.

Hardon, Anita, and Eileen Moyer. 2014. "Anthropology of AIDS: Modes of Engagement." *Medical Anthropology* 33(4): 255–262. doi:10.1080/01459740.2014.889132.

Hardon, Anita, and Deborah Posel. 2012. "Secrecy as Embodied Practice: Beyond the Confessional Imperative." *Culture, Health & Sexuality* 14(Suppl 1): S1–S13. doi:10.1080/13691058.2012.726376.

Hardon, Anita, Eva Vernooij, Grace Bongololo-Mbera, Peter Cherutich, Alice Desclaux, David Kyaddondo, Odette Ky-Zerbo, et al. 2012. "Women's Views on Consent, Counseling, and Confidentiality in PMTCT: A Mixed-Methods Study in Four African Countries." *BMC Public Health* 12: art. 26. doi:10.1186/1471-2458-12-26.

Hatzenbuehler, Mark L., Jo C. Phelan, and Bruce G. Link. 2013. "Stigma as a Fundamental Cause of Population Health Inequalities." *American Journal of Public Health* 103(5): 813–821. doi:10.2105/AJPH.2012.301069.

Haugerud, Angelique. 1995. *The Culture of Politics in Modern Kenya.* Cambridge: Cambridge University Press.

Hecht, Robert, Anita Alban, Kate Taylor, Sarah Post, Nina B. Andersen, and Ryan Schwarz. 2006. "Putting It Together: AIDS and the Millennium Development Goals." *PLoS Medicine* 3(11): e455. doi:10.1371/journal.pmed.0030455.

Hershey, Megan. 2019. *Whose Agency: The Politics and Practice of Kenya's HIV-Prevention NGOs.* Madison: University of Wisconsin Press.

Hirsch, Jennifer S., Richard G. Parker, and Peter Aggleton. 2007. "Social Aspects of Antiretroviral Therapy Scale-Up: Introduction and Overview." *AIDS* 21(Suppl 5): S1–S4. doi:10.1097/01.aids.0000298096.51728.7d.

Hirsch, Jennifer S., Holy Wardow, Daniel Jordan Smith, Harriet M. Phinney, Shanti Parikh, and Constance A. Nathanson, eds. 2009. *The Secret: Love, Marriage, and HIV.* Nashville, TN: Vanderbilt University Press.

Hodgson, Dorothy, and Sheryl A. McCurdy, eds. 2001. *"Wicked" Women and the Reconfiguration of Gender in Africa.* Portsmouth, NH: Heinemann.

HRW (Human Rights Watch). 2001. "Kenya: In the Shadow of Death: HIV/AIDS and Children's Rights in Kenya." New York: Human Rights Watch. https://www.hrw.org/reports/2001 /kenya/.

Humphreys, Michael, and Tony Watson. 2009. "From 'Writing Up Ethnographic Research' to 'Writing Ethnography.'" In *Organizational Ethnography: Studying the Complexities of Everyday Life*, edited by Sierk Ybema, Dvora Yanow, Harry Wels, and Fran H. Kemsteeg, 40–55. Thousand Oaks, CA: Sage.

Hunter, Mark, 2002. "The Materiality of Everyday Sex: Thinking beyond 'Prostitution.'" *African Studies* 61(1): 99–120. doi:10.1080/00020180220140091.

Hunter, Mark. 2007. "The Changing Political Economy of Sex in South Africa: The Significance of Unemployment and Inequalities to the Scale of the AIDS Pandemic." *Social Science & Medicine* 64(3): 689–700. doi:10.1016/j.socscimed.2006.09.015.

Hunter, Mark. 2010. *Love in the Time of AIDS: Inequality, Gender, and Rights in South Africa*. Durban, South Africa: University of KwaZulu-Natal Press.

Iliffe, John. 2006. *The African AIDS Epidemic: A History*. Athens: Ohio University Press.

Jackson, Denis J., Joel P. Rakwar, Barbara A. Richardson, Krupali Mandaliya, Bhavna H. Chohan, Job J. Bwayo, Jeckoniah Ndinya-Achola, et al. 1997. "Decreased Incidence of Sexually Transmitted Diseases among Trucking Company Workers in Kenya: Results of a Behavioural Risk-Reduction Programme." *AIDS* 11(7): 903–990. doi:10.1097/00002030-199707000-00010.

Jackson, Lynette A. 2002. "'When in the White Man's Town': Zimbabwean Women Remember Chibeura." In *Women in African Colonial Histories: An Introduction*, edited by Susan Geiger, Nakanyike Musisi, and Jean Marie Allman, 119–218. Bloomington: Indiana University Press.

Jackson, Michael, and Ivan Karp, eds. 1990. *Personhood and Agency: The Experience of Self and Other in African Society*. Washington, DC: Smithsonian Institution Press.

Jacoby, Ann. 1994. "Felt versus Enacted Stigma: A Concept Revisited: Evidence from a Study of People with Epilepsy in Remission." *Social Science & Medicine* 38(2): 269–274. doi:10.1016 /0277-9536(94)90396-4.

Janz, Bruce. 2002. "Janz on Mbembe, 'On the Postcolony.'" *H-Africa*, March. https://networks .h-net.org/node/28765/reviews/32781/janz-mbembe-postcolony.

Jasanoff, Sheila, ed. 2004. *States of Knowledge: The Co-production of Science and the Social Order*. London: Routledge.

Jenkins, Rachel, Caleb Othieno, Stephen Okeyo, Julyan Aruwa, James Kingora, and Ben Jenkins. 2013. "Health System Challenges to Integration of Mental Health Delivery in Primary Care in Kenya: Perspectives of Primary Care Health Workers." *BMC Health Services Research* 13: article 368. doi:10.1186/1472-6963-13-368.

Kaler, Amy, and Susan Watkins. 2010. "Asking God about the Date You Will Die: HIV Testing as a Zone of Uncertainty in Rural Malawi." *Demographic Research* 23: article 32, 905–932. https://www.demographic-research.org/volumes/vol23/32/23-32.

Kalofonos, Ippolytos Andreas. 2010. "'All I Eat Is ARVs': The Paradox of AIDS Treatment Interventions in Central Mozambique." *Medical Anthropology Quarterly* 24(3): 363–380. doi:10.1111/j.1548-1387.2010.01109.x.

Kamungi, Prisca Mbura. 2009. "The Politics of Displacement in Multiparty Kenya." *Journal of Contemporary African Studies* 27(3): 345–364. doi:10.1080/02589000903166713.

Kane, Stephanie. 1998. *AIDS Alibis: Sex, Drugs, and Crime in the Americas*. Philadelphia: Temple University Press.

Karatzas, Nicolaos, Trevor Peter, Sailly Dave, Clare Fogarty, Nandi Belinsky, and Nitika Pant Pai. 2019. "Are Policy Initiatives Aligned to Meet UNAIDS 90-90-90 Targets Impacting HIV Testing and Linkages to Care? Evidence from a Systematic Review." *PLoS One* 14(6): e0216936. doi:10.1371/journal.pone.0216936.

Karp, Ivan. 2002. "Development and Personhood: Tracing the Contours of a Moral Discourse." In *Critically Modern: Alternatives, Alterities, Anthropologies*, edited by Bruce Knauft, 82–104. Bloomington: Indiana University Press.

Kaufman, Carol E., and Stavros E. Stavrou. 2004. "'Bus Fare Please': The Economics of Sex and Gifts among Young People in Urban South Africa." *Culture, Health & Sexuality* 6(5): 377–391. doi:10.1080/13691050410001680492.

Kemp, Christopher G., Brooke A. Jarrett, Churl-Su Kwon, Lanxin Song, Nathalie Jetté, Jaime C. Sapag, Judith Bass, et al. 2019. "Implementation Science and Stigma Reduction Interventions in Low- and Middle-Income Countries: A Systematic Review." *BMC Medicine* 17(6). doi:10.1186/s12916-018-1237-x.

Kenworthy, Nora. 2017. *Mistreated: The Political Consequences of the Fight against AIDS in Lesotho*. Nashville, TN: Vanderbilt University Press.

Kenworthy, Nora, Matthew Thomann, and Richard Parker. 2018. "From a Global Crisis to the 'End of AIDS': New Epidemics of Signification." *Global Public Health* 13(8): 960–971. doi: 10.1080/17441692.2017.1365373.

Kenyan Ministry of Health. 2014. *Kenya HIV Prevention Revolution Road Map: Count Down to 2030*. Nairobi: National AIDS Control Council. https://reliefweb.int/sites/reliefweb.int /files/resources/Kenya_HIV_Prevention_Revolution_Road_Map.pdf.

Kenyatta, Jomo. 1962. *Facing Mount Kenya*. New York: Vintage Books.

Kidder, Tracy. 2003. *Mountains beyond Mountains: The Quest of Dr. Paul Farmer, a Man Who Would Cure the World*. New York: Random House.

Kielmann, Karina. 1997. "'Prostitution,' 'Risk,' and 'Responsibility': Paradigms of AIDS Prevention and Women's Identities in Thika, Kenya." In *The Anthropology of Infectious Disease: International Health Perspectives*, edited by Marcia Inhorn and Peter Brown, 375–412. London: Routledge.

Kim, Young Soo. 2015. "World Health Organization and Early Global Response to HIV/ AIDS: Emergence and Development of International Norms." *Journal of International and Area Studies* 22(1): 19–40. https://www.jstor.org/stable/43490278.

Kimanga, Davies O., Samuel Ogola, Mamo Umuro, Anne Ng'ang'a, Lucy Kimondo, Patrick Murithi, James Muttunga, et al. 2014. "Prevalence and Incidence of HIV Infection, Trends, and Risk Factors among Persons Aged 15–64 Years in Kenya: Results from a Nationally Representative Study." *Journal of Acquired Immune Deficiency Syndromes* 66(Suppl 1): S13–S26. doi:10.1097/QAI.0000000000000124.

Kleinman, Arthur. 1988. *The Illness Narratives: Suffering, Healing & The Human Condition*. New York: Basic Books.

Kleinman, Arthur. 2006. *What Really Matters: Living a Moral Life amidst Uncertainty and Danger*. New York: Oxford University Press.

Kleinman, Arthur. 2009. "Global Mental Health: A Failure of Humanity." *The Lancet* 374(9690): 603–604. doi:10.1016/S0140-6736(09)61510-5.

Knight, Lindsay. 2008. *UNAIDS: The First 10 Years*. Geneva: UNAIDS (Joint United Nations Programme on HIV/AIDS). https://data.unaids.org/pub/report/2008/jc1579_first_10 _years_en.pdf.

Kurth, Ann E., Charles M. Cleland, Don C. Des Jarlais, Helgar Musyoki, John A. Lizcano, Nok Chhun, and Peter Cherutich. 2015. "HIV Prevalence, Estimated Incidence, and Risk Behaviors among People Who Inject Drugs in Kenya." *Journal of Acquired Immune Deficiency Syndromes* 70(4): 420–427. doi:10.1097/QAI.0000000000000769.

Kyaddondo, David, Rhoda K. Wanyenze, John Kinsman, and Anita Hardon. 2012. "Home-Based HIV Counseling and Testing: Client Experiences and Perceptions in Eastern Uganda." *BMC Public Health* 12: 966. doi:10.1186/1471-2458-12-966.

Landsman, Gail Heidi. 2009. *Reconstructing Motherhood and Disability in the Age of "Perfect" Babies*. New York: Routledge.

Langley, Myrtle S. 1979. *The Nandi of Kenya: Life Crisis Rituals in a Period of Change*. London: C. Hurst.

Langwick, Stacey A. 2011. *Bodies, Politics, and African Healing: The Matter of Maladies in Tanzania*. Bloomington: Indiana University Press.

Lassiter, Eric. 2005. *The Chicago Guide to Collaborative Ethnography*. Chicago: University of Chicago Press.

Levine, Ruth, Ngaire Woods, Danielle Kuczynski, and Devi Sridhar. 2009. "UNAIDS: Preparing for the Future: Report of the UNAIDS Leadership Transition Working Group." Washington, DC: Center for Global Development. https://www.cgdev.org/sites/default/files/1421429_file_CGD_GEG_UNAIDS_FINAL.pdf.

Lingappa, Jairam R., Erin Kahle, Nelly Mugo, Andrew Mujugira, Amalia Magaret, Jared Baeten, Elizabeth A. Bukusi, et al. 2009. "Characteristics of HIV-1 Discordant Couples Enrolled in a Trial of HSV-2 Suppression to Reduce HIV-1 Transmission: The Partners Study." *PLoS One* 4(4): e5272. doi:10.1371/journal.pone.0005272.

Link, Bruce G., and Jo Phelan. 2014. "Stigma Power." *Social Science & Medicine* 103(February): 24–32. doi:10.1016/j.socscimed.2013.07.035.

Link, Bruce G., and Jo C. Phelan. 2001. "Conceptualizing Stigma." *Annual Review of Sociology* 27: 363–385. doi:10.1146/annurev.soc.27.1.363.

Link, Bruce G., and Jo C. Phelan. 2017. "Labeling and Stigma." In *A Handbook for the Study of Mental Health: Social Contexts, Theories, and Systems*, 3rd ed., edited by Teresa L. Scheid and Eric R. Wright, 393–408. New York: Cambridge University Press.

Liu, Shao-hua. 2009. "Contested AIDS Stigmatization in Southwest China." *Human Organization* 68(4): 395–405. doi:10.17730/humo.68.4.7337165480066855.

Livingston, Julie. 2012. *Improvising Medicine: An African Oncology Ward in an Emerging Cancer Epidemic*. Durham, NC: Duke University Press.

Lock, Margaret, and Vinh-Kim Nguyen. 2010. *An Anthropology of Biomedicine*. Malden, MA: Wiley-Blackwell.

Lock, Margaret, and Nancy Scheper-Hughes. 1996. "A Critical-Interpretive Approach in Medical Anthropology: Rituals and Routines of Discipline and Dissent." In *Medical Anthropology: Contemporary Theory and Method*, edited by Carolyn F. Sargent and Thomas M. Johnson, 41–70. Westport, CT: Praeger.

Lonsdale, John. 1992. "The Moral Economy of Mau Mau: Wealth, Poverty & Civic Virtue in Kikuyu Political Thought." In *Unhappy Valley: Conflict in Kenya & Africa*, edited by Bruce Berman and John Lonsdale, 315–504. London: James Currey.

Lorch, Donatella. 1993. "After Years of Ignoring AIDS Epidemic, Kenya Has Begun Facing Up to It." *New York Times*, December 18. https://www.nytimes.com/1993/12/18/world/after-years-of-ignoring-aids-epidemic-kenya-has-begun-facing-up-to-it.html.

Lynch, Gabrielle. 2011. *I Say to You: Ethnic Politics and the Kalenjin in Kenya*. Chicago: University of Chicago Press.

Macha, Ndesanjo. 2012. "Kenya: Schoolgirl Skirts—How Short Is Too Short?" *GlobalVoices*, July 26. https://globalvoices.org/2012/07/26/kenya-netizens-debate-culture-modenirty-and-miniskirts/.

"Male Edifice Crumbles as Women Rise." 2012. *Daily Nation*, February 18.

Manderson, Lenore. 2014. "Telling Points." In *Disclosure in Health and Illness*, edited by Mark Davis and Lenore Manderson, 1–15. New York: Routledge.

Manderson, Lenore, Elizabeth Cartwright, and Anita Hardon. 2016. *The Routledge Handbook of Medical Anthropology*. New York: Routledge.

Manderson, Lenore, Mark Davis, Chip Colewell, and Tanja Ahlin. 2015. "On Secrecy, Disclosure, the Public, and the Private in Anthropology: An Introduction to Supplement 12." *Current Anthropology* 56(S12): S183–S190. doi:10.1086/683302.

Mann, Jonathan. 1987. "The World Health Organisation's Global Strategy for the Prevention and Control of AIDS." *Western Journal of Medicine* 147(6): 732–734.

Mann, Jonathan, Daniel J. M. Tarantola, and Thomas W. Netter, eds. 1992. *AIDS in the World 1992*. Cambridge, MA: Harvard University Press.

Marcus, George, and Michael Fischer. 1999. *Anthropology as Cultural Critique: An Experimental Moment in the Human Sciences*. Chicago: University of Chicago Press.

Marsland, Rebecca, and Ruth Prince. 2012. "What Is Life Worth? Exploring Biomedical Interventions, Survival, and the Politics of Life." *Medical Anthropology Quarterly* 26(4): 453–469. doi:10.1111/maq.12001.

Martin, Faith, Thadeus Kiwanuka, Rachel Kawuma, Flavia Zalwango, and Janet Seeley. 2013. "Tasks and Strategies of Self-Management of Living with Antiretroviral Therapy in Uganda." *AIDS Patient Care and STDs* 27(12): 697–706. doi:10.1089/apc.2013.0254.

Massey, Doreen, 1994. *Space, Place, and Gender*. Cambridge: Polity Press.

Masyuko, Sarah, Irene Mukui, Olivia Njathi, Maureen Kimani, Patricia Oluoch, Joyce Wamicwe, Jane Mutegi, et al. 2018. "Pre-Exposure Prophylaxis Rollout in a National Public Sector Program: The Kenyan Case Study." *Sexual Health* 15(6): 578–586. doi:10.1071/SH18090.

Mattes, Dominik. 2011. "'We Are Just Supposed to Be Quiet': The Production of Adherence to Antiretroviral Treatment in Urban Tanzania." *Medical Anthropology* 30(2): 158–182. doi: 10.1080/01459740.2011.552454.

Mattes, Dominik. 2014. "Caught in Transition: The Struggle to Live a 'Normal' Life with HIV in Tanzania." *Medical Anthropology* 33(4): 270–287. doi:10.1080/01459740.2013.877899.

Mattes, Dominik. 2019. *Fierce Medicines, Fragile Socialities: Grounding Global HIV Treatment in Tanzania*. New York: Berghahn Books.

Mazanderani, Fadhila, and Sara Paparini. 2015. "The Stories We Tell: Qualitative Research Interviews, Talking Technologies and the 'Normalisation' of Life with HIV." *Social Science & Medicine* 131(April): 66–73. doi:10.1016/j.socscimed.2015.02.041.

Mbembe, Achille, 2001. *On the Postcolony*. Berkeley: University of California Press.

Mbembe, Achille, 2006. "On Politics as a Form of Expenditure." In *Law and Disorder in the Postcolony*, edited by Jean Comaroff and John L. Comaroff, 299–336. Chicago: University of Chicago Press.

Mbugua, G. G., L. N. Muthami, C. W. Mutura, S. A. Oogo, P. G. Waiyaki, C. P. Lindan, and N. Hearst. 1995. "Epidemiology of HIV Infection among Long Distance Truck Drivers in Kenya." *East African Medical Journal* 72(8): 515–518.

McCormick, Joseph B., and Susan Fisher-Hoch. 1996. *Level 4: Virus Hunters of the CDC: Tracking Ebola and the World's Deadliest Viruses*. Atlanta, GA: Turner.

McCoy, David, and Guddi Singh. 2014. "A Spanner in the Works? Anti-Politics in Global Health Policy: Comment on 'A Ghost in the Machine? Politics in Global Health Policy.'" *International Journal of Health Policy and Management* 3(3): 151–153. doi:10.15171/ijhpm.2014.77.

McGrath, Janet W., Margaret S. Winchester, David Kaawa-Mafigiri, Eddy Walakira, Florence Namutiibwa, Judith Birungi, George Ssendegye, et al. 2014. "Challenging the Paradigm: Anthropological Perspectives on HIV as a Chronic Disease." *Medical Anthropology* 33(4): 303–317. doi:10.1080/01459740.2014.892483.

McHenry, Megan Song, Winstone M. Nyandiko, Michael L. Scanlon, Lydia J. Fischer, Carole I. McAteer, Josephine Aluoch, Violet Naanyu, et al. 2017. "HIV Stigma: Perspectives from Kenyan Child Caregivers and Adolescents Living with HIV." *Journal of the International Association of Providers of AIDS Care* 16(3): 215–225. doi:10.1177/2325957416668995.

McKay, Ramah. 2018. *Medicine in the Meantime: The Work of Care in Mozambique.* Durham, NC: Duke University Press.

Mendenhall, Emily. 2017. "Syndemics: A New Path for Global Health Research." *The Lancet* 389(10072): 889–891. doi:10.1016/S0140-6736(17)30602-5.

Mendenhall, Emily, Gregory Barnabas Omondi, Edna Bosire, Gitonga Isaiah, Abednego Musau, David Ndetei, and Victoria Mutiso. 2015. "Stress, Diabetes, and Infection: Syndemic Suffering at an Urban Kenyan Hospital." *Social Science & Medicine* 146(December): 11–20. doi:10.1016/j.socscimed.2015.10.015.

Merson, Michael, and Stephen Inrig. 2018. *The AIDS Pandemic: Searching for a Global Response.* Cham, Switzerland: Springer International Publishing.

Mills, Edward J., Celestin Bakanda, Josephine Birungi, Keith Chan, Nathan Ford, Curtis L. Cooper, Jean B. Nachega, et al. 2011. "Life Expectancy of Persons Receiving Combination Antiretroviral Therapy in Low-Income Countries: A Cohort Analysis from Uganda." *Annals of Internal Medicine* 155(4): 209–216. doi:10.7326/0003-4819-155-4-201108160-00358.

Mills, Edward J., Chris Beyrer, Josephine Birungi, and Mark R. Dybul. 2012. "Engaging Men in Prevention and Care for HIV/AIDS in Africa." *PLoS Medicine* 9: e1001167. doi:10.1371/journal.pmed.1001167.

Mkandawire, Thandika. 2002. "Globalisation, Equity and Social Development." *African Sociological Review* 6(1): 115–137. doi:10.4314/asr.v6i1.23205.

Mkhwanazi, Nolwazi. 2016. "Medical Anthropology in Africa: The Trouble with a Single Story." *Medical Anthropology* 35(2): 193–202. doi:10.1080/01459740.2015.1100612.

Mojola, Sanyu A. 2014. *Love, Money, and HIV: Becoming a Modern African Woman in the Age of AIDS.* Oakland: University of California Press.

Mol, Annemarie. 2008. *The Logic of Care: Health and the Problem of Patient Choice.* New York: Routledge.

Moore, Alexander, and Ronald LeBron. 1986. "The Case for a Haitian Origin of the AIDS Epidemic." In *The Social Dimension of AIDS: Method and Theory*, edited by Douglas Feldman and Thomas Johnson, 77–93. New York: Praeger.

Morton, Andrew. 1998. *Moi: The Making of an African Statesman.* London: Michael O'Mara Books.

Moyer, Eileen. 2012. "*Faidha gani?* What's the Point: HIV and the Logics of (Non)-Disclosure among Young Activists in Zanzibar." *Culture, Health & Sexuality* 14(Suppl 1): S67–S79. doi:10.1080/13691058.2012.662524.

Moyer, Eileen. 2015. "The Anthropology of Life after AIDS: Epistemological Continuities in the Age of Antiretroviral Therapy." *Annual Review of Anthropology* 44: 259–275. doi:10.1146/annurev-anthro-102214-014235.

Moyer, Eileen, and Anita Hardon. 2014. "A Disease Unlike Any Other? Why HIV Remains Exceptional in the Age of Treatment." *Medical Anthropology* 33(4): 263–269. doi:10.1080/01459740.2014.890618.

Moyer, Eileen, and Emmy Igonya. 2018. "Queering the Evidence: Remaking Homosexuality and HIV Risk to 'End AIDS' in Kenya." *Global Public Health* 13(8): 1007–1019. doi:10.1080/17441692.2018.1462841.

MSF (Médecins sans Frontières). 2009. *HIV/AIDS Treatment in Developing Countries: The Battle for Long-Term Survival Has Just Begun.* Geneva: MSF.

Mweru, Maureen. 2010. "Why Are Kenyan Teachers Still Using Corporal Punishment Eight Years after a Ban on Corporal Punishment?" *Child Abuse Review* 19(4): 248–258. doi:10.1002/car.1121.

NACC (National AIDS Control Council). 2005. *Kenya National HIV/AIDS Stategic Plan (KNASP) 2005/06–2009/10.* Nairobi: Office of the President of the Republic of Kenya.

http://www.ilo.org/wcmsp5/groups/public/---ed_protect/---protrav/---ilo_aids
/documents/legaldocument/wcms_127530.pdf.

NACC (National AIDS Control Council). 2008. *UNGASS 2008: United Nations General Assembly Special Session on HIV and AIDS: Country Report—Kenya*. Nairobi: Office of the President of the Republic of Kenya. http://data.unaids.org/pub/report/2008/kenya_2008_country_progress_report_en.pdf.

NACC (National AIDS Control Council). 2009. *Kenya HIV Prevention Response and Modes of Transmission Analysis*. Nairobi: NACC. http://siteresources.worldbank.org/INTHIVAIDS/Resources/375798-1103037153392/KenyaMOT22March09Final.pdf.

NACC (National AIDS Control Council). 2010. *UNGASS 2010: Country Report for Kenya*. Nairobi: Office of the President of the Republic of Kenya. http://data.unaids.org/pub/Report/2010/kenya_2010_country_progress_report_en.pdf.

NACC/NASCOP (National AIDS Control Council/National AIDS and STI Control Programme). 2012. *Kenya AIDS Epidemic Update 2012*. Nairobi: Ministry of Health.

NASCOP (National AIDS and STI Control Programme). 1999. *AIDS in Kenya*. 5th ed. Nairobi: Ministry of Health.

NASCOP (National AIDS and STI Control Programme). 2012. *Kenya AIDS Indicator Survey 2012*. Nairobi: Ministry of Health. http://nascop.or.ke/library/3d/Preliminary%20Report%20for%20Kenya%20AIDS%20indicator%20survey%202012.pdf.

NASCOP (National AIDS and STI Control Programme). 2017. *Framework for the Implementation of Pre-Exposure Prophylaxis of HIV in Kenya*. https://www.prepwatch.org/wp-content/uploads/2017/05/Kenya_PrEP_Implementation_Framework.pdf.

NASCOP/NACC (National AIDS and STI Control Programme and National AIDS Control Council). 2013. *Geographic Mapping of Most at Risk Populations for HIV (MARPS) in Kenya, June 2012*. https://www.icop.or.ke/wp-content/uploads/2016/09/Kenya-mapping-report-NASCOP-and-UoM-2013.pdf.

Ndege, Samson, Sierra Washington, Alice Kaaria, Wendy Prudhomme-O'Meara, Edwin Were, Monica Nyambura, Alfred K. Keter, et al. 2016. "HIV Prevalence and Antenatal Care Attendance among Pregnant Women in a Large Home-Based HIV Counseling and Testing Program in Western Kenya." *PloS One* 11(1): e0144618. doi:10.1371/journal.pone.0144618.

Negin, Joel, Makandwe Nyirenda, Janet Seeley, and Portia Mutevedzi. 2013. "Inequality in Health Status among Older Adults in Africa: The Surprising Impact of Anti-Retroviral Treatment." *Journal of Cross-Cultural Gerontology* 28: 491–493. doi:10.1007/s10823-013-9215-4.

NEPHAK (National Empowerment Network of People Living with HIV and AIDS in Kenya). 2012. *Positive Health, Dignity and Prevention in Kenya*. Nairobi: NEPHAK. https://www.gnpplus.net/assets/wbb_file_updown/2117/2012_Kenyan_PHDP_Report_2012_-_Web_Version.pdf.

Ng'ang'a, Pauline W. 2011. "Prevalence of Anxiety and Depression among HIV/AIDS Patients Attending the Comprehensive Care Centre (CCC), Kenyatta National Hospital (KNH)." MS thesis, University of Nairobi. http://erepository.uonbi.ac.ke/handle/11295/3790.

Nguyen, Vinh-Kim. 2010. *Republic of Therapy: Triage and Sovereignty in West Africa's Time of AIDS*. Durham, NC: Duke University Press.

Niehaus, Isak. 2014. "Treatment Literacy, Therapeutic Efficacy, and Antiretroviral Drugs: Notes from Bushbuckridge, South Africa." *Medical Anthropology* 33(4): 351–366. doi:10.1080/01459740.2013.802319.

Ochs, Elinor, and Lisa Capps. 1996. "Narrating the Self." *Annual Review of Anthropology* 25: 19–43. doi:10.1146/annurev.anthro.25.1.19.

Okuro, Samwel O. 2009. "Daniel arap Moi and the Politics of HIV and AIDS in Kenya, 1983–2002." *African Journal of AIDS Research* 8(3): 275–283. doi:10.2989/AJAR.2009.8.3.4.925.

Oware, Phoene M. 2020. "Informal Social Protection Actors: A Focus on Women Self-Help Groups in Kenya." *International Social Work* 63(5): 612–625. doi:10.1177/0020872820940013.

Parikh, Shanti. 2009. "Going Public." In *The Secret: Love, Marriage, and HIV*, edited by Jennifer S. Hirsch, Holly Wardlow, Daniel Jordan Smith, Harriet M. Phinney, Shanti Parikh, and Constance A. Nathanson, 168–196. Nashville, TN: Vanderbilt University Press.

Parker, Richard. 2001. "Sexuality, Culture, and Power in HIV/AIDS Research." *Annual Review of Anthropology* 30: 163–179. doi:10.1146/annurev.anthro.30.1.163.

Parker, Richard, and Peter Aggleton. 2003. "HIV/AIDS-Related Stigma and Discrimination: A Conceptual Framework and Implications for Action." *Social Science & Medicine* 57(1): 13–24. doi:10.1016/S0277-9536(02)00304-0.

Parmet, Wendy E. 2008. "Stigma, Hysteria, and HIV." *Hastings Center Report* 38(5): 57. doi:10.1353/hcr.0.0059.

Parsitau, Seleina. 2009. "'Keep Holy Distance and Abstain till He Comes': Interrogating a Pentecostal Church's Engagements with HIV/AIDS and the Youth in Kenya." *Africa Today* 56(1): 45–64. doi:10.2979/aft.2009.56.1.44.

Parsons, Talcott. 1951. *The Social System*. Glencoe, IL: Free Press.

Patterson, Amy. 2018. *Africa and Global Health Governance: Domestic Politics and International Structures*. Baltimore, MD: Johns Hopkins University Press.

Patton, Cindy. 1990. *Inventing AIDS*. New York: Routledge.

Patton, Cindy. 2002. *Globalizing AIDS*. Minneapolis: University of Minnesota Press.

Pebody, Roger. 2019. "How Did Kenya Build Africa's Largest PrEP Programme?" NAM. https://www.aidsmap.com/news/jan-2019/how-did-kenya-build-africas-largest-prep-programme.

Penn, David L., and Patrick W. Corrigan. 2002. "The Effects of Stereotype Suppression on Psychiatric Stigma." *Schizophrenia Research* 55(3): 269–276. doi:10.1016/S0920-9964(01)00207-9.

PEPFAR (U.S. President's Emergency Plan for AIDS Relief). 2008. *The Power of Partnerships: The U.S. President's Emergency Plan for AIDS Relief: 2008 Annual Report to Congress*. https://www.state.gov/wp-content/uploads/2019/08/PEPFAR-2008-Annual-Report-to-Congress.pdf.

PEPFAR (U.S. President's Emergency Plan for AIDS Relief). 2014. *PEPFAR 3.0: Controlling the Epidemic: Delivering on the Promise of an AIDS-Free Generation*. Washington, DC: Office of the Global AIDS Coordinator. https://www.avac.org/sites/default/files/resource-files/pepfar3.pdf.

PEPFAR (U.S. President's Emergency Plan for AIDS Relief). 2017. *PEPFAR 2017 Annual Report to Congress*. https://reliefweb.int/sites/reliefweb.int/files/resources/267809.pdf.

PEPFAR (U.S. President's Emergency Plan for AIDS Relief). 2019. *PEPFAR 2019 Annual Report to Congress*. https://www.state.gov/wp-content/uploads/2019/09/PEPFAR2019ARC.pdf.

Pescosolido, Bernice, Jack Martin, Annie Lang, and Sigryn Olafsdottir. 2008. "Rethinking Theoretical Approaches to Stigma: A Framework Integrating Normative Influences on Stigma (FINIS)." *Social Science & Medicine* 67(3): 431–440. doi:10.1016/j.socscimed.2008.03.018.

Pescosolido, Bernice, Jack K. Martin, Scott J. Long, Tait R. Medina, Jo C. Phelan, and Bruce Link. 2010. "'A Disease Like Any Other'? A Decade of Change in Public Reactions to Schizophrenia, Depression, and Alcohol Dependence." *American Journal of Psychiatry* 167: 1321–1330. doi:10.1176/appi.ajp.2010.09121743.

Petryna, Adriana. 2002. *Life Exposed: Biological Citizens after Chernobyl*. Princeton, NJ: Princeton University Press.

Pfeiffer, Elizabeth J., and Harrison M. K. Maithya. 2018. "Bewitching Sex Workers, Blaming Wives: HIV/AIDS, Stigma, and the Gender Politics of Panic in Western Kenya." *Global Public Health* 13(2): 234–248. doi:10.1080/17441692.2016.1215484.

Pfeiffer, Elizabeth J., and Harrison M. K. Maithya. 2021. "The Cultural Politics of Secrecy during HIV Home Counselling and Testing Campaigns in Kenya." *Culture, Health & Sexuality* 23(7): 867–882. doi:10.1080/13691058.2020.1736632.

Pfeiffer, Elizabeth J., Harrison M. K. Maithya, Mary Ott, and Kara Wools-Kaloustian. 2017. "Dangerous Bodies, Unpredictable Minds: HIV/AIDS, Mental Disorders, and Stigma Syndemics in Western Kenya." In *Foundations of Biosocial Health: Stigma and Illness Interactions*, edited by Shir Lerman, Bayla Ostrach, and Merrill Singer, 133–156. Lanham, MD: Lexington Books.

Pigg, Stacy Leigh. 1992. "Inventing Social Categories through Place: Social Representations and Development in Nepal." *Comparative Studies in Society and History* 34(3): 491–513. doi:10.1017/S0010417500017928.

Piot, Charles. 1999. *Remotely Global: Village Modernity in West Africa*. Chicago: University of Chicago Press.

Piot, Peter, Francis A. Plummer, Marie-Anne Rey, Elisabeth N. Ngugi, Christine Rouzioux, Josiah O. Ndinya-Achola, Gaby Veracauteren, et al. 1987. "Retrospective Seroepidemiology of AIDS Virus Infection in Nairobi Populations." *Journal of Infectious Diseases* 155(6): 1108–1112. doi:10.1093/infdis/155.6.1108.

Piot, Peter, Henri Taelman, Kapita Bila Minlangu, N. Mbendi, K. Ndangi, Kayembe Kalambayi, Chris Bridts, et al. 1984. "Acquired Immunodeficiency Syndrome in a Heterosexual Population in Zaire." *The Lancet* 324(8394): 65–69. doi:10.1016/S0140 -6736(84)90241-1.

Poulin, Michelle. 2007. "Sex, Money, and Premarital Partnerships in Southern Malawi." *Social Science & Medicine* 65(11): 2383–2393. doi:10.1016/j.socscimed.2007.05.030.

Prince, Ruth. 2012. "HIV and the Moral Economy of Survival in an East African City." *Medical Anthropology Quarterly* 26(4): 534–556. doi:10.1111/maq.12006.

Prince, Ruth. 2014. "Precarious Projects: Conversions of (Biomedical) Knowledge in an East African City." *Medical Anthropology* 33(1): 68–83. doi:10.1080/01459740.2013.833918.

Prince, Ruth, and Rebecca Marsland. 2013. *Making and Unmaking Public Health in Africa: Ethnographic and Historical Perspectives*. Athens: Ohio University Press.

"Putting HIV-Positive People at the Centre of Prevention." 2010. *The New Humanitarian*, May 28. http://www.irinnews.org/report/89280/kenya-putting-hiv-positive-people-at-the-centre -of-prevention.

Rao, Deepa, Ahmed Elshafei, Minh Nguyen, Mark L. Hatzenbuehler, Sarah Frey, and Vivian F. Go. 2019. "A Systematic Review of Multi-Level Stigma Interventions: State of the Science and Future Directions." *BMC Medicine* 17(41). doi:10.1186/s12916-018-1244-y.

Rasmussen, Louise Mubanda. 2013. "Counselling Clients to Follow 'the Rules' of Safe Sex and ARV Treatment." *Culture, Health & Sexuality* 15(Suppl 4): S537–S552. doi:10.1080/1369105 8.2013.809606.

Raviola, Guiseppe, Machoki M'Imunya, Esther Mwaikambo, and Mary Jo DelVecchio Good. 2002. "HIV, Disease Plague, Demoralization, and 'Burnout': Resident Experience of the Medical Profession in Nairobi, Kenya." *Culture, Medicine and Psychiatry* 26: 55–86. doi:10.1023 /A:1015289132151.

Reed, Joel Christian. 2018. *Landscapes of Activism: Civil Society, HIV and AIDS Care in Northern Mozambique*. New Brunswick, NJ: Rutgers University Press.

Reid, Graeme. 2010. "Gossip, Rumour and Scandal: The Circulation of AIDS Narratives in a Climate of Silence and Secrecy." In *Morality, Hope and Grief: Anthropologies of AIDS in Africa*, edited by Hansjörg Dilger and Ute Luig, 192–217. New York: Berghahn Books.

Reid, Richard J. 2009. *A History of Modern Africa: 1800 to the Present*. Malden, MA: Wiley Blackwell.

Rhodes, Tim, Merrill Singer, Philippe Bourgois, Samuel R. Friedman, and Steffanie A. Strath-dee. 2005. "The Social Structural Production of HIV Risk among Injecting Drug Users." *Social Science & Medicine* 61(5): 1026–1044. doi:10.1016/j.socscimed.2004.12.024.

Riessman, Catherine Kohler. 1993. *Narrative Analysis*. Newbury Park, CA: Sage.

Rispel, Laetitia C., Allanise Cloete, and Carol A. Metcalf. 2015. "'We Keep Her Status to Our-selves': Experiences of Stigma and Discrimination among HIV-Discordant Couples in South Africa, Tanzania, and Ukraine." *SAHARA-J: Journal of Social Aspects of HIV/AIDS* 12(1): 10–17. doi:10.1080/17290376.2015.1014403.

Robertson, Claire. 1996. "Transitions to Kenyan Patriarchy: Attempts to Control Nairobi Area Traders, 1920–1963." In *Courtyards, Markets, City Streets*, edited by Kathleen Sheldon, 47–72. Boulder, CO: Westview Press.

Rödlach, Alexander. 2006. *Witches, Westerners, and HIV: AIDS & Cultures of Blame in Africa*. Walnut Creek, CA: Left Coast Press.

Rosaldo, Michelle Z. 1980. *Knowledge and Passion: Ilongot Notions of Self & Social Life*. Cam-bridge: Cambridge University Press.

Rosenbrock, Rolf, Francoise Dubois-Arber, Martin Moers, Patrice Pinell, Doris Schaeffer, and Michel Setbon. 2000. "The Normalization of AIDS in Western European Countries." *Social Science & Medicine* 50(11): 1607–1629. doi:10.1016/S0277-9536(99)00469-4.

Russell, Steve, Faith Martin, Flavia Zalwango, Stella Namukwaya, Ruth Nalugya, Richard Muhumuza, Joseph Katongole, et al. 2016. "Finding Meaning: HIV Self-Management and Wellbeing among People Taking Antiretroviral Therapy in Uganda." *PloS One* 11(1): e0147896. doi:10.1371/journal.pone.0147896.

Russell, Steven, and Janet Seeley. 2010. "The Transition to Living with HIV as a Chronic Con-dition in Rural Uganda: Working to Create Order and Control When on Antiretroviral Therapy." *Social Science & Medicine* 70(3): 375–382. doi:1016/j.socscimed.2009.10.039.

Russell, Steven, Janet Seeley, Enoch Ezati, Nafuna Wamai, Willy Were, and Rebecca Bunnell. 2007. "Coming Back from the Dead." *Health Policy Planning* 22(5): 344–347. doi:10.1093/heapol/czm023.

Ryan, Gery W., and H. Russell Bernard. 2003. "Techniques to Identify Themes." *Field Methods* 15(1): 85–109. doi:10.1177/1525822X02239569.

Scheper-Hughes, Nancy, and Philippe Bourgois, eds. 2004. *Violence in War and Peace: An Anthology*. Malden, MA: Wiley-Blackwell.

Schmidt, Siegmar, and Gichira Kibara. 2002. *Kenya on the Path toward Democracy? An Interim Evaluation: A Qualitative Assessment of Political Developments in Kenya between 1990 and June 2002*. Nairobi: Konrad Adenauer Foundation.

Schoepf, Brooke G. 1992a. "AIDS, Sex, and Condoms: African Healers and the Reinvention of Tra-dition in Zaire." *Medical Anthropology* 14(2–4): 225–242. doi:10.1080/01459740.1992.9966073.

Schoepf, Brooke G. 1992b. "Women at Risk: Case Studies from Zaire." In *The Time of AIDS: Social Analysis, Theory, and Method*, edited by Gilbert Herdt and Shirley Lindenbaum, 259–286. London: Sage.

Schoepf, Brooke G. 2001. "International AIDS Research in Anthropology: Taking a Critical Perspective on the Crisis." *Annual Review of Anthropology* 30(1): 335–361. doi:10.1146/annurev.anthro.30.1.335.

Schoepf, Brooke G. 2010. "Assessing AIDS Research in Africa: Twenty-Five Years Later." *Afri-can Studies Review* 53(1): 105–142. doi:10.1353/arw.0.0252.

Schroeder, Richard. 1999. *Shady Practices: Agroforestry and Gender Politics in the Gambia*. Berkeley: University of California Press.

Setel, Philip W. 1999. *A Plague of Paradoxes: AIDS, Culture, and Demography in Northern Tan-zania*. Chicago: University of Chicago Press.

Shelton, James D., Daniel T. Halperin, Vinand Nantulya, Malcolm Potts, and Helene D. Gayle. 2004. "Partner Reduction Is Crucial for Balanced 'ABC' Approach to HIV Prevention." *BMJ* 328(April 8): 891–893. doi:10.1136/bmj.328.7444.891.

Singer, Merrill, and Scott Clair. 2003. "Syndemics and Public Health: Reconceptualizing Disease in Bio-Social Context." *Medical Anthropology Quarterly* 17(4): 423–441. doi:10.1525/maq.2003.17.4.423.

Smith, Daniel Jordan. 2014. *AIDS Doesn't Show Its Face: Inequality, Morality, and Social Change in Nigeria.* Chicago: University of Chicago Press.

Smith, Daniel Jordan. 2017. *To Be a Man Is Not a One-Day Job: Masculinity, Money, and Intimacy in Nigeria.* Chicago: University of Chicago Press.

Smith, James Howard. 2008. *Bewitching Development: Witchcraft and the Reinvention of Development in Neoliberal Kenya.* Chicago: University of Chicago Press.

Smith, James Howard. 2011. "Making Peace with the Devil: The Political Life of Devil Worship Rumors in Kenya." In *Displacing the State: Religion and Conflict in Neoliberal Africa,* edited by James Howard Smith and Rosalind I. J. Hackett, 49–81. Notre Dame, IN: University of Notre Dame Press.

Smith, Julia H., and Alan Whiteside. 2010. "The History of AIDS Exceptionalism." *Journal of the International AIDS Society* 13(1): 1–47. doi:10.1186/1758-2652-13-47.

Sontag, Susan. 1989. *AIDS and Its Metaphors.* New York: Farrar, Straus and Giroux.

Squire, Corinne. 2015. "Partial Secrets." *Current Anthropology* 56(S12): S201–S210. doi:10.1086/683299.

Stangl, Anne L., Valerie A. Earnshaw, Carmen H. Logie, Wim van Brakel, Leickness C. Simbayi, Iman Barré, and John F. Dovidio. 2019. "The Health Stigma and Discrimination Framework: A Global, Crosscutting Framework to Inform Research, Intervention Development, and Policy on Health-Related Stigmas." *BMC Medicine* 17: article 31. https://bmcmedicine.biomedcentral.com/articles/10.1186/s12916-019-1271-3.

Steenberg, Bent. 2020. "Patients and Personhood: Perceptions of HIV in Mozambican Immigrants in South Africa." *Medical Anthropology* 39(3): 211–224. doi:10.1080/01459740.2019.1677646.

Stoebenau, Kirsten, Lori Heise, Joyce Wamoyi, and Natalia Bobrova. 2016. "Revisiting the Understanding of 'Transactional Sex' in Sub-Saharan Africa: A Review and Synthesis of the Literature." *Social Science & Medicine* 168(November): 186–197. doi:10.1016/j.socscimed.2016.09.023.

Stoeltje, Beverly. 2009. "Asante Traditions and Female Self-Assertion: Sister Abena's Narrative." *Research in African Literatures* 40(1): 27–41.

Swendeman, Dallas, Barbara L Ingram, and Mary Jane Rotheram-Borus. 2009. "Common Elements in Self-Management of HIV and Other Chronic Illnesses: An Integrative Framework." *AIDS Care* 21(10): 1321–1334. doi:10.1080/09540120902803158.

Syvertsen, Jennifer L., Kawango Agot, Spala Ohaga, Steffanie A. Strathdee, Carol S. Camlin, Eunice Omanga, Petronilla Odonde, et al. 2015. "Evidence of Injection Drug Use in Kisumu, Kenya: Implications for HIV Prevention." *Drug and Alcohol Dependence* 151: 262–266. doi:10.1016/j.drugalcdep.2015.02.037.

Talle, Aud. 1995. "Bar Workers at the Border." In *Young People at Risk: Fightings AIDS in Northern Tanzania,* edited by Knut-Inge Klepp, Paul M. Biswalo, and Aud Talle, 18–30. Oslo: Scandinavian University Press.

Thomas, Felicity. 2008. "Indigenous Narratives of HIV/AIDS: Morality and Blame in a Time of Change." *Medical Anthropology* 27(3): 227–256. doi:10.1080/01459740802222716.

Thomas, Lynn M. 2003. *Politics of the Womb: Women, Reproduction, and the State in Kenya.* Berkeley: University of California Press.

Thomas, Lynn M., and Jennifer Cole. 2009. "Introduction: Thinking through Love in Africa." In *Love in Africa*, edited by Jennifer Cole and Lynn M. Thomas, 1–30. Chicago: University of Chicago Press.

Throup, David. 2003. "The Kenya General Election: December 27, 2002." *Africa Notes* 14 (January): 1–9. https://csis-website-prod.s3.amazonaws.com/s3fs-public/legacy_files /files/media/csis/pubs/anotes_0301b.pdf.

Treichler, Paula. 1999. *How to Have Theory in an Epidemic: Cultural Chronicles of AIDS*. Durham, NC: Duke University Press.

Tsing, Anna Lowenhaupt. 2005. *Friction: An Ethnography of Global Connection*. Princeton, NJ: Princeton University Press.

"*Tunaomba serikali ije itusaidie na tatizohili*" (We Beg the Government to Come and Rescue Us from This Problem). 2012. Cartoon in *Daily Nation*, February 27.

Turner, Victor. 1967. *The Forest of Symbols: Aspects of Ndembu Ritual*. Ithaca, NY: Cornell University Press.

Turshen, Meredeth. 1999. *Privatizing Health Services in Africa*. New Brunswick, NJ: Rutgers University Press.

"U=U Taking Off in 2017." 2017. *The Lancet* 4 (11): e475. doi:10.1016/S2352-3018(17)30183-2.

UN (United Nations). 2015. "Transforming Our World: The 2030 Agenda for Sustainable Development." https://sustainabledevelopment.un.org/content/documents/21252030% 20Agenda%20for%20Sustainable%20Development%20web.pdf.

UN (United Nations). 2016. "We Can End Poverty: Millennium Development Goals and beyond 2015." https://www.un.org/millenniumgoals/.

UN (United Nations). 2020. "Goals: 5: Achieve Gender Equality and Empower All Women and Girls." https://sdgs.un.org/goals/goal5#progress_and_info.

UNAIDS (Joint United Nations Programme on HIV/AIDS). 2000. *Report on the Global HIV/AIDS Epidemic*. Geneva: UNAIDS. https://data.unaids.org/pub/report/2000/2000 _gr_en.pdf.

UNAIDS (Joint United Nations Programme on HIV/AIDS). 2003. "Fact Sheet: Stigma and Discrimination." Geneva: UNAIDS. https://data.unaids.org/publications/fact-sheets03 /fs_stigma_discrimination_en.pdf.

UNAIDS (Joint United Nations Programme on HIV/AIDS). 2016. *Global AIDS Update 2016*. https://www.unaids.org/sites/default/files/media_asset/global-AIDS-update-2016_en.pdf.

UNAIDS (Joint United Nations Programme on HIV/AIDS). 2017. *Ending AIDS: Progress towards the 90-90-90 Targets*. Geneva: UNAIDS. http://www.unaids.org/sites/default/files /media_asset/Global_AIDS_update_2017_en.pdf.

UNAIDS (Joint United Nations Programme on HIV/AIDS). 2018. *UNAIDS Data 2018*. Geneva: UNAIDS. https://www.unaids.org/sites/default/files/media_asset/unaids-data -2018_en.pdf.

UNAIDS (Joint United Nations Programme on HIV/AIDS). 2019. *Communities at the Centre: Defending Rights, Breaking Barriers, Reaching People with HIV Services*. Geneva: UNAIDS. https://www.unaids.org/sites/default/files/media_asset/2019-global-AIDS-update_en.pdf.

UNAIDS (Joint United Nations Programme on HIV/AIDS). 2020a. "Global HIV and AIDS Statistics—Fact Sheet." https://www.unaids.org/en/resources/fact-sheet.

UNAIDS (Joint United Nations Programme on HIV/AIDS). 2020b. *Seizing the Moment: Tackling Entrenched Inequalities to End Epidemics*. Geneva: UNAIDS. https://www.unaids .org/sites/default/files/media_asset/2020_global-aids-report_en.pdf.

UNAIDS (Joint United Nations Programme on HIV/AIDS). 2021. "Discriminatory Attitudes towards People Living with HIV Declining in Some Regions, Rebounding in Others."

Update, January 25. https://www.unaids.org/en/resources/presscentre/featurestories/2021/january/20210125_discriminatory-attitudes.

UNICEF-WHO Joint Committee on Health Policy. 1989. "Report on WHO Global Programme on AIDS (GPA)." https://apps.who.int/iris/bitstream/handle/10665/61713/JC27-UNICEF-WHO-89.9-eng.pdf?sequence=1&isAllowed=y.

Urban, Greg. 2001. *Metaculture: How Culture Moves through the World*. Minneapolis: University of Minnesota Press.

USDOS (U.S. Department of State). 2018. "Remembering the 1998 Embassy Bombings." https://www.state.gov/remembering-the-1998-embassy-bombings-2/.

Ushie, Boniface Ayanbekongshie, Kenneth Juma, Grace Kimemia, Maggie Magee, Emily Maistrellis, Terry McGovern, and Sara E. Casey. 2020. "Foreign Assistance or Attack? Impact of the Expanded Global Gag Rule on Sexual and Reproductive Health and Rights in Kenya." *Sexual and Reproductive Health Matters* 28(3): 23–38. doi:10.1080/26410397.2020.1794412.

Vaughan, Megan. 1991. *Curing Their Ills: Colonial Power and African Illness*. Stanford, CA: Stanford University Press.

Wacquant, Loïc. 2007. *Urban Outcasts: A Comparative Sociology of Advanced Marginality*. Malden, MA: Wiley.

Walker, Liz. 2020. "Problematising the Discourse of 'Post-AIDS.'" *Journal of Medical Humanities* 41(2): 95–105. doi:10.1007/s10912-017-9433-9.

Wambuii, Henry. 2006. *Politics of HIV/AIDS and Implications for Democracy in Kenya*. Lewiston, NY: Edwin Mellen Press.

Wamoyi, Joyce S., Kirsten Stoebenau, Natalia Bobrova, Tanya Abramsky, and Charlotte Watts. 2016. "Transactional Sex and Risk for HIV Infection in Sub-Saharan Africa: A Systematic Review and Meta-Analysis." *Journal of the International AIDS Society* 19(1): 20992. doi:10.7448/IAS.19.1.20992.

Watkins, Susan Cotts, Ann Swidler, and Crystal Biruk. 2011. "Hearsay Ethnography: A Method for Learning about Responses to Health Interventions." In *The Handbook of the Sociology of Health, Illness, and Healing*, edited by Bernice A. Pescosolido, Jack K. Martin, Jane D. McLeod, and Anne Rogers, 431–445. New York: Springer.

Watts, Michael. 2006. "Empire of Oil: Capitalist Dispossession and the Scramble for Africa." *Monthly Review* 58(4): 1–17. doi:10.14452/MR-058-04-2006-08_1.

Weisner, Thomas S., Candice Bradley, and Philip L. Kilbride, eds. 1997. *African Families and the Crisis of Social Change*. Westport, CT: Bergin & Garvey.

West, Robin. 1992. *Narrative, Authority, and Law*. Ann Arbor: University of Michigan Press.

White, Luise. 1990. *The Comforts of Home: Prostitution in Colonial Nairobi*. Chicago: University of Chicago Press.

White, Luise. 2000. *Speaking with Vampires: Rumor and History in Colonial Africa*. Berkeley: University of California Press.

WHO (World Health Organization). 1988. *Guidelines for the Development of a National AIDS Prevention and Control Programme*. Geneva: WHO. https://apps.who.int/iris/handle/10665/39721.

WHO (World Health Organization). 1989. *Global Strategy for the Prevention and Control of AIDS: Report by the Director-General*. EB85/20. Geneva: WHO Executive Board. https://apps.who.int/iris/bitstream/handle/10665/163481/EB85_20_eng.pdf?sequence=1&isAllowed=y.

WHO (World Health Organization). 1999. *The World Health Report 1999: Making a Difference*. Geneva: WHO. https://www.who.int/whr/1999/en/whr99_en.pdf?ua=1.

WHO (World Health Organization). 2007. *Guidance on Provider-Initiated HIV Testing and Counselling in Health Facilities.* https://apps.who.int/iris/bitstream/handle/10665/43688/9789241595568_eng.pdf?sequence=1&isAllowed=y.

WHO (World Health Organization). 2012. *Service Delivery Approaches to HIV Testing and Counselling (HTC): A Strategic HTC Programme Framework.* Geneva: WHO. https://apps.who.int/iris/bitstream/handle/10665/75206/9789241593877_eng.pdf?sequence=1&isAllowed=y.

WHO (World Health Organization). 2015. "Treat All People Living with HIV, Offer Antiretrovirals as Additional Prevention Choice for People at 'Substantial' Risk." https://www.who.int/news/item/30-09-2015-treat-all-people-living-with-hiv-offer-antiretrovirals-as-additional-prevention-choice-for-people-at-substantial-risk.

WHO (World Health Organization). 2020. "Ebola: North Kivu/Ituri, Democratic Republic of the Congo, August 2018–June 2020." https://www.who.int/emergencies/situations/Ebola-2019-drc-.

WHO (World Health Organization). 2021a. "Estimated Number of People (All Ages) Living with HIV." https://www.who.int/data/gho/data/indicators/indicator-details/GHO/estimated-number-of-people-(all-ages)-living-with-hiv.

WHO (World Health Organization). 2021b. "Human Rights." https://www.who.int/health-topics/human-rights#tab=tab_1.

WHO (World Health Organization). 2021c. "Why the HIV Epidemic Is Not Over." https://www.who.int/news-room/spotlight/why-the-hiv-epidemic-is-not-over.

WHO/UNAIDS/UNICEF (World Health Organization, Joint United Nations Programme on HIV/AIDS, United Nations Children's Fund). 2009. *Towards Universal Access: Scaling Up Priority HIV/AIDS Interventions in the Health Sector: Progress Report 2009.* Geneva: WHO. https://data.unaids.org/pub/report/2009/20090930_tuapr_2009_en.pdf.

WHO/UNAIDS/UNICEF (World Health Organization, Joint United Nations Programme on HIV/AIDS, United Nations Children's Fund). 2011. *Global HIV/AIDS Response: Epidemic Update and Health Sector Progress towards Universal Access: Progress Report 2011.* https://apps.who.int/iris/bitstream/handle/10665/44787/9789241502986_eng.pdf?sequence=1&isAllowed=y.

Whyte, Susan Reynolds. 1997. *Questioning Misfortune: The Pragmatics of Uncertainty in Eastern Uganda.* Cambridge: Cambridge University Press.

Whyte, Susan Reynolds. 2002. "Subjectivities and Subjunctivities: Hoping for Health in Eastern Uganda." In *Postcolonial Subjectivities in Africa*, edited by Richard Werbner, 171–190. London: Zed Books.

Whyte, Susan Reynolds. 2012. "Chronicity and Control: Framing 'Noncommunicable Diseases' in Africa." *Anthropology & Medicine* 19(1): 63–74. doi:10.1080/13648470.2012.660465.

Whyte, Susan Reynolds, ed. 2014. *Second Chances: Surviving AIDS in Uganda.* Durham, NC: Duke University Press.

Whyte, Susan Reynolds, and Benedicte Ingstad. 1995. "Disability and Culture: An Overview." In *Disability and Culture*, edited by Benedicte Ingstad and Susan Reynolds Whyte, 3–37. Berkeley: University of California Press.

Wilhelm-Solomon, Matthew. 2013. "The Priest's Soldiers: HIV Therapies, Health Identities, and Forced Encampment in Northern Uganda." *Medical Anthropology* 32(3): 227–246. doi:10.1080/01459740.2012.709891.

Wilkinson, Richard, and Michael Marmot, eds. 2003. *Social Determinants of Health: The Solid Facts.* 2nd ed. Copenhagen: World Health Organization Europe.

Wilson, Anika. 2012. "Of Love Potions and Witch Baskets: Domesticity, Mobility, and Occult Rumors in Malawi." *Western Folklore* 71(2): 149–173.

Winchester, Margaret S., Janet W. McGrath, David Kaawa-Mafigiri, Florence Namutiibwa, George Ssendegye, Amina Nalwoga, Emily Kyarikunda, et al. 2017. "Routines, Hope, and Antiretroviral Treatment among Men and Women in Uganda." *Medical Anthropology Quarterly* 31(2): 237–256. doi:10.1111/maq.12301.

Wipper, Audrey. 1975. "The Maendeleo ya Wanawake Organzation: The Co-Optation of Leadership." *African Studies Review* 18(3): 99–120. doi:10.2307/523724.

World Bank. 2021. "Population, Total—Kenya." https://data.worldbank.org/indicator/SP .POP.TOTL?locations=KE&most_recent_value_desc=false.

Wyrod, R. 2016. *AIDS and Masculinity in the African City: Privilege, Inequality, and Modern Manhood.* Berkeley: University of California Press.

Yang, Lawrence Hsin, Arthur Kleinman, Bruce G. Link, Jo C. Phelan, Sing Lee, and Byron Good. 2007. "Culture and Stigma: Adding Moral Experience to Stigma Theory." *Social Science & Medicine* 64(7): 1524–1535. doi:10.1016/j.socscimed.2006.11.013.

INDEX

ABC model, 9; and PEPFAR funding, 41
"abstinence, be faithful, or use condoms."
See ABC model
advertisements seeking relationships,
166–167
AIDS (acquired immunodeficiency syndrome): biomedicalization of, 149; dis-
proportionate distribution of, 32–33; as a
global crisis, 8, 42; and globalization, 5; as a
human rights issue, 7–8; improvements in
understanding, 41; in Kenya, 30, 36, 37–38;
origin of, 33, 36, 183n1 (chap. 1); society's
pretreatment response to, 30, 34; United
States' early information on, 33. See also
ending AIDS; HIV
AIDS, death from: denying, 32; graphic
description of, 33–34; Mahali's citizens'
pre-ART reactions to, 29–30
"AIDS carrier," 95
AIDS exceptionalism. See HIV
exceptionalism
AIDS industry: certificate training in, 121;
navigating employment with, 71, 119–120;
people's desired attachment to, 21; priorities of, 3
AIDS Support Organization (Uganda), 7
anthropologists: "in the middle of things,"
1–2; and storytelling, xxi
"anti-politics machine," global health as an,
20, 177
antiretroviral therapy. See ART
ART (antiretroviral therapy): equitable
access to, 41; fear of being cut off from, 65;
hiding use of, 134, 135 fig. 5.2; percentages
of people taking, 42; prohibitive cost of, 8;
transforms HIV from fatal to treatable
chronic condition, 5, 65; transforms
stigma, 133–137, 138
Ashforth, Adam, on post-2007 election
fighting, 63–64

Bakhtin, Mikhail, on statements never being
independent, 22

behaviors, changing, to control spread of
HIV, x, 6, 8–9, 36, 58, 128, 130
Benton, Adia, on vertical and horizontal
global health programs, 21
"biological citizenship," 166
biomedicalization: cannot fix societal problems, 23, 85; loses perceived worth in
Kenya, 37; success in reducing HIV infection rates, 21. See also TasP
biosocial approach to healing, 149
blame: cast inadvertently on individuals for
contracting HIV, 129; from clinic as a de-
faulter, 132–133; gendered dimensions of,
68–70, 103, 108, 119, 157–167; for HIV linked
to ethnicity, 71–72; placed on individuals
for structural conditions, 84, 139, 154. See
also List, the
bridewealth, 129
burden, becoming a, 130, 132

CD4+ T cells, 46
chai, xv, 53, 96, 161
chapatis, 123, 169
chronic disease model/paradigm, 138,
174–178; attempts to normalize HIV,
86–87; complicates stigma, 85; contributes
to public stigma, 94; keeps people from
feeling/being "normal," 25; as narratives/
discourses, 123; as one-size-fits-all model,
127; and socialization for social spaces,
133, 143
colonial period in Kenya, 56–58
colonial policies: early, 56; later, 58; in postcolonial times, 41, 61
colonists' attitude toward Africans, 13, 57–58
Comaroff, Jean and John, on personhood,
149–150
commercial sex worker (CSW), use of term,
183n2 (intro.)
Comprehensive Care Center. See HIV clinic
confidentiality: as an enemy to eradicating
AIDS, 93–94; as key component in HIV
testing initiatives by WHO, 93–94; in

ABOUT THE AUTHOR

ELIZABETH J. PFEIFFER is an assistant professor of anthropology at Rhode Island College. Her work has been published in a variety of peer-reviewed journals, including *Culture, Health & Sexuality, Global Public Health, African Studies Review, Medicine Anthropology Theory,* and *Sexually Transmitted Diseases.*

Available titles in the Medical Anthropology:
Health, Inequality, and Social Justice series:

Printed in the United States
by Baker & Taylor Publisher Services